AF339277

CONTACT LENSES

CONTACT LENSES

EDITED BY

JAMES V. AQUAVELLA M.D.

Clinical Professor of Ophthalmology
Director, Cornea Research Laboratory
University of Rochester School of Medicine and Dentistry
Rochester, New York

GULLAPALLI N. RAO M.D.

Clinical Associate Professor of Ophthalmology
University of Rochester Medical Center
Rochester, New York
Director
L. V. Prasad Eye Institute
Hyderabad, India

15 CONTRIBUTORS

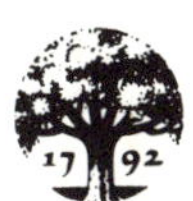

J. B. LIPPINCOTT COMPANY   Philadelphia

London   Mexico City   New York   St. Louis   São Paulo   Sydney

Developmental Editor: Sanford Robinson
Manuscript Editor: Virginia M. Barishek
Indexer: Alexandra Weir
Design Director: Tracy Baldwin
Design Coordinator: Earl Gerhart
Designer: Adrianne Onderdonk Dudden
Production Supervisor: Kathleen Dunn
Production Coordinator: Susan Hess
Compositor: TAPSCO, Inc.
Printer/Binder: R. R. Donnelley & Sons Company

Copyright © 1987, by J. B. Lippincott Company. All rights reserved. No part of this book may be used or reproduced in any manner whatsoever without written permission except for brief quotations embodied in critical articles and reviews. Printed in the United States of America. For information write J. B. Lippincott Company, East Washington Square, Philadelphia, Pennsylvania 19105.

6 5 4 3 2 1

Library of Congress Cataloging-in-Publication Data

Contact lenses.

  Bibliography.
  Includes index.
  1. Contact lenses. I. Aquavella, James V.,
DATE. II. Rao, Gullapalli N. [DNLM: 1. Contact
Lenses. WW 355 C7558]
RE977.C6C589 1987   617.7'523   86-10321
ISBN 0-397-50655-4

The authors and publisher have exerted every effort to ensure that drug selection and dosage set forth in this text are in accord with current recommendations and practice at the time of publication. However, in view of ongoing research, changes in government regulations, and the constant flow of information relating to drug therapy and drug reactions, the reader is urged to check the package insert for each drug for any change in indications and dosage and for added warnings and precautions. This is particularly important when the recommended agent is a new or infrequently employed drug.

CONTRIBUTORS

James V. Aquavella, M.D.
Clinical Professor of Ophthalmology
Director, Cornea Research Laboratory
University of Rochester
School of Medicine and Dentistry
Rochester, New York

**Mr. Noel A. Brennan, M.Sc.Optom.,
F.A.A.O.**
Lecturer
Department of Optometry
University of Melbourne
Parkville, Victoria, Australia

**Dr. Nathan Efron, B.Sc.Optom., Ph.D.,
F.A.A.O.**
Lecturer
Department of Optometry
University of Melbourne
Parkville, Victoria, Australia

James M. Gordon, M.D.
Clinical Assistant Professor of
Ophthalmology
Washington University School of
Medicine
St. Louis, Missouri

Sidney J. Hanish, M.D.
Assistant Professor of Ophthalmology
Director of Low Vision Clinic
Washington University
St. Louis, Missouri

Jeffrey K. Harris, M.D.
Clinical Assistant Professor of
Ophthalmology
University of Rochester Medical Center
Rochester, New York

Brien A. Holden, Ph.D., F.A.A.O.
Associate Professor and Director
Cornea and Contact Lens Research Unit
School of Optometry
University of New South Wales
Kensington, New South Wales,
Australia

Thomas John, M.D.
Clinical Fellow, Cornea Service
Massachusetts Eye and Ear Infirmary
Department of Ophthalmology,
Harvard Medical School
Research Associate
Eye Research Institute of Retina
Foundation
Boston, Massachusetts
Postdoctoral Associate
Department of Applied Biological
Science
Massachusetts Institute of Technology
Cambridge, Massachusetts

Emily Kenyon, O.D.
Research Associate
The Morton D. Sarver Center for
Research in Cornea and Contact
Lens
School of Optometry
University of California, Berkeley
Berkeley, California

William B. Orenberg, M.D.
Corneal Fellow and Instructor
University of Rochester Medical Center
Rochester, New York

Kenneth A. Polse, O.D., M.S., F.A.A.O.
Professor
The Morton D. Sarver Center for
Research in Cornea and Contact
Lens
School of Optometry
University of California, Berkeley
Berkeley, California

Gullapalli N. Rao, M.D.
Clinical Associate Professor of
 Ophthalmology
University of Rochester Medical Center
Rochester, New York
Director
L. V. Prasad Eye Institute
Hyderabad, India

Jagjit S. Saini, M.D.
Assistant Professor of Ophthalmology
Post Graduate Institute of Medical
 Education and Research
Chandigarh, India

Ms. Helen A. Swarbrick, M.Sc.
Research Optometrist
Cornea and Contact Lens Research Unit
School of Optometry
University of New South Wales
Kensington, New South Wales,
 Australia

Alan Tomlinson, Ph.D.
Professor of Optometry
Southern California College of
 Optometry
Fullerton, California

PREFACE

Contact lens technology has undergone significant change over the past several years. The development of hydrophilic and oxygen-permeable materials has necessitated the development of new techniques for fitting. Although contact lenses enable large numbers of individuals to have comfortable vision without spectacles, it is increasingly apparent that they do have the potential for harm. Consequently, the interrelation between corneal physiology and the physical properties of contact lens materials is extremely important. To minimize contact lens complications, both practitioners and patients must be educated in the proper techniques for cleaning, disinfection, and storage. A comprehensive approach involving the efforts of manufacturers, fitters, and ancillary staff is necessary. All patients must be properly informed of their responsibilities in wearing contact lenses, and have access to appropriate care should a problem arise. We have attempted to portray these different aspects of contact lenses to provide a comprehensive picture of the field to the reader.

The editors would like to take this opportunity to thank all of the contributors for their diligence in adhering to the schedules and for the overall excellent quality of the material submitted. The efforts of Miss Helen Theodor and Mrs. Catherine Pultorak in organizing and retyping the manuscripts are truly appreciated.

Gullapalli N. Rao, M.D.
James V. Aquavella, M.D.

CONTENTS

1 The Contact Lens: Physiological Considerations 1
Brien A. Holden, Noel A. Brennan, Nathan Efron, and Helen A. Swarbrick

2 Fitting Techniques for Gas-Permeable Rigid Lenses 39
James M. Gordon and Sidney J. Hanish

3 Hydrogel Lenses: Aphakia 47
William B. Orenberg and Gullapalli N. Rao

4 Hydrogel Lenses: Cosmetic 70
Thomas John

5 Contact Lens Correction of Presbyopia 115
Alan Tomlinson

6 Therapeutic Contact Lenses 140
James V. Aquavella

7 Special Refractive Problems 164
Kenneth A. Polse and Emily Kenyon

8 Extended-Wear Contact Lenses 188
Gullapalli N. Rao

9 Complications of Contact Lenses 195
Gullapalli N. Rao and Jagjit S. Saini

10 Solutions for Cleaning, Disinfection, and Storage 226
Jeffrey K. Harris

Appendix: Bibliography 263

Index 265

THE CONTACT LENS: PHYSIOLOGICAL CONSIDERATIONS

BRIEN A. HOLDEN, NOEL A. BRENNAN, NATHAN EFRON, and HELEN A. SWARBRICK

Since the advent of the soft, flexible hydrogel lens, the attention of the clinician has moved from the geometrical considerations involved in fitting rigid lenses to assessment of the overall physiological impact of the contact lens on the cornea and adjacent tissues.

The relative simplicity of fitting a hydrogel lens, especially a thin flexible lens, has enabled the clinician to obtain an acceptable, comfortable lens fitting with ease. It was soon realized, however, that initial comfort was not a good guide to prolonged success. Edema and striae, vascularization, loss of sensitivity, and even endothelial changes were soon recorded by astute clinicians and researchers. After some lively debate, it became clear that the earlier thick hydrogel lenses severely restricted oxygen flow to the cornea, to an even greater extent than polymethyl methacrylate (PMMA) lenses.

As researchers began to understand the nature of the effects of restricted oxygen availability, manipulation of lens water content and thickness to improve the oxygen transmissibility of hydrogel lenses became the new basis for "fitting" these lenses.

Altering base curve and diameter seemed to have little effect in varying this aspect of lens performance. However, as we have learned more recently, the fit of hydrogel lenses plays a subtle but important role in determining the success of these lenses, especially for extended wear. Hydrogel lens material properties and design are significant factors in clearing debris that collects behind the lens, and in providing tear-carried metabolites essential for maintaining epithelial growth and repair during extended wear.

This chapter will review current knowledge about the effects of contact lenses on the physiology of the cornea and adjacent tissues.

THE NORMAL CORNEAL ENVIRONMENT

Although a full account of the physiological requirements of the cornea is beyond the scope of this chapter, it is pertinent to review aspects that are particularly relevant to contact lens fitting.

SUPPLY OF METABOLITES

Oxygen

Like other tissues of the body, the cornea requires energy for various functions such as the maintenance of normal cellular integrity, cell division and tissue repair. Several authors have demonstrated that the cornea is dependent on oxygen for carbohydrate metabolism,[39,41,44] and that this supply comes from atmospheric oxygen through the tears.[87,161,179] Little oxygen is supplied by other routes.[57,127,169]

Corneal oxygen availability is reduced by almost two thirds when the eye is closed; that is, from 20.9% O_2 (the volumetric concentration of oxygen in the atmosphere) to approximately 8% O_2.[46,99] Under closed lid conditions, oxygen is supplied to the cornea from the capillary plexus of the superior palpebral conjunctiva, and possibly from the atmosphere through an imperfect palpebral aperture seal.[46]

The relative oxygen consumption (per unit tissue volume) of epithelium:stroma:endothelium is 10:1:50.[65] There has been considerable debate whether the endothelium obtains its oxygen supply from the atmosphere[11,12,13] or the aqueous.[51,57,115,146,169,200] This is an important question because it is known that corneal hydration is essentially controlled by the pump-leak mechanism located in the endothelium.[128,147]

The intact epithelium is a major barrier to the influx of water into the cornea,[145] and plays a minor role in the active pumping of water from the cornea.[167] Interference with the pathways of metabolites required for epithelial and endothelial metabolism may restrict these functions. Sweeney and co-workers have provided evidence of neural influence on epithelial metabolism.[186] This could explain why the cornea of an aphakic eye, in which innervation has been disturbed by surgery, has a lower oxygen uptake rate than the cornea of a phakic eye.

The minimum level of oxygen required by the cornea has been the subject of considerable interest in the literature; some of the estimates of the "critical oxygen requirement" are given in Table 1-1. It is difficult to compare the results of some studies because different criteria have been used to define corneal dysfunction. Recent studies, which have used more appropriate experimental designs, suggest that the cornea needs in excess of 10% O_2 to avoid dysfunction. The results of Holden and co-workers are given in Figure 1-1; they demonstrated that an average precorneal oxygen tension of 10% O_2 is required to prevent corneal edema.[100] However, individual critical oxygen requirements vary considerably.

Glucose and Glycogen

The principal metabolic substrates utilized in the epithelium are glucose and glycogen. Glucose is obtained principally from the aqueous humor, although up to 10% of the corneal glucose supply may be obtained from the tears and the limbal vasculature.[52,68] Large glycogen stores also have been observed in epithelial cells.

TABLE 1-1 Estimates of the Minimum Oxygen Requirement of the Cornea

Authors	Year	Critical Oxygen Tension (%)	Criterion
Polse, Mandell[161]	1970	1.5–2.5	Corneal swelling
Uniacke et al[195]	1972	5.0	LDH reactivity Epithelial swelling Glycogen depletion
Hill et al[89]	1974	4.0	SDH reactivity
Carney[28a]	1974	2.0	Corneal swelling
Mandell, Farrell[126a]	1980	3.0	Corneal swelling
Millodot, O'Leary[143]	1980	8.0	Corneal sensitivity
Hamano et al[76]	1983	13.2	Lactate accumulation Epithelial mitotic rate
Holden et al[100]	1984	10.1	Corneal swelling

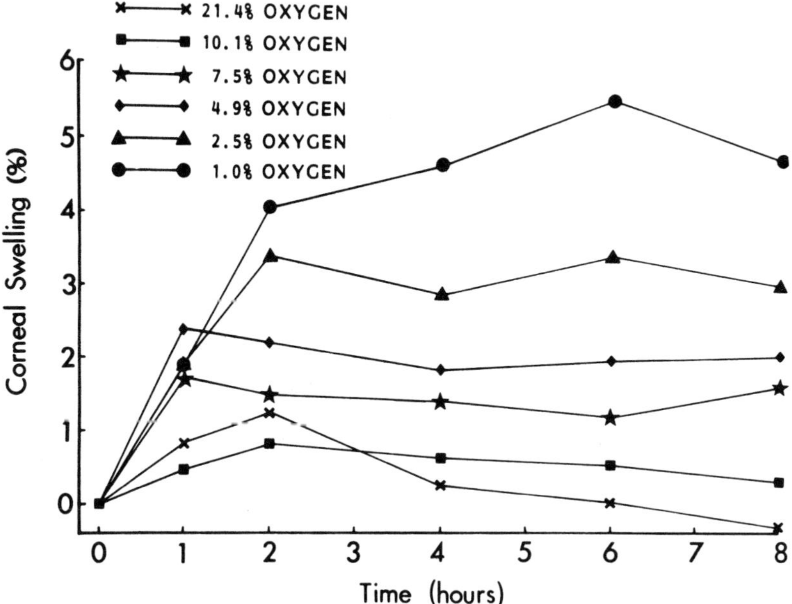

Figure 1-1   Average corneal swelling versus time for a range of precorneal oxygen concentrations. Gas-goggles were used to expose the cornea to gases of various oxygen tensions over an 8-hour period. Eight human subjects were used. (Holden BA, Sweeney DF, Sanderson G: The minimum precorneal oxygen tension to avoid corneal edema. Invest Ophthalmol Vis Sci 25:476, 1984)

Glucose and glycogen are metabolized in the epithelium by three pathways:

1. Embden–Meyerhof anaerobic glycolysis, which breaks down glucose and glycogen to lactate in the absence of oxygen, yielding two moles of high-energy adenosine triphosphate (ATP) for each mole of glucose.

2. The tricarboxylic acid cycle (TCA or Krebs cycle), which yields carbon dioxide and water from aerobic breakdown of pyruvate or lactate. This cycle produces 36 moles of ATP per mole of glucose.

3. The hexose monophosphate shunt, which converts hexose to pentose for use in the synthesis of nucleic acids. This pathway eventually yields 1 mole of ATP per mole of glucose.

Although only 15% of the glucose substrate is metabolized aerobically, the rest being converted to lactate, the high energy yield of the TCA cycle makes this the major source of energy for epithelial metabolic processes.

Amino acids, vitamins, minerals, and other substances required for corneal metabolism appear to be derived from the aqueous.[52]

REMOVAL OF METABOLIC BY-PRODUCTS

Just as a pathway for metabolites is required for normal corneal function, a pathway for the removal of metabolic by-products is also necessary. Accumulation of a by-product may result in a concentration of the substance that is toxic to the cornea. The by-products that must be cleared from the cornea include lactate, carbon dioxide, water, and necrotic cellular matter.

Carbon Dioxide

Carbon dioxide is highly permeable in corneal tissue (about 20 times that of oxygen.)[52] Fatt concluded that the transport of carbon dioxide in the cornea is determined by the carbon dioxide tensions in the aqueous humor and tear film, and not by metabolism in the corneal tissue. Because the carbon dioxide tension is 55 mmHg in the aqueous humor and essentially zero in the air-saturated tear film, a flux is expected to occur in the anterior direction across the cornea.[52,54]

Experimental evidence supports the expectation of Fatt.[52] Redslob and Tremblay measured the efflux of carbon dioxide from the surface of the rabbit cornea by passing carbon dioxide-free air over the cornea and analyzing the resultant gas.[165] They arrived at a value of 24 μl/h for the whole cornea. Carbon dioxide efflux was measured by Fatt and co-workers in the human cornea by mounting a carbon dioxide electrode in a contact lens.[59] Their finding of 21 μl/h for the whole cornea (corresponding to 16 μl/cm^{2}h) was in good agreement with the earlier work of Redslob and Tremblay.[165]

Lactate

The rabbit cornea produces about 0.9 μM/cm^{2}h lactate when perfused or incubated *in vitro* under aerobic conditions. In an anaerobic environment, lactate production is increased to a rate of 1.2 μM/cm²h.[129] This is reflected in human studies by the increased ratio of lactate dehydrogenase to malate dehydrogenase in the tears upon awakening, indicating a shift towards anaerobic metabolism under closed-eye conditions.[69]

Further studies on perfused tissue indicate that conversion to lactate accounts for 84% of all glucose used by the cornea.[65,129] Fatt points out that the production of lactate is usually an indication that cells are not receiving sufficient oxygen for complete oxidation of glucose.[52] Because the cornea is a thin tissue bathing in an oxygen-rich fluid, Fatt considers the high rate of lactate production in the cornea to be an "unresolved problem in corneal physiology." Lactate produced in the cornea is removed principally across the endothelium into the aqueous humor.[112]

Cellular Debris

The normal cornea has a relatively rapid turnover of epithelial cells. Those at the surface are sloughed off, and so a pathway must be available for the disposal of this unwanted material. Normally the lids, tears, and lacrimal drainage system provide this route for removal.

TEMPERATURE

Hill and Leighton used a lens-mounted thermistor to measure the temperature of the cornea in the relaxed, open eye; this was found to be 32.1°C.[88] Using Mapstone's bolometer, a device that monitors infrared radiation, Fatt and Chaston found the temperature of the cornea to be somewhat higher, 33°C to 36°C.[56] The temperature of the corneal surface increases beneath the closed eyelid to lie within the range 35.6°C to 36.5°C.[56] Holden and Sweeney, using a lens-mounted thermistor, found the temperature of the superior palpebral conjunctiva to be 36.2°C.[99]

Corneal temperature can become a significant consideration in contact lens wear, in view of the demonstration by Freeman and Fatt of the dependence of corneal metabolic activity upon corneal temperature.[66] Increased temperatures will increase metabolic activity, resulting in a higher corneal oxygen demand.

TEAR CHEMISTRY

The role of the precorneal tear film in maintaining normal corneal function is poorly understood; however, the areas of tear pH and osmolarity have received some attention.

Using a closed chamber temperature-stabilized microelectrode system, Carney and Hill found that human tear pH usually exhibits cyclic patterns of change about a mean of 7.45 ± 0.16 in the open eye.[30] Following 6 to 8 hours of eyelid closure, the pH of the tears was found to decrease slightly (7.21 ± 0.16); it took 3 to 4 hours to return to average open-eye levels. This relative stability of tear pH reflects the significant, although limited, buffering capacity of the tears.[31]

Terry and Hill used a precision thermocouple hygrometer to determine the diurnal variation in the osmotic pressure of tears.[187] They reported a shift in tear tonicity from 0.97% ± 0.02% NaCl in the waking eye to 0.89% ± 0.01% NaCl following sleep periods of 6 to 8 hours.

ALTERATION TO THE CORNEAL ENVIRONMENT INDUCED BY CONTACT LENSES

RESTRICTION OF METABOLITES: OXYGEN

Many studies have shown that both hard and soft contact lenses present a formidable barrier to the oxygen available to the cornea.[60,87,163,179] A decreased partial pressure of oxygen at the anterior corneal surface results in a decreased flow into the cornea.[152]

The available evidence suggests that this is the major way in which a contact lens restricts the flow of metabolites into the corneal epithelium.

The Open Eye

During contact lens wear, oxygen can reach the cornea in two ways: by diffusion through the lens, and by circulation of oxygen-rich tears under the lens, driven by a lid-activated tear pump.

DIFFUSION THROUGH THE LENS

The rate at which oxygen diffuses through a gas-permeable contact lens is given by the formula:

$$j = (P_1 - P_2)Dk/L$$

where D is the diffusivity and k is the solubility of oxygen in the lens material, L is the lens thickness, and P_1 and P_2 are the oxygen tensions at the anterior and posterior lens surfaces.[60] The term Dk is known as the oxygen permeability of the lens material, and the term Dk/L as the oxygen transmissibility of the contact lens itself.

Various authors have estimated the level of oxygen at the corneal surface under contact lenses of various known oxygen transmissibilities.[47] The variability in these estimates can be attributed to the varying methods used, which include mathematical modelling, clinically derived measures based on the edema response to lens wear, and the epithelial oxygen uptake rate following lens removal.[47,50,54,55,57,83,160] Nevertheless, all studies agree that lenses with greater oxygen transmissibility allow more oxygen to reach the cornea.

TEAR PUMPING

The oxygen supply reaching the cornea is supplemented to some extent by circulation under the lens of oxygen dissolved in the tears; this circulation is maintained by a lid-activated tear pump. With PMMA lenses, which are virtually impermeable to oxygen, this is the major route for supplying oxygen to the central cornea.

An estimated 10% to 20% exchange of tears occurs under a rigid lens with each blink. This has been demonstrated using flame photometry and oxygen sensor techniques.[38,58] However, considerably less tear circulation occurs under hydrogel lenses due to their greater flexibility; Polse estimates a tear exchange of only 1% with each blink.[159] That the tear pump does not supplement corneal oxygenation under a hydrogel lens to any significant extent was verified by Efron and Carney (Figs. 1-2, 1-3).[48]

The Closed Eye

Under closed-eye conditions, the cornea receives its oxygen supply from the capillary network of the palpebral conjunctiva. The oxygen availability is considerably lower than when the eye is open (8% Po_2 versus 20.9% Po_2). Therefore, the flow of oxygen through a contact lens worn under closed-eye conditions is considerably reduced. Efron and Carney have measured oxygen levels at the corneal surface under these conditions in the human eye, and have concluded that overnight wear of present-generation hydrogel

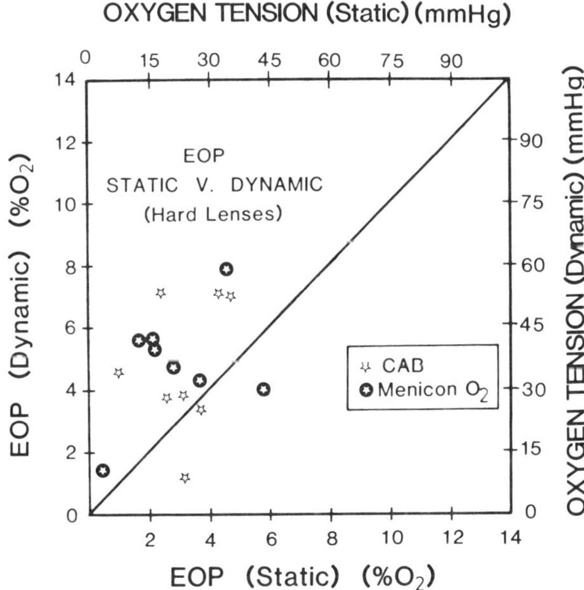

Figure 1-2 Matched static versus dynamic EOP values for hard gas-permeable lenses. EOP values were obtained by measuring epithelial oxygen uptake rate immediately following lens removal. Each data point represents the mean of six pairs of data for a single subject. (Efron N, Carney LG: Effect of blinking on the level of oxygen beneath hard and soft gas-permeable contact lenses. J Am Optom Assoc 54:229, 1983. Reproduced with permission from the *Journal of the American Optometric Association*.)

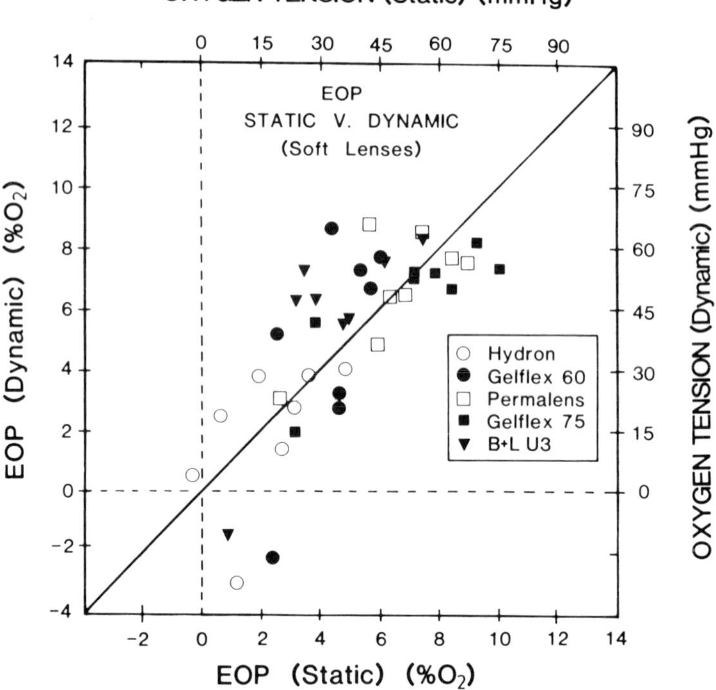

Figure 1-3 Matched static versus dynamic EOP values for hydrogel lenses. EOP values were obtained by measuring epithelial oxygen uptake rate immediately following lens removal. Each data point represents the mean of six pairs of data for a single subject. (Efron N, Carney LG: Effect of blinking on the level of oxygen beneath hard and soft gas-permeable contact lenses. J Am Optom Assoc 54:229, 1983. Reproduced with permission from the *Journal of the American Optometric Association.*)

lenses reduces oxygen availability at the epithelial surface below safe minimum levels to ensure corneal integrity.[46]

Although there is no tear circulation due to lid action during closed-eye lens wear, it has been suggested that circulation may occur during the "rapid eye movement" phase of sleep. However, Benjamin and Rasmussen have shown that such a mechanism is unlikely.[18]

RESTRICTION OF OUTFLOW OF METABOLIC BY-PRODUCTS

Carbon Dioxide

Fatt has stated that the transmissibility of carbon dioxide through a hydrogel contact lens is 20 times greater than that of oxygen.[53] This suggests that carbon dioxide efflux is not significantly restricted by the presence of a hydrogel contact lens. However, there is some evidence to suggest that a significant rise in precorneal P_{CO_2} occurs beneath hydrogel lenses. Using a Radiometer carbon dioxide electrode, Holden found that a 38% water hydroxyethyl methacrylate (HEMA) lens, 0.15 mm thick, created a carbon dioxide partial pressure of 50 mmHg beneath the lens (Fig. 1-4).[95] Such a rise in P_{CO_2} would be expected to decrease the pH of the precorneal tear film, as occurs during eyelid closure.

Cellular Debris

The corneal epithelium continually is replenishing cells by mitosis; these cells are produced at the basal layer and move towards the surface until they are eventually sloughed off and washed away in the tears.

During rigid lens wear, this cellular debris is readily flushed out from behind the lens. However, debris is more likely to become trapped behind a hydrogel lens because of the lower rate of tear exchange. Enzymes released during breakdown of this cellular matter have the potential to provoke a toxic response in the epithelium. This mechanism has been implicated in the "red eye" reaction seen in some extended lens wearers.[208]

TEMPERATURE

The temperature of the cornea may be altered during contact lens wear; this effect becomes more significant in the closed eye.[56,84] The rate of epithelial metabolism is largely dependent on ambient temperature.[66] Thus, although the changes in corneal temperature under a contact lens are small, the fine balance of oxygen supply and corneal oxygen demand under the closed lid may be upset by these changes. Further research is needed to clarify this situation.

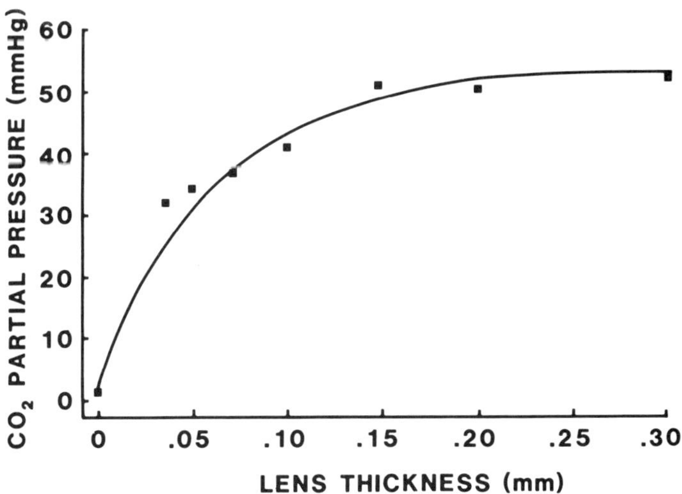

Figure 1-4 Carbon dioxide partial pressure beneath HEMA lenses of varying center thicknesses. (Holden BA: unpublished data, 1985)

TEAR CHEMISTRY

The major short-term changes in the tear film during contact lens wear are a hypotonic shift and a slight decrease in tear pH. These changes, however, must be considered against a pattern of diurnal variation, which includes a shift toward hypertonicity and acidity during sleep. Changes in tear film chemistry may affect the permeability of the epithelium to certain molecules or ions. This is evidenced by an increase in glucose levels in the tears following hypotonic challenge,[40] and an alteration in the sodium and chloride transport properties of the cornea as the pH falls.[61] These effects on transport properties, and hence on transcorneal potential of the cornea, may alter corneal hydration; indeed, the osmotic effect alone may cause significant corneal swelling.[201] In addition, an acidic environment may decrease corneal oxygen consumption.[29]

Although these effects are significant, the extent to which epithelial function is compromised by altered tear chemistry during contact lens wear is generally masked by the more prominent effects of decreased oxygen availability.

STRUCTURAL AND FUNCTIONAL CHANGES IN THE CORNEA INDUCED BY CONTACT LENS WEAR

CORNEAL EPITHELIUM

Short-Term Changes

METABOLIC CHANGES

Contact lens-induced epithelial hypoxia causes a decrease in the rate of aerobic metabolism and a consequent increase in the rate of anaerobic metabolism in the corneal epithelium. This leads to an increase in the concentration of lactate in the epithelium and stroma.[180] It has been suggested that this increase in lactate concentration may osmotically induce a net flow of water into the cornea, leading to corneal edema.[112]

With contact lens wear, stores of glycogen in the epithelium are reduced.[77,85,178,180,194] This is apparently not due to depletion of epithelial glucose, because more than sufficient glucose is available from the aqueous to maintain metabolism even under conditions of total anoxia.[188] It has been suggested that the mild epithelial trauma associated with lens wear may by itself stimulate epithelial glycogen mobilization.[189] It is also possible that a "rate-limiting" enzyme such as hexokinase restricts the rate of entry of glucose into the epithelial metabolic cycles, because it has been shown that glycogen stores may be depleted with gas-induced hypoxia alone.[189]

The concentration in the epithelium of various metabolic enzymes has been found to alter under hypoxic conditions. Lactate dehydrogenase (LDH), which catalyzes the formation of lactate, becomes concentrated in the basal cell layer.[108] Levels of succinic dehydrogenase (SDH), a Krebs cycle enzyme, have also been found to alter in response to hypoxic stress.[89] These alterations in enzyme levels and distribution reflect the change in the nature of metabolic activity with oxygen deprivation, and have been found to parallel other physiological changes such as corneal edema and depletion of glycogen stores.[195]

PHYSICAL CHANGES

As well as inducing changes in the local environment, a contact lens may have a direct mechanical effect on the corneal epithelium. The most obvious mechanical stimulants are those that cause interruption of the epithelial surface and produce staining, such as lens imperfections, lens coatings, foreign bodies under the lens, normal lens rubbing, and in soft lenses the bevel region of the lens periphery.[110] More subtle changes due to a mechanical effect also have been suggested. Hamano has reported a loosening of tight junctions between cells and a decrease in surface microvilli, which occur primarily with hard lens wear.[74] Kwok has attributed a decrease in transcorneal potential to the leakage caused by this mechanical effect.[116] In addition, epithelial permeability to various molecules would be increased, which could account for the increased levels of certain substances, such as glucose, in the tears during lens wear.[40,106] Another subtle change, which has been partially attributed to a mechanical effect, is the mobilization of glycogen.[189] However, the clinical significance of these effects is uncertain.

Histologically, the epithelial changes believed to be due to hypoxia during contact lens wear include accumulation of fluid in both intercellular and intracellular spaces, with shrinkage and shape change of cells, the formation of lipid-like bodies in cells, and the disappearance of certain cell junctions.[19] Lambert and Klyce have found intercellular accumulation of fluid, but without thickness changes.[118] Other authors have suggested that the epithelium swells with hypoxia.[192,193] More recent evidence contradicts this finding, suggesting that the increased epithelial thickness found by Uniacke and co-workers was possibly an artifact of the histological procedure.[202,203]

EPITHELIAL MITOSIS

Hamano and Hori have demonstrated that HEMA contact lenses can cause a 94.3% suppression of epithelial mitosis in the rabbit cornea.[75] These authors attributed this dramatic change to lens-induced alterations in epithelial metabolism, which are likely to result in a decrease in energy available for normal cell division.

TRANSCORNEAL POTENTIAL

Because anaerobic metabolism produces less energy than aerobic metabolism, ATP levels fall during contact lens wear.[189] The consequent decrease in cation pumping produces a fall in the transcorneal potential,[78,116] which is associated with an increase in intracellular edema.[67]

Long-Term Changes

EPITHELIAL THINNING

As mentioned earlier, a decreased level of metabolism appears to lead to a decrease in the rate of cell mitosis. If the rate of cell production decreases but the rate of cell death and removal at the anterior surface remains constant, the number of corneal cells would decrease continually. Because the epithelium does remain intact, certain compensations must be taking place. First of all, cell life would be expected to increase, because the turnover rate has necessarily decreased. As a result, the cells at the anterior surface of a contact lens wearer's epithelium may not be as functionally resistant as those in a non-wearer. This phenomenon has been observed and described as an increase in epithelial fragility.[144,155] Secondly, the epithelium would be expected to reach a new steady-state thickness as the rate of cell production and cell loss reaches a new equilibrium. A thinning has been observed in the epithelium of long-term extended lens wearers.[101] As shown in Figure 1-5, recovery to normal epithelial thickness occurs within approximately 1 month following cessation of lens wear.[101]

EPITHELIAL OXYGEN CONSUMPTION

A decrease in the epithelial oxygen consumption rate of contact lens wearers has been reported recently (Fig. 1-6).[101] This change could be associated

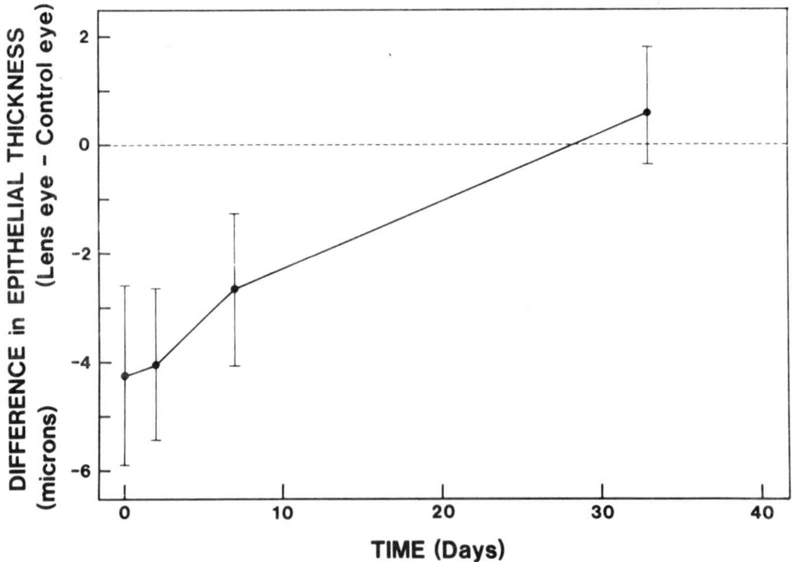

Figure 1-5 Changes in epithelial thickness of the lens-wearing eye relative to the control eye (*dotted line*), after ceasing hydrogel extended lens wear. The subjects had worn a lens in one eye only for an average of 5 years. Data on day 0 were obtained within 2 hours of lens removal. Error bars represent the standard error. (Holden BA, Sweeney DF, Vannas A et al: Effects of long-term extended contact lens wear on the human cornea. Invest Ophthalmol Vis Sci 26:1489, 1985)

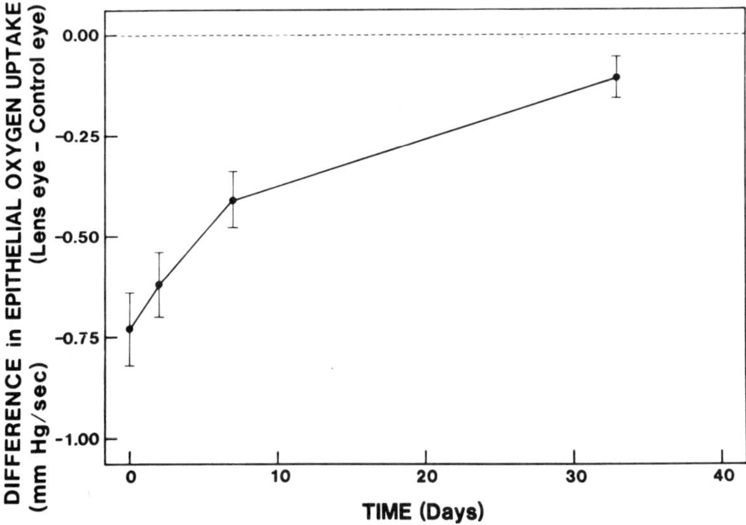

Figure 1-6 Changes in epithelial oxygen uptake rate of the lens-wearing eye relative to the control eye (*dotted line*), after ceasing hydrogel extended lens wear. The subjects had worn a lens in one eye only for an average of 5 years. Data on day 0 were obtained within 2 hours of lens removal. Error bars represent the standard error. (Holden BA, Sweeney DF, Vannas A et al: Effects of long-term extended contact lens wear on the human cornea. Invest Ophthalmol Vis Sci 26:1489, 1985)

with either an overall reduction in the number of epithelial cells or a reduction in cell metabolic activity. Both the epithelial thickness and oxygen consumption rate return to normal within 30 days of cessation of extended lens wear, indicating that changes in epithelial function produced by long-term lens wear are reversible.

EPITHELIAL MICROCYSTS

A more commonly reported change in long-term extended lens wearers is the occurrence of epithelial microcysts.[101,103,208] As shown in Figure 1-7, these appear as pockets of increased refractive index, approximately 10 μm to 90 μm in size.[103] Microcysts are believed to be collections of disorganized encapsulated cellular material. They are rarely observed in daily wear but usually appear with extended hydrogel lens wear after 3 months.

After ceasing lens wear, the number of microcysts increases at first, and then slowly decreases (Fig. 1-8).[101] The initial increase is attributed to a resurgence in epithelial mitotic activity as the cornea resumes normal levels of aerobic respiration, causing an initial rapid movement of microcysts towards the surface. In the absence of further microcystic development, the number of microcysts decreases as the remainder are pushed to the surface.

CORNEAL SENSITIVITY

Changes in corneal sensitivity during contact lens wear have been well documented. Both soft and hard lenses have been shown to cause an in-

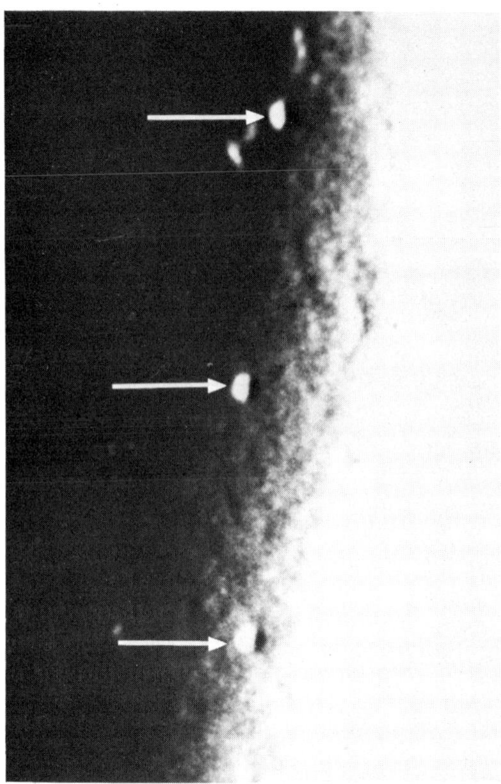

Figure 1-7 Slit-lamp photograph of epithelial microcysts (*arrows*) in the corneal epithelium of a lens-wearing eye. Note that the microcysts display reversed illumination; that is, the distribution of light within the microcysts is opposite to that of the background. This suggests that microcysts represent pockets of cellular debris. (Holden BA, Sweeney DF, Vannas A et al: Effects of long-term extended contact lens wear on the human cornea. Invest Ophthalmol Vis Sci 26:1489, 1985)

crease in the corneal touch threshold, with hard lenses producing the greater effect.[138,140] The length of wear is also an important factor in determining the magnitude of sensitivity loss.[139] After cessation of wear, sensitivity follows a slow process of recovery, which may also be dependent on the length of wear.[140]

Studies on the etiology of decreased corneal sensitivity with lens wear have implicated hypoxia as the cause.[143] However, reduced sensitivity can occur in the absence of edema,[141] and may also occur in the presence of a mechanical stimulus without hypoxia.[158] A proposed mechanism for reduced sensitivity during contact lens wear is a decrease in the concentration of the neurotransmitter acetylcholine with hypoxia.[142]

Although initially it may seem that reduced corneal sensitivity results in increased tolerance to the presence of a lens, consideration of the etiology of the change suggests that the reduction is not simply a mechanical adaptation. In fact, reduction in corneal sensitivity during contact lens wear may

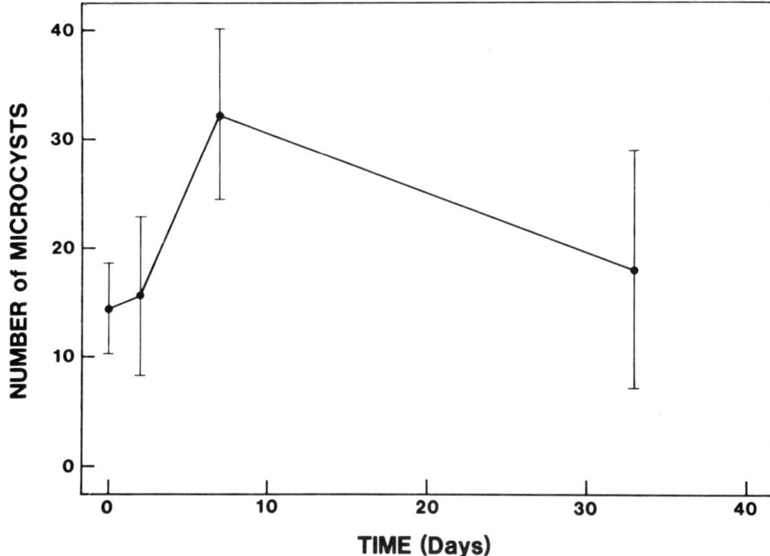

Figure 1-8 Changes in the number of epithelial microcysts in the lens-wearing eye after ceasing hydrogel extended lens wear. Data for day 0 were obtained within 2 hours of lens removal. Error bars represent the standard error. (Holden BA, Sweeney DF, Vannas A et al: Effects of long-term extended contact lens wear on the human cornea. Invest Ophthalmol Vis Sci 26:1489, 1985)

have clinical consequences. Awareness of foreign bodies is reduced, and susceptibility to corneal abrasions and other possible complications may increase. Hence, increased corneal touch threshold is an important complication of contact lens wear.

EPITHELIAL FRAGILITY

O'Leary and Millodot described how a Cochet–Bonnet esthesiometer can be used to measure epithelial fragility; that is, the mechanical strength of the epithelium.[155] They demonstrated that both hard and soft contact lens wear significantly reduce the damage threshold of the epithelium. Epithelial hypoxia has been suggested as the cause of increased epithelial fragility during lens wear.[155]

CORNEAL STROMA

Short-Term Changes

EDEMA

Although the oxygen tension in the stroma may drop to nearly zero with contact lens wear,[74] this tissue does not appear to suffer directly from hypoxia. The absence of a direct hypoxic effect may be attributed to the low oxygen requirement of the tissue, due to its relatively low metabolic rate.[169]

Nevertheless, the stroma shows one of the most prominent effects of reduced oxygen levels at the anterior cornea through its swelling response.[180] In some contact lens wearers the stroma may swell by up to 30% of its original thickness.[22,123] Increased corneal thickness is due to an increased level of hydration of the stromal tissue.[79] However, it seems that this is not so much a direct effect of hypoxia on the stroma as on the epithelium.

The mechanisms of stromal swelling have been the subject of great interest in the ophthalmic literature. The cornea has a strong tendency to take up water; to remain in a deturgescent state requires an active pumping mechanism, the major component of which is situated in the endothelium.[91–93,128,131,132,147] When corneal thickness is stable, the efflux of water pumped out by the endothelium is equal to the influx of water by passive diffusion.

Initial theories on the increase of stromal hydration with hypoxia postulated that a decrease in the endothelial pump rate occurred due to a lowered metabolic rate in the endothelium with hypoxia, or from an inhibitory effect of lactate.[169,178] However, no direct evidence has been presented to indicate that endothelial pump activity is reduced under hypoxic conditions. Stevenson and co-workers suggest that the endothelial pump rate is relatively constant regardless of the level of corneal edema; this view is supported by the findings of Baum and co-workers.[15,184] However, it has been noted that the *in vitro* cornea deswells more rapidly following hydration than would be expected if the endothelial pump rate was constant, suggesting that pump activity increases with hydration.[42,92,113] This question still needs to be resolved.

Because the endothelial pump rate is either constant or increases with hydration, and the epithelium contributes little to the active removal of water from the cornea,[167] the increase in hydration with hypoxia must be due to an increase in the passive diffusion of water across the endothelium or epithelium. Flow rate through a membrane is proportional to the pressure gradient and inversely proportional to the resistance of the membrane. Therefore, an increased flow of water into the cornea would be due either to an increase in the osmotic pressure of the stroma, or to a decrease in the strong barriers that the epithelium and endothelium present to water flow.[145] The first possibility has been strongly implicated as the mechanism for corneal edema during hypoxia. According to the theory of Klyce, lactate, a by-product of anaerobic metabolism in the corneal epithelium, diffuses only slowly through the stromal tissue and into the anterior chamber.[112] As a result, the concentration of lactate in the stroma increases under hypoxic conditions and provides sufficient osmotic pressure to explain the rise in corneal hydration.[113] Several authors have observed an increase in corneal lactate levels with contact lens wear or hypoxia.[119,151,166,178]

Daily Lens Wear The amount of corneal edema that develops during hydrogel contact lens wear is primarily determined by the lens oxygen transmissibility (Dk/L). Holden and Mertz have demonstrated that lenses of low

Dk/L can induce up to 9% edema during daily wear.[96] On the other hand, these authors showed that corneal edema can be avoided if the lens Dk/L is greater than 24.1×10^{-9} (cm $\times$ ml O_2)/(s $\times$ ml $\times$ mmHg). The relationship between lens Dk/L and corneal swelling is given in Figure 1-9. The amount of swelling induced by a rigid gas-permeable lens will generally be less than that induced by a hydrogel lens of the same Dk/L because the rigid lens tear pump provides additional oxygen to the cornea.

Extended Lens Wear When hydrogel contact lenses are worn on an extended-wear basis, the cornea experiences a cyclic edema response that parallels the wake/sleep cycle (Fig. 1-10). Holden and co-workers found that the mean overnight corneal swelling upon awakening ranged from 9.7% to 15.1%, depending on the Dk/L of the lens worn.[97] The mean contact lens-induced edema 12 hours after awakening varied from 1.6% to 5.8% for the various lenses; considerable individual variations in these responses were noted.

The critical hydrogel lens Dk/L needed to limit overnight corneal swelling to 4% (the level experienced without a contact lens in place) was found to be 87.0×10^{-9} (cm $\times$ ml O_2)/(s $\times$ ml $\times$ mmHg) (Fig. 1-11).[96] This "ideal" level of oxygen transmissibility is not possible with current hydrogel materials but can be met with silicone elastomers or very high Dk/L gas-perme-

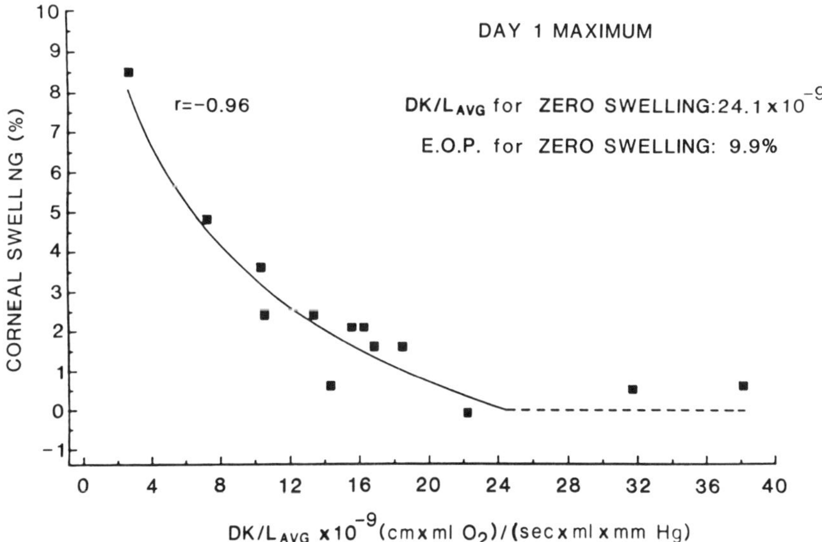

Figure 1-9 Maximum corneal swelling (%) versus average lens oxygen transmissibility (Dk/L_{avg}) for 13 lens types worn on a daily-wear basis. Dk/L_{avg} values were calculated using published polymer oxygen permeability (Dk) data or manufacturers' specifications, and measured lens thickness. Critical Dk/L_{avg} and EOP values necessary to reduce daily-wear swelling to zero are also shown. (Holden BA, Mertz GW: Critical oxygen levels to avoid corneal edema for daily and extended wear contact lenses. *Invest Ophthalmol Vis Sci* 25:1161, 1984)

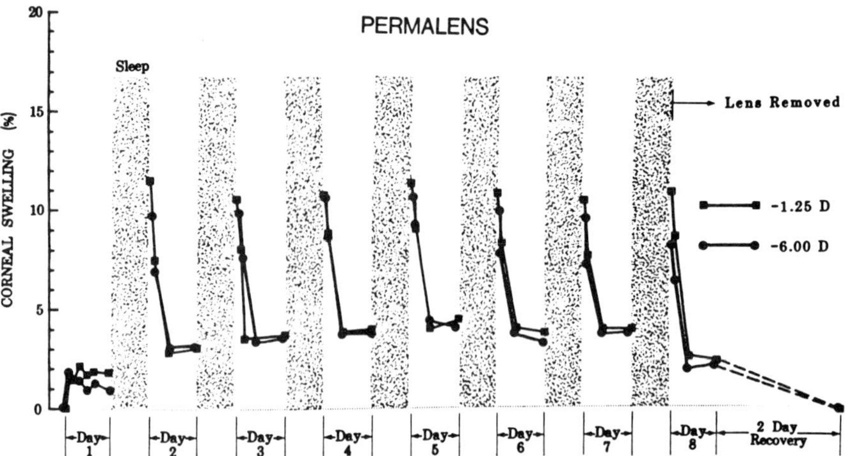

Figure 1-10 Corneal swelling versus time for five unadapted subjects wearing Cooper Permalens contact lenses continuously for a period of 1 week. All subjects wore a −1.25 D lens in one eye and a −6.00 D lens in the other eye. (Holden BA, Mertz GW, McNally JJ: Corneal swelling response to contact lenses worn under extended wear conditions. Invest Ophthalmol Vis Sci 24:218, 1983)

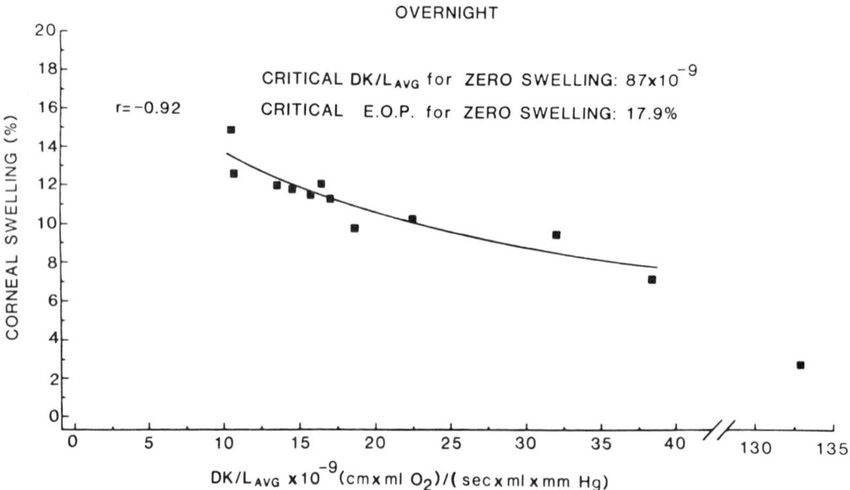

Figure 1-11 Overnight corneal swelling (%) versus average lens oxygen transmissibility (Dk/L_{avg}) for 12 lens types. Dk/L_{avg} values were calculated using published polymer oxygen permeability (Dk) data or manufacturers' specifications, and measured lens thickness. Critical Dk/L_{avg} and EOP values necessary to reduce overnight swelling to the 4% experienced without a lens in place are also shown. (Holden BA, Mertz GW: Critical oxygen levels to avoid corneal edema for daily and extended wear contact lenses. Invest Ophthalmol Vis Sci 25:1161, 1984)

able materials. Holden and Mertz have suggested an interim criterion for acceptance of hydrogel lenses for extended wear: a Dk/L that will achieve zero residual swelling, that is, the Dk/L required to allow the cornea to return to normal thickness soon after eye opening following sleep with lenses.[96] The Dk/L criterion for zero residual swelling was found to be 34.3 $\times$ 10^{-9} (cm $\times$ ml O$_2$)/(s $\times$ ml $\times$ mmHg) (Fig. 1-12).

From a physiological standpoint, rigid gas-permeable contact lenses may better satisfy the prerequisites for extended wear. Such lenses would be expected to induce similar overnight edema responses to hydrogel materials, but have the added advantage of greater flushing action for the removal of tear debris from behind the lens upon awakening.[156] Preliminary clinical studies suggest that rigid lenses are a promising extended-wear alternative.

STRIAE IN THE POSTERIOR STROMA

The relative contributions of the epithelium and endothelium as the entry site of fluid during corneal swelling have not been determined. Bergmanson and Chu have found greater edema in the posterior stroma with contact lens wear, suggesting that the endothelium is the major entry site.[19] However, other studies have demonstrated that the posterior stroma has a greater capacity to swell than the anterior stroma, which may explain these findings.[121,204] This differential swelling capacity probably gives rise to the striate corneal lines seen during contact lens wear, which appear to be caused by a

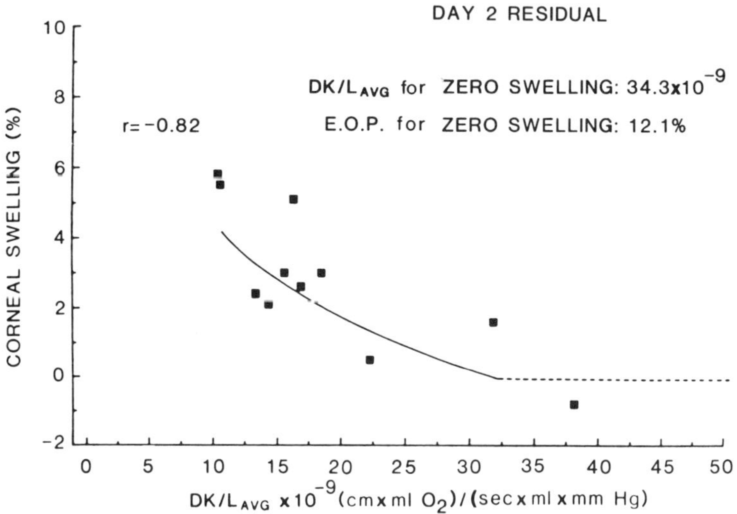

Figure 1-12 Residual overnight corneal swelling (%) versus average lens oxygen transmissibility (Dk/L_{avg}) for 11 lens types. Dk/L_{avg} values were calculated using published polymer oxygen permeability (Dk) data or manufacturers' specifications, and measured lens thickness. Critical Dk/L_{avg} and EOP values necessary to reduce residual overnight swelling to zero are also shown. (Holden BA, Mertz GW: Critical oxygen levels to avoid corneal edema for daily and extended wear contact lenses. Invest Ophthalmol Vis Sci 25:1161, 1984)

buckling of the posterior stroma and Descemet's membrane.[171,198] This phenomenon is found with edema, and although the result of decreased oxygen availability, it is probably directly due to the swelling effect.[162,163]

ULTRASTRUCTURAL CHANGES

The only observed change in the stromal tissue that may be caused directly by insufficient oxygen is a degeneration and possible death of keratocytes.[19] Even so, these changes may be secondary to other factors such as toxic levels of lactate or chronic edema. Therefore, the short-term stromal changes that have been observed are probably due more to epithelial alterations than a reaction of the stroma to hypoxia.

Long-Term Changes

STROMAL THINNING

Corneal swelling during contact lens wear tends to increase in magnitude during the first week of wear. After reaching a peak at about this time, the cornea tends to return towards baseline thickness, and in many cases may become thinner than before commencement of lens wear.[120,173] The course of corneal swelling varies between individuals, and in isolated cases, chronic corneal thickening occurs.[153,173]

Holden and co-workers found that a small but significant amount of stromal thinning had occurred in a group of unilateral contact lens patients after 5 years of extended wear (Fig. 1-13).[101] They hypothesized that chronic corneal edema causes an alteration of function in the keratocytes. Consequently, the production of collagen, glycoproteins, and proteoglycans is reduced, less stromal tissue is produced, and stromal thinning results. Alternatively the action of lactate, which accumulates in the stroma under hypoxic conditions, on the mucopolysaccharide ground substance may lead to some dissolution of stromal tissue.

INFILTRATES

Although infiltration of polymorphonucleocytes (PMNs) into the corneal epithelium with contact lens wear is more frequent, stromal infiltrates have more serious clinical consequences.[105] Infiltrates are generally associated with the "red eye" response, and may be induced by several factors.[208] A number of reports link the occurrence to pathogenic stimuli, whether actual bacterial infections, viral conditions, or as a response to endotoxins due to the presence of pathogens on the contact lens.[9,43,105] Other reports implicate preservatives used in the lens maintenance procedure.[21,149] Zantos and Holden have proposed that debris trapped under the lens during extended wear can provide a stimulus to infiltrates.[208] This debris may be from necrotic epithelial cells, from which certain enzymes may be released.[94] These enzymes may act as a chemical stimulus to the entry of PMN cells into the cornea.

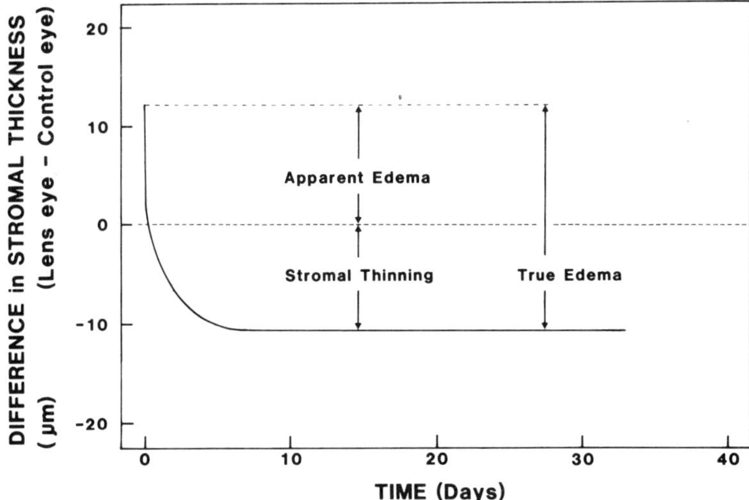

Figure 1-13 Changes in stromal thickness of the lens-wearing eye relative to the control eye (*dotted line*), after ceasing hydrogel extended lens wear. The subjects had worn a lens in one eye only for an average of 5 years. The apparent edema on lens removal, the true edema, and stromal thinning after lens-induced edema has subsided are indicated. (Holden BA, Sweeney DF, Vannas A et al: Effects of long-term extended contact lens wear on the human cornea. Invest Ophthalmol Vis Sci 26:1489, 1985)

VASCULARIZATION

The presence of blood vessels invading the cornea is a sign that the tissue is under some stress.[133] Thus, vascularization induced by contact lens wear indicates that the fitting, maintenance, or mode of wear of the lens is inappropriate. Contact lens-induced vascularization is one of the most frequent complications of lens wear.[170] Although vascularization is observed in daily lens wear, it occurs most frequently in cosmetic extended wear or therapeutic and aphakic wear.[37,82,154,172,177,182,199] The cause of vascularization is uncertain, but the etiology appears to be multifactorial.

The intact stroma is resistant to vessel infiltration. The integrity of the stroma depends on mucopolysaccharides, especially hyaluronosulphuric acid, which may be an antivascular factor.[170] Degeneration of the stroma may be initiated by collagenase, fibrinolysin, or hyaluronidase.[34,35] This softening of the stroma may promote vessel infiltration, although on its own may not provide the stimulus to initiate vessel growth.

Stromal edema may also be a predisposing factor to stromal softening and vessel growth, although the relationship may be casual rather than causal.[14,33,62,134] Thoft and co-workers believe that edema has a role in facilitating vascularization, but on its own the presence of edema is not a sufficient stimulus.[190] Just as edema accompanies new vessel growth, factors producing edema such as hypoxia and lactate accumulation have also been reported in association with vascularization.[8,45,122] However, even in the presence of these conditions, other mediators may be necessary to produce vessel proliferation.

Leucocytic infiltration has been observed as a precursor to vascularization.[104,111] Although this may be the stimulant in some cases, the presence of leucocytes is not essential for vessel growth.[49,105]

Epithelial chemistry has been suggested by several authors as a mediating influence on vessel growth. It has been proposed that the intact epithelium provides a growth inhibitor that suppresses the collagenolytic activity of keratocytes.[17,130] Some stimulus or corneal injury may neutralize this inhibition process; or the injury may stimulate release of a vasogenic factor or metabolites that can promote collagenolysis.[17,49,62,70,210] Such injury could be provided by trauma during contact lens wear,[36] or by the occlusive effects of the lens on oxygen flow.[170]

Other suggested vasogenic factors are prostaglandin E_2 (PGE_2), Michaelson's factor, or tumor angiogenic factor.[16,170]

In conclusion, a contact lens could have an etiological role in the induction of stromal vascularization by means of a number of possible mechanisms: mechanical, chemical, or physiological. Thus, it has not been possible to identify the specific feature of contact lenses that promotes corneal vascularization.

CORNEAL ENDOTHELIUM

Short-Term Changes

ENDOTHELIAL BLEBS

In the first few minutes after the insertion of a contact lens, regions of the endothelium cease to reflect specularly when viewed with the slit-lamp (Fig. 1-14).[207] These dark lines and spots, known as *blebs,* constitute a maximum proportion of the endothelial area at 15 to 40 minutes after lens insertion.[10,175,197] With continued wear the magnitude of the bleb response decreases, suggesting an adaptation process.

The loss of the specular reflection from the areas of the endothelium, which appear as blebs, is due to localized bulging of the posterior endothelial surface.[196]

Although lens-induced hypoxia has been suggested as the primary cause of the bleb response, Holden and co-workers have demonstrated that blebs can be produced independently of precorneal hypoxia.[102] These authors suggest that local environmental changes such as a reduction in pH due to lactate or carbonic acid accumulation may induce these transient changes. They also found that blebs could be induced in the absence of increased corneal hydration, suggesting that this response does not compromise endothelial pump or barrier function, at least in the short term.

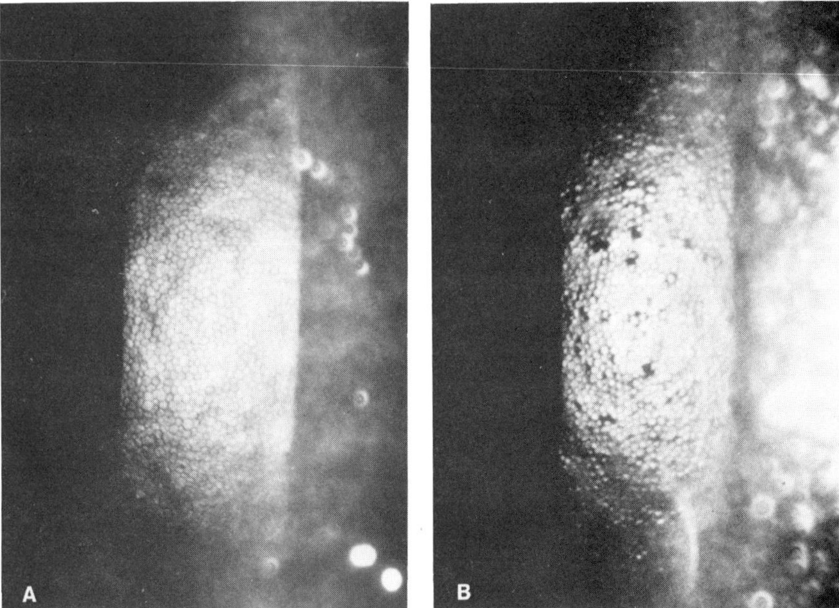

Figure 1-14 A typical endothelial bleb response. The stimulus in this case was a thick HEMA contact lens. *(A)* Prior to lens insertion, endothelial bleb response, expressed as a percentage of the area covered by blebs, is 0.18%. *(B)* Peak response to stimulus (5.40% of area under blebs). (Holden BA, Williams L, Zantos SG: The etiology of transient endothelial changes in the human cornea. Invest Ophthalmol Vis Sci 26:1354, 1985)

Long-Term Changes

CELL DENSITY

Because the corneal endothelium is a monolayer of cells, and apparently a nonregenerating tissue in humans, a decrease in cell numbers due to any source would be of concern. Decreased cell density occurs with age and with surgical procedures interfering with the cornea.[24,98,117,205,206] It is also possible that contact lens wear may reduce cell numbers. Caldwell and co-workers have reported a decreased cell density during hard contact lens wear that exceeds the usual decrease with age, although their data are not convincing because of an inadequate control group.[27] Others have not found a significantly reduced cell density in wearers of hard, soft, and extended-wear lenses.[26,90,101,174]

POLYMEGATHISM

Although endothelial cell density may not be affected by contact lens wear, there have been a number of reports that indicate some alteration of the endothelium with contact lens wear. Cell morphology is fairly uniform throughout the endothelium in normal corneas, but this uniformity of size and shape may be lost during contact lens wear.[26,90,101,174] Variation in cell size is known as *polymegathism* (Fig. 1-15), and variation in cell shape as *pleomorphism.*

The reasons for these changes are uncertain. Because the effects of contact lens wear on the oxygen tension at the endothelium are disputed, the role of endothelial hypoxia is questionable. Other factors, such as an increase in the lactate concentration or decrease in *p*H in the vicinity of the endothelium, may have some long-term effects. Contrary to the popular belief that the human corneal endothelium does not regenerate, it has been suggested that polymegathism may be an indication that mitosis is occurring.[90] Reduction of polymegathism after cessation of long-term contact lens wear is not significant after 1 month (Fig. 1-16), and a return to pre-lens-wearing levels may never occur.[101]

The effects of polymegathism are uncertain. Sweeney and co-workers have demonstrated that corneas with higher degrees of polymegathism show greater levels of corneal swelling and a slower rate of deswelling following hypoxic stress.[185] However, further research into this and other aspects of endothelial function with contact lens wear is indicated.

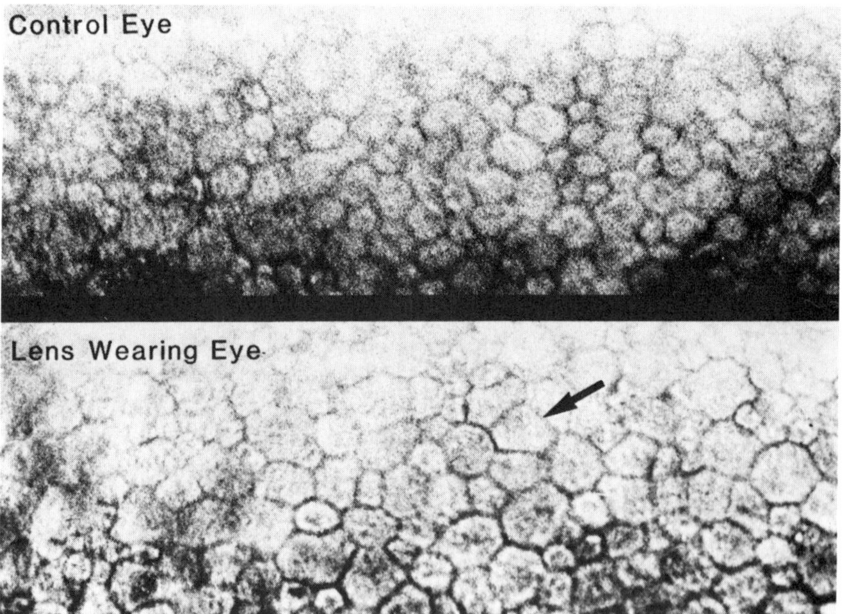

Figure 1-15   Endothelial photograph of non-lens-wearing eye (*top*) and lens-wearing eye (*bottom*) of a patient who had worn a hydrogel lens on an extended-wear basis in one eye only for 79 months. A greater variation in endothelial cell size (polymegathism) is evident in the lens-wearing eye. Also evident in that eye are a number of rosette formations (*arrow*); these are thought to occur following injury of a single endothelial cell, whereby neighboring cells radiate towards the center of the damaged cell. (Holden BA, Sweeney DF, Vannas A et al: Effects of long-term extended contact lens wear on the human cornea. Invest Ophthalmol Vis Sci 26:1489, 1985)

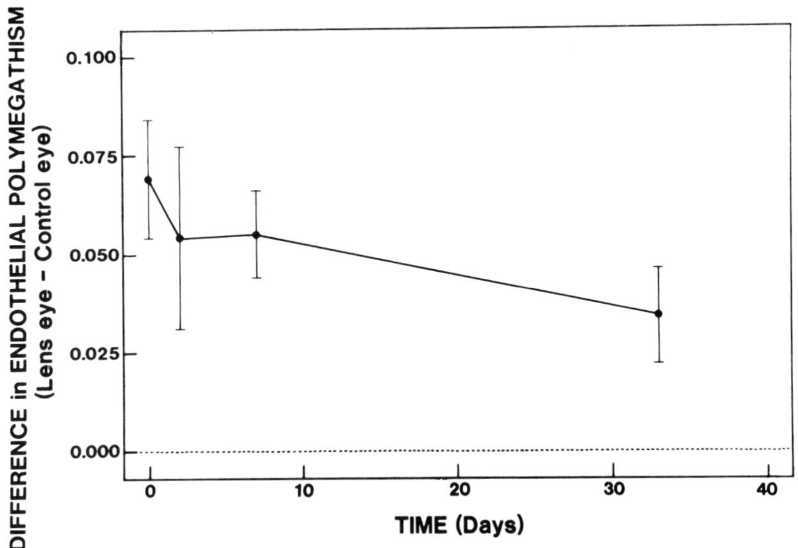

Figure 1-16 Changes in endothelial polymegathism (coefficient of variation of mean cell area) of the lens-wearing eye relative to the control eye (*dotted line*) after ceasing hydrogel extended lens wear. The subjects had worn a lens in one eye only for an average of 5 years. Data on day 0 were obtained within 2 hours of lens removal. Error bars represent the standard error. Although lens-induced polymegathism appears to decrease over the 33-day recovery period, this trend was not statistically significant. (Holden BA, Sweeney DF, Vannas A et al: Effects of long-term extended contact lens wear on the human cornea. Invest Ophthalmol Vis Sci 26:1489, 1985)

ENDOTHELIAL BEDEWING

Endothelial bedewing may be described as either a cluster of fluid droplets or a constellation of leucocytes deposited on the surface of the corneal endothelium. This phenomenon has been reported in association with chronic intolerance to contact lens wear and active inflammation of the anterior part of the eye.[136,209]

The coincidence of chronic intolerance to contact lens wear and endothelial bedewing is a matter for speculation at this stage. It is possible that corneal edema accompanying chronic or acute overwear of contact lenses may stimulate a response from the anterior uvea, leading to a release of inflammatory cells into the aqueous and their subsequent deposition on the posterior corneal surface.[136]

However, the relationship between endothelial bedewing and contact lens intolerance does not appear to be obligatory, because not all intolerant lens wearers show endothelial bedewing, and bedewing has been observed in successful contact lens wearers and non-contact lens wearers. In addition, it would seem that intolerance to lens wear and endothelial bedewing need not follow the same time course.[136]

STRUCTURAL AND FUNCTIONAL CHANGES IN OTHER ANTERIOR OCULAR STRUCTURES INDUCED BY CONTACT LENS WEAR

CONJUNCTIVA

Short-Term Changes

HYPEREMIA

Although the conjunctiva would appear to be a useful indicator of adverse reactions to contact lens wear, it has received comparatively little attention. Conjunctival injection often occurs soon after the insertion of a contact lens, probably as a foreign body reaction. It occurs with poor lens fits, probably in response to hypoxia or the mechanical effect of the lens, and accompanies corneal edema.[191] It also has been attributed to a toxic reaction to chemicals used in the lens cleaning procedure.[21,109,149,150] The mechanism is probably similar to that observed in other tissues of the body where a defense response is initiated.

Limbal injection is a common finding in contact lens wearers, and has been attributed to a number of factors, including damaged or dirty lenses, adverse reactions to preservatives, hay fever, eyestrain, toxic environmental conditions, and lack of sleep.[134,135] Chronic limbal injection may be a precursor to corneal vascularization.[134]

Long-Term Changes

GIANT PAPILLARY CONJUNCTIVITIS

Although giant papillary conjunctivitis (GPC) is a long-term complication of contact lens wear, its occurrence is not necessarily correlated with time of wear.[164] It has been found in daily and extended wearers of both hard and soft lenses.[7,37,125,181] Reports on frequency vary, but in our experience it would appear to occur more frequently than 0.35%, as reported in the large study by Price and co-workers.[164] The condition causes discharge or excess mucus secretion, itching, and lens intolerance.[7,72] GPC presents a clinical picture of conjunctival papillae and a mucus coating, usually on the upper tarsal conjunctiva. This appearance is quite similar to that observed in vernal conjunctivitis, but there are various distinguishing characteristics.[1,2,4,80]

The conjunctival surface of patients with GPC is morphologically different from that of normal contact lens wearers, which is again different from that of non-contact lens wearers.[7,71,73] There appears to be some continuity between these changes; asymptomatic wearers have the usual conjunctival epithelial cell covering of villi isolated to the center of the cell, whereas this effect is more pronounced in GPC sufferers.[168] The reduced number of villi and the mucus secretion may be due in part to the mechanical effect of the contact lens on the conjunctiva, and may be aggravated further by a rough contact lens surface such as occurs with contact lens deposits.[114,168] Histologically, few uncharacteristic inflammatory cells are observed in normal contact lens wearers, whereas abnormal inflammatory cells may be found with GPC.[3,5,6] No qualitative difference has been found between the surface coatings on lenses worn by patients with GPC and those worn by asymptomatic wearers.[63,64] Combined with other similarities between the two groups, this suggests that individual factors initiate the condition.

In addition, a number of lens-related factors may be involved such as design, amount of coating, and chemicals used in lens maintenance.[148] Although the problem is generally solved by ceasing lens wear, a complete refit may enable the asymptomatic continuation of wear.

SUPERIOR LIMBIC KERATOCONJUNCTIVITIS

Contact lens-induced superior limbic keratoconjunctivitis is a syndrome of contact lens intolerance manifested by changes involving the superior cornea and upper tarsal and bulbar conjunctiva. This condition has been observed in patients wearing soft, and occasionally hard gas-permeable, contact lenses.[137,176,183] The clinical signs typically include a crescent or wedge-shaped area of epithelial haze in the superior third of the cornea, which is sharply demarcated from the uninvolved cornea. Hyperemia and staining of the bulbar conjunctiva in the area of the superior limbus also occur. Papillae are often present in the upper tarsal conjunctiva.

Although the etiology of the syndrome is unclear, it has been suggested that it may represent an intolerance to thimerosal, exacerbated by mechanical irritation from the bevel edge of a soft contact lens.[23] Following cessation of lens wear, the symptoms generally improve rapidly; however, in some cases the superior cornea does not recover normal appearance, and the associated contact lens intolerance is persistent for weeks or months.

CLUMPING OF MICROVILLI

As mentioned previously, certain changes may occur in the conjunctiva of asymptomatic lens wearers. All contact lens wearers have altered upper tarsal conjunctival surfaces, probably due to the mechanical effects of the lens. The changes include clumping of surface microvilli in the center of the epithelial cells, and prominence of the cell borders.[168] The clinical significance of these changes is uncertain.

Of other cases where the conjunctiva is involved, there is usually an associated complication. Conjunctival hyperemia occurs in the red-eye response to debris under lenses, or corneal infiltration.[94,208] In these cases there is probably no direct effect on the conjunctiva, and its reaction is the usual vascular response to tissue injury.

EYELIDS

Lid Sensitivity

The initial discomfort of contact lens wear is caused mainly by rubbing of the lids, particularly the upper lid, on the lens. Adaptation is relatively quick, and with hard lens wear, is partly due to a loss of sensitivity of the lid margins.[124] The initial acceptance of soft lenses is greater than for hard lenses as a result of the larger diameter and thinner edge, which minimizes lid contact.[126] In fact, soft lens comfort can be improved by increasing lens diameter.[28] Alterations to edge thickness are of more questionable value, probably because the top edge of a soft contact lens remains under the top lid at all times, and the rubbing of this lid on the lens induces the discomfort.[81] Edge lift has been suggested as a factor in determining lens comfort during hard lens wear, although varying base curve to alter edge lift in soft lenses does not affect comfort.[107]

Blinking

The eyelids perform the very important function during contact lens wear of rewetting the anterior lens surface during each blink, and so changes that may affect this function are important. The work of Hill and Carney indicates that there is an increased blink rate with both hard and soft lens wearers, with a decreased frequency of long interblink periods.[32,86] The blink rate is affected more in hard lens wearers.[25] These changes may be more prominent during the early period of wear, but reduce in magnitude as the lid margins become less sensitive to the mechanical effects of the lens.[124]

UVEA

The uveal tract may also react to contact lens wear. This is usually associated with acute corneal conditions.[20,94,157,177] Therefore, it is accompanied by marked symptoms such as photophobia, pain, and visual loss, and signs of epithelial decompensation, conjunctival hyperemia, stromal infiltrates, epithelial microcysts, endothelial bedewing, circumcorneal injection, lid swelling, and corneal edema. The response may be initiated by a severe hypoxic reaction, infection, overwear, or chemical toxicity.

CONCLUSION

This chapter has reviewed the vast array of changes to the anterior ocular structures that are induced by contact lenses. Although the etiology of many of these changes remains unclear, a factor that is frequently implicated is tissue hypoxia. We now have a good idea of the effects of oxygen deprivation on corneal physiology, and guidelines for providing adequate corneal oxygen availability, so that the fitting and design of contact lenses can be optimized to alleviate lens-induced hypoxic stress. Filling this prescription may be difficult, but this has stimulated a tremendous proliferation of promising new lens materials.

There is a need, however, to investigate more fully other physiological aspects of lens wear that have been largely ignored in the literature. For example, the entrapment of cellular debris behind hydrogel lenses appears to be a major factor in the etiology of adverse reactions to extended hydrogel lens wear. The nature of the trapped debris, the mechanism by which cellular debris initiates an adverse response, the minimum tear exchange needed to clear debris, and the identification of lens design features that can prevent debris buildup are questions that need to be studied.

The ability of carbon dioxide to escape from a contact lens-wearing cornea is another unresolved problem of considerable importance. The desirable levels and types of lens coating to ensure continuing lens compatibility with the adjacent tissues are also yet to be determined. Certainly, it is clear that contact lenses are a complex problem demanding an ever-increasing input from specialists in other disciplines, such as ocular physiologists, surface and polymer chemists, biochemists, physicists, and engineers.

REFERENCES

1. Abelson MB, Soter NZ, Simon MA et al: Histamine in human tears. Am J Ophthalmol 83:417, 1977
2. Allansmith MR, Baird RS: Percentage of degranulated mast cells in vernal conjunctivitis and giant papillary conjunctivitis associated with contact lens wear. Am J Ophthalmol 91:71, 1981
3. Allansmith MR, Baird RS, Greiner JV: Number and type of inflammatory cells in contact lens wear. Am J Ophthalmol 87:171, 1979
4. Allansmith MR, Baird RS, Greiner JV: Vernal conjunctivitis and contact lens associated giant papillary conjunctivitis compared and contrasted. Am J Ophthalmol 87:544, 1979
5. Allansmith MR, Greiner JV, Baird RS: Number of inflammatory cells in normal conjunctiva. Am J Ophthalmol 86:250, 1978
6. Allansmith MR, Korb DR, Greiner JV: Giant papillary conjunctivitis in contact lens wearers: History. Ophthalmology 85:766, 1978
7. Allansmith MR, Korb DR, Greiner JV et al: Giant papillary conjunctivitis in contact lens wearers. Am J Ophthalmol 83:687, 1977
8. Ashton N: Neovascularization in ocular disease. Trans Ophthalmol Soc UK 81:145, 1961
9. Backman HA: A preliminary investigation of the aging of soft contact lenses. Int Contact Lens Clin 7:40, 1980
10. Barr JT, Schoessler JP: Corneal endothelial response to rigid contact lenses. Am J Optom Physiol Opt 57:267, 1980
11. Barr RE, Hennessey M, Murphy VG: Diffusion of oxygen at the endothelial surface of the rabbit cornea. J Physiol 270:1, 1977
12. Barr RE, Roetman EL: Oxygen gradients in the anterior chamber of anesthetized rabbits. Invest Ophthalmol 13:386, 1974
13. Barr RE, Silver IA: Effects of corneal environment on oxygen tension in the anterior chambers of rabbits. Invest Ophthalmol 12:140, 1973
14. Baum JL, Martola E: Corneal edema and corneal vascularization. Am J Ophthalmol 65:881, 1968
15. Baum JP, Maurice DM, McCarey BE: The active and passive transport of water across the corneal endothelium. Exp Eye Res 39:335, 1984

16. BenEzra D: Neovasculogenic ability of prostaglandins, growth factors, and synthetic chemoattractants. Am J Ophthalmol 86:455, 1978

17. BenEzra D, Tanishima T: Possible regulatory mechanisms in the cornea. Arch Ophthalmol 96:1891, 1978

18. Benjamin W, Rasmussen MA: The closed lid tear pump: Oxygenation? Int Eyecare 1:251, 1985

19. Bergmanson JPG, Chu LW-F: Corneal response to rigid contact lens wear. Br J Ophthalmol 66:667, 1982

20. Binder PS: Extended wear of soft contact lenses. Contact Intraoc Lens Med J 5:60, 1979

21. Binder PS, Rasmussen DM, Gordon M: Keratoconjunctivitis and soft contact lens solutions. Arch Ophthalmol 99:87, 1981

22. Binder PS, Worthen DM: Clinical evaluation of continuous wear hydrophilic lenses. Am J Ophthalmol 83:549, 1977

23. Boruchoff SA, Bajart AM: The superior limbic manifestations of contact lens intolerance. In Dabezies OH (ed): Contact Lenses: The CLAO Guide to Basic Science and Clinical Practice, pp 44.1–44.3. Orlando, Grune & Stratton, 1984

24. Bourne WM, Kaufman HE: Specular microscopy of human corneal endothelium *in vivo*. Am J Ophthalmol 81:319, 1976

25. Brown M, Chinn S, Fatt I et al: The effect of soft and hard contact lenses on blink rate, amplitude and length. J Am Optom Assoc 44:254, 1973

26. Caillau S, Cochet P: Hornhautenendothel und kontaklinsen. Contactologia 5:32, 1983

27. Caldwell DR, Kastl PR, Dabezies OH et al: The effect of long-term hard lens wear on corneal endothelium. Contact Intraoc Lens Med J 8:87, 1982

28. Callender M: An evaluation of Bausch & Lomb ultra-thin soflens (Polymacon) contact lenses. Can J Optom 41:79, 1979

28a. Carney LG: Studies on the Basis of Ocular Changes During Contact Lens Wear. Ph.D. thesis, University of Melbourne, Australia, 1974

29. Carney LG, Efron N: pH ambient et flux d'oxygene corneen. J Fr Ophthalmol 3:125, 1980

30. Carney LG, Hill RM: Human tear pH. Arch Ophthalmol 94:821, 1976

31. Carney LG, Hill RM: Human tear buffering capacity. Arch Ophthalmol 97:951, 1979

32. Carney LG, Hill RM: Variation in blinking behavior during soft lens wear. Int Contact Lens Clin 11:250, 1984

33. Cogan DG: Corneal vascularization. Invest Ophthalmol 1:253, 1962

34. Collin HB: Lymphatic drainage of 131 I-albumin from the vascularized cornea. Invest Ophthalmol 9:146, 1970

35. Collin HB: Ultrastructure of lymphatic vessels in the vascularized rabbit cornea. Exp Eye Res 10:207, 1970

36. Collin HB: Limbal vascular response prior to corneal vascularization. Exp Eye Res 16:443, 1973

37. Coon LJ, Miller JP, Meier RF: Overview of extended wear contact lenses. J Am Optom Assoc 50:745, 1979

38. Cuklanz HD, Hill RM: Oxygen requirements of corneal contact lens systems. Am J Optom Arch Am Acad Optom 46:228, 1969

39. Dallos J: Sattler's veil. Br J Ophthalmol 30:607, 1946

40. Daum KM, Hill RM: Human tears: Glucose instabilities. Acta Ophthalmol 62:472, 1984

41. De Roetth A Jr: Respiration of the cornea. AMA Arch Ophthalmol 44:666, 1950
42. Dikstein S, Maurice DM: The active control of corneal hydration. Israel J Med Sci 8:1523, 1972
43. Dohlman CH, Buruchoff SA, Mobilia EF: Complications in use of soft contact lenses in corneal disease. Arch Ophthalmol 90:367, 1973
44. Duane TD: Metabolism of the cornea. AMA Arch Ophthalmol 41:736, 1949
45. Duffin RM, Weissman BA, Ueda J: Complications of extended wear hard contact lenses on rabbits. Int Contact Lens Clin 9:101, 1982
46. Efron N, Carney LG: Oxygen levels beneath the closed eyelid. Invest Ophthalmol Vis Sci 18:93, 1979
47. Efron N, Carney LG: Models of oxygen performance for the static, dynamic and closed-lid wear of hydrogel contact lenses. Aust J Optom 64:223, 1981
48. Efron N, Carney LG: Effect of blinking on the level of oxygen beneath hard and soft gas-permeable contact lenses. J Am Optom Assoc 54:229, 1983
49. Eliason JA: Leukocytes and experimental corneal vascularization. Invest Ophthalmol Vis Sci 17:1087, 1978
50. Fatt I: Steady-state distribution of oxygen and carbon dioxide in the *in vivo* cornea. II. The open eye in nitrogen and the covered eye. Exp Eye Res 7:413, 1968
51. Fatt I: Oxygen pathways to a cornea covered by a contact lens. Contacto 21:4, 1977
52. Fatt I: The cornea. In Physiology of the Eye: An Introduction to the Vegetative Functions, pp 92–188. Boston, Butterworths, 1978
53. Fatt I: Gas transmission properties of soft contact lenses. In Ruben M (ed): Soft Contact Lenses: Clinical and Applied Technology, pp 83–110. London, Baillière Tindall, 1978
54. Fatt I, Bieber MT: The steady-state distribution of oxygen and carbon dioxide in the *in vivo* cornea. I. The open eye in air and the closed eye. Exp Eye Res 7:103, 1968
55. Fatt I, Bieber MT, Pye SD: Steady-state distribution of oxygen and carbon dioxide in the *in vivo* cornea of an eye covered by a gas-permeable contact lens. Am J Optom Arch Am Acad Optom 46:3, 1969
56. Fatt I, Chaston J: Temperature of a contact lens on the eye. Int Contact Lens Clin 7:195, 1980
57. Fatt I, Freeman RD, Lin D: Oxygen distribution in the cornea: A re-examination. Exp Eye Res 18:357, 1974
58. Fatt I, Hill RM: Oxygen tension under a contact lens during blinking: A comparison of theory and experimental observation. Am J Optom Arch Am Acad Optom 47:50, 1970
59. Fatt I, Hill RM, Takahashi GH: Carbon dioxide efflux from the human cornea *in vivo*. Nature 203:738, 1964
60. Fatt I, St. Helen R: Oxygen tension under an oxygen-permeable contact lens. Am J Optom Arch Am Acad Optom 48:545, 1971
61. Fischer FH, Schmitz L, Hoff W et al: Sodium and chloride transport in the isolated human cornea. Pflugers Arch 373:179, 1978
62. Folca PJ: Corneal vascularization induced experimentally with corneal extracts. Br J Ophthalmol 53:827, 1969

63. Fowler SA, Allansmith MR: The surface of the continuously worn contact lens. Arch Ophthalmol 98:1233, 1980

64. Fowler SA, Greiner JV, Allansmith MR: Soft contact lenses from patients with giant papillary conjunctivitis. Am J Ophthalmol 88:1056, 1979

65. Freeman RD: Oxygen consumption by the component layers of the cornea. J Physiol 225:15, 1972

66. Freeman RD, Fatt I: Environmental influences on ocular temperature. Invest Ophthalmol 12:596, 1973

67. Friend J: Biochemistry of ocular surface epithelium. Int Ophthalmol Clin 19:73, 1979

68. Friend J: Physiology of the cornea: Metabolism and biochemistry. In Smolin G, Thoft RA (eds): The Cornea: Scientific Foundations and Clinical Practice, pp 17–21. Boston, Little, Brown & Co, 1983

69. Fullard RJ, Carney LG: Human tear enzyme changes as indicators of the corneal response to anterior hypoxia. Acta Ophthalmol 63:678, 1985

70. Graymore C, Ashton N, McCormick A: Alloxan and lactic acid dehydrogenase activity of the cornea. Br J Ophthalmol 52:677, 1968

71. Greiner JV, Covington HI, Allansmith MR: Surface morphology of the human upper tarsal conjunctiva. Am J Ophthalmol 83:892, 1977

72. Greiner JV, Covington HI, Allansmith MR: Surface morphology of giant papillary conjunctivitis in contact lens wearers. Am J Ophthalmol 85:242, 1978

73. Greiner JV, Covington HI, Korb DR et al: Conjunctiva in asymptomatic contact lens wearers. Am J Ophthalmol 86:403, 1978

74. Hamano H: Fundamental research on the effects of contact lenses on the eye. In Ruben M (ed): Soft Contact Lenses: Clinical and Applied Technology, pp 121–142. London, Baillière Tindall, 1978

75. Hamano H, Hori M: Effect of contact lens wear on the mitoses of corneal epithelial cells: Preliminary report. CLAO J 9:133, 1983

76. Hamano H, Hori M, Hamano T et al: Effects of contact lens wear on mitosis of corneal epithelium and lactate content in aqueous humor of rabbit. Jpn J Ophthalmol 27:451, 1983

77. Hamano H, Hori H, Hirayama K: The effects of hard and soft contact lenses on rabbit corneas. Contacto 16:26, 1972

78. Hamano H, Kikkawa Y: Corneal potential as influenced by the contact lens. Contacto 12:23, 1968

79. Hedbys BO, Mishima S: The thickness–hydration relationship of the cornea. Exp Eye Res 5:221, 1966

80. Henriquez AS, Kenyon KR, Allansmith MR: Mast cell ultrastructure: Comparison in contact lens-associated giant papillary conjunctivitis and vernal conjunctivitis. Arch Ophthalmol 99:1266, 1981

81. Hernandez V, Tomlinson A: The effects of soft lens edge thickness. Contact Lens Forum 8:77, 1983

82. Highman VN: High water content soft contact lenses for continuous wear. Contact Lens J 5:21, 1976

83. Hill RM: Oxygen requirements at the cornea with flexible lenses. In Bitonte JL, Keates RH (eds): Symposium on the Flexible Lens. St Louis, CV Mosby, 1972

84. Hill RM: How the cornea takes the heat. Int Contact Lens Clin 5:302, 1978

85. Hill RM, Augsburger A, Uniacke CA: Oxygen permeable hard contact lenses. Contact Lens J 3:40, 1972

86. Hill RM, Carney LG: The effects of hard lens wear on blinking behavior. Int Contact Lens Clin 11:242, 1984
87. Hill RM, Fatt I: How dependent is the cornea on the atmosphere? J Am Optom Assoc 35:873, 1964
88. Hill RM, Leighton AJ: Temperature changes of human cornea and tears under a contact lens. 1. The relaxed open eye, and the natural and forced closed eye conditions. Am J Optom Arch Am Acad Optom 42:9, 1965
89. Hill RM, Rengstorff RH, Petrali JP et al: Critical oxygen requirement of the corneal epithelium as indicated by succinic dehydrogenase reactivity. Am J Optom Physiol Opt 51:331, 1974
90. Hirst LW, Auer C, Cohn J et al: Specular microscopy of hard contact lens wearers. Ophthalmology 91:1147, 1984
91. Hodson S: Evidence for a bicarbonate-dependent sodium pump in corneal endothelium. Exp Eye Res 11:20, 1971
92. Hodson S: The regulation of corneal hydration by a salt pump requiring the presence of sodium and bicarbonate ions. J Physiol 236:271, 1974
93. Hodson S, Miller F: The bicarbonate ion pump in the endothelium which regulates the hydration of rabbit cornea. J Physiol 263:563, 1976
94. Holden BA: Ocular changes associated with the extended wear of contact lenses. Ophthalmic Optician 23:140, 1983
95. Holden BA: Unpublished data, 1985
96. Holden BA, Mertz GW: Critical oxygen levels to avoid corneal edema for daily and extended wear contact lenses. Invest Ophthalmol Vis Sci 25:1161, 1984
97. Holden BA, Mertz GW, McNally JJ: Corneal swelling response to contact lenses worn under extended wear conditions. Invest Ophthalmol Vis Sci 24:218, 1983
98. Holden BA, Polse KA, Fonn D et al: Effects of cataract surgery on corneal function. Invest Ophthalmol Vis Sci 22:343, 1982
99. Holden BA, Sweeney DF: The oxygen tension and temperature of the superior palpebral conjunctiva. Acta Ophthalmol 63:100, 1985
100. Holden BA, Sweeney DF, Sanderson G: The minimum precorneal oxygen tension to avoid corneal edema. Invest Ophthalmol Vis Sci 25:476, 1984
101. Holden BA, Sweeney DF, Vannas A et al: Effects of long-term extended contact lens wear on the human cornea. Invest Ophthalmol Vis Sci 26:1489, 1985
102. Holden BA, Williams L, Zantos SG: The etiology of transient endothelial changes in the human cornea. Invest Ophthalmol Vis Sci 26:1354, 1985
103. Humphreys JA, Larke JR, Parrish ST: Microepithelial cysts observed in extended contact lens wearing subjects. Br J Ophthalmol 64:888, 1980
104. Inomata H, Smelser GK, Polach FM: Corneal vascularization in experimental uveitis and graft rejection. Invest Ophthalmol 10:840, 1971
105. Josephson JE, Caffery BE: Infiltrative keratitis in hydrogel lens wearers. Int Contact Lens Clin 6:47, 1979
106. Kilp H: Biochemistry. In Ruben M (ed): Soft Contact Lenses: Clinical and Applied Technology, pp 111–120. London, Baillière Tindall, 1978
107. Kimball D, Mandell RB: Clinical performance of ultrathin lenses. Int Contact Lens Clin 1:99, 1974
108. King JE, Augsburger A, Hill RM: Quantifying the distribution of lactic acid dehydrogenase in the corneal epithelium with oxygen deprivation. Am J Optom Arch Am Acad Optom 48:1016, 1971

109. Kline LN, DeLuca TJ: Thermal versus chemical disinfection. Int Contact Lens Clin 5:260, 1978

110. Kline LN, DeLuca TJ: Corneal staining. Int Ophthalmol Clin 21:13, 1981

111. Klintworth GK: The contribution of morphology to our understanding of the pathogenesis of experimentally produced corneal vascularization. Invest Ophthalmol Vis Sci 16:281, 1977

112. Klyce SD: Stromal lactate accumulation can account for corneal edema osmotically following epithelial hypoxia in the rabbit. J Physiol 321:49, 1981

113. Klyce SD, Russell SR: Numerical solution of coupled transport equations applied to corneal hydration dynamics. J Physiol 292:107, 1979

114. Korb DR, Greiner JV, Finnemore VM: Treatment of contact lenses with papain: Increase in wearing time in keratoconic patients with giant papillary conjunctivitis. Arch Ophthalmol 101:48, 1983

115. Kwan M, Niinikoski J, Hunt TK: *In vivo* measurements of oxygen tension in the cornea, aqueous humor, and anterior lens of open eye. Invest Ophthalmol 11:108, 1972

116. Kwok S: Review: The effects of contact lens wear on the electrophysiology of the corneal epithelium. Aust J Optom 66:138, 1983

117. Laing RA, Sandstrom M, Berrospi A et al: Changes in corneal endothelium as a function of age. Exp Eye Res 22:587, 1976

118. Lambert SR, Klyce SD: The origins of Sattler's veil. Am J Ophthalmol 91:51, 1981

119. Langham M: Utilization of oxygen by the component layers of the living cornea. J Physiol 177:461, 1952

120. Lebow KA, Plishka K: Ocular changes associated with extended wear contact lenses. Int Contact Lens Clin 7:11, 1980

121. Lee D, Wilson G: Non-uniform swelling properties of the corneal stroma. Current Eye Res 1:457, 1981

122. Levene R, Shapiro A, Baum J: Experimental corneal vascularization. Arch Ophthalmol 70:242, 1963

123. Liebowitz HM, Laing RA, Sandstrom M: Continuous wear of hydrophilic contact lenses. Arch Ophthalmol 89:309, 1973

124. Lowther GE, Hill RM: Sensitivity threshold of the lower lid margin in the course of adaptation to contact lenses. Am J Optom Arch Am Acad Optom 45:587, 1968

125. Mackie IA, Wright P: Giant papillary conjunctivitis (secondary vernal) in association with contact lens wear. Trans Ophthalmol Soc UK 98:3, 1978

126. Mandell RB: Why are gel lenses comfortable? Int Contact Lens Clin 1:30, 1974

126a. Mandell RB, Farrell R: Corneal swelling at low atmospheric oxygen pressures. Invest Ophthalmol Vis Sci 19:697, 1980

127. Maurice DM: The cornea and sclera. In Davson H (ed): The Eye, Vol 1b, Vegetative Physiology and Biochemistry, pp 1–158. London, Academic Press, 1984

128. Maurice DM: The location of the fluid pump in the cornea. J Physiol 221:43, 1972

129. Maurice DM, Riley MV: The cornea. In Graymore CN (ed): Biochemistry of the Eye, pp 1–103. New York, Academic Press, 1970

130. Maurice DM, Zauberman H, Michaelson IC: The stimulus to neovascularization in the cornea. Exp Eye Res 5:168, 1966

131. Mayes KR, Hodson S: An *in vivo* demonstration of the bicarbonate ion pump of rabbit corneal endothelium. Exp Eye Res 28:699, 1979
132. McCarey BE, Edelhauser HF, Van Horn DL: Functional and structural changes in the corneal endothelium during *in vitro* perfusion. Invest Ophthalmol 12:410, 1973
133. McMonnies CW: Contact lens-induced corneal vascularisation. Int Contact Lens Clin 10:12, 1983
134. McMonnies CW: Risk factors in the etiology of contact lens induced corneal vascularization. Int Contact Lens Clin 11:286, 1984
135. McMonnies CW, Chapman-Davies A, Holden BA: Vascular response to contact lens wear. Am J Optom Physiol Opt 59:10, 1982
136. McMonnies CW, Zantos SG: Endothelial bedewing of the cornea in association with contact lens wear. Br J Ophthalmol 63:478, 1979
137. Miller RA, Brightbill FS, Slama S: Superior limbic keratoconjunctivitis in soft contact lens wearers. Cornea 1:293, 1982
138. Millodot M: Effect of soft lenses on corneal sensitivity. Acta Ophthalmol 52:603, 1974
139. Millodot M: Effect of the length of wear of contact lenses on corneal sensitivity. Acta Ophthalmol 54:721, 1976
140. Millodot M: Long term wear of hard contact lenses and corneal integrity. Contacto 22:7, 1978
141. Millodot M: Clinical evaluation of an extended wear lens. Int Contact Lens Clin 11:16, 1984
142. Millodot M, O'Leary DJ: Loss of corneal sensitivity with lid closure in humans. Exp Eye Res 29:417, 1979
143. Millodot M, O'Leary DJ: Effect of oxygen deprivation on corneal sensitivity. Acta Ophthalmol 58:434, 1980
144. Millodot M, O'Leary DJ: Corneal fragility and its relationship to sensitivity. Acta Ophthalmol 59:820, 1981
145. Mishima S, Hedbys BO: The permeability of the corneal epithelium and endothelium to water. Exp Eye Res 6:10, 1967
146. Mishima S, Kaye GI, Takahashi GH et al: The function of the corneal endothelium in the regulation of corneal hydration. In Langham ME (cd): The Cornea, pp 207–235. Baltimore, Johns Hopkins Press, 1969
147. Mishima S, Kudo T: *In vivo* incubation of rabbit cornea. Invest Ophthalmol 6:329, 1967
148. Molinari JF: The clinical management of giant papillary conjunctivitis. Am J Optom Physiol Opt 58:886, 1981
149. Mondino BJ, Groden LR: Conjunctival hyperemia and corneal infiltrates with chemically disinfected soft contact lenses. Arch Ophthalmol 98:1767, 1980
150. Morgan JF: Complications associated with contact lens solutions. Ophthalmology 86:1107, 1979
151. Morley N, McCulloch C: Corneal lactate and pyridine nucleotides (PNS) with contact lenses. AMA Arch Ophthalmol 66:379, 1961
152. Natsumeda NH, Fatt I: Corneal swelling and oxygen flux through a soft contact lens. Am J Optom Physiol Opt 58:590, 1981
153. Nirankari VS, Baer JC: Persistent corneal edema in aphakic eyes from daily-wear and extended-wear contact lenses. Am J Ophthalmol 98:329, 1984
154. Nirankari VS, Karesh J, Lakhanpal V et al: Deep stromal vascularization

associated with cosmetic, daily-wear contact lenses. Arch Ophthalmol 101:46, 1983

155. O'Leary DJ, Millodot M: Abnormal epithelial fragility in diabetes and in contact lens wear. Acta Ophthalmol 59:827, 1981

156. O'Neal MR, Polse KA, Sarver MD: Corneal responses to rigid and hydrogel lenses during eye closure. Invest Ophthalmol Vis Sci 25:837, 1984

157. Paullisky CJ, Alexander A: Aphakia, uveitis and extended contact lens wear. Am J Optom Physiol Opt 61:289, 1984

158. Polse KA: Etiology of corneal sensitivity changes accompanying contact lens wear. Invest Ophthalmol Vis Sci 17:1202, 1978

159. Polse KA: Tear flow under hydrogel contact lenses. Invest Ophthalmol Vis Sci 18:409, 1979

160. Polse KA, Decker M: Oxygen tension under a contact lens. Invest Ophthalmol Vis Sci 18:188, 1979

161. Polse KA, Mandell RB: Critical oxygen tension at the corneal surface. Arch Ophthalmol 84:505, 1970

162. Polse KA, Mandell RB: Etiology of corneal striae accompanying hydrogel lens wear. Invest Ophthalmol 15:553, 1976

163. Polse KA, Sarver MD, Harris MG: Corneal edema and vertical striae accompanying the wearing of hydrogel lenses. Am J Optom Physiol Opt 52:185, 1975

164. Price MJ, Morgan JF, Willis WE et al: Tarsal conjunctival appearance in contact lens wearers. Contact Intraoc Lens Med J 8:16, 1982

165. Redslob E, Tremblay JL: Etude sur les echanges gazeux a la surface de l'oeil. Annals Oculist 170:415, 1933 (cited by Maurice DM, Riley MV, 1970)

166. Reim M, Baeck H, King P et al: Aqueous humor and corneal stroma metabolite levels under various conditions. Ophthalmic Res 3:241, 1972

167. Remiach PS, Candia OA, Alvarez LJ: Energetic requirements of transepithelial Na and Cl transport in the isolated bullfrog cornea. Exp Eye Res 29:637, 1979

168. Richmond PP, Allansmith MR: Giant papillary conjunctivitis. Int Ophthalmol Clin 21:65, 1981

169. Riley MV: Glucose and oxygen utilization of the cornea. Exp Eye Res 8:193, 1969

170. Ruben M: Corneal vascularization. Int Ophthalmol Clin 21:27, 1981

171. Sarver MD: Striate lines among patients wearing hydrophilic contact lenses. Am J Optom Arch Am Acad Optom 48:762, 1971

172. Schecter DR, Emery JM, Soper JW: Corneal vascularization in therapeutic soft lens wear. Contact Intraoc Lens Med J 1:141, 1975

173. Schoessler JP, Barr JT: Corneal thickness changes with extended contact lens wear. Am J Optom Physiol Opt 57:729, 1980

174. Schoessler JP, Woloschak MJ: Corneal endothelium in veteran PMMA contact lens wearers. Int Contact Lens Clin 8:19, 1981

175. Schoessler JP, Woloschak MJ, Mauger TF: Transient endothelial changes produced by hydrophilic contact lenses. Am J Optom Physiol Opt 59:764, 1982

176. Sendele DD, Kenyon KR, Mobilia EF et al: Superior limbic keratoconjunctivitis in contact lens wearers. Ophthalmology 90:616, 1983

177. Slatt B, Stein HA: Complications of prolonged wear hydrogel lenses. Contact Intraoc Lens Med J 5:82, 1979

178. Smelser GK, Chen DK: Physiological changes in cornea induced by contact lenses. AMA Arch Ophthalmol 53:676, 1955

179. Smelser GK, Ozanics V: Importance of atmospheric oxygen for maintenance of the optical properties of the human cornea. Science 115:140, 1952

180. Smelser GK, Ozanics V: Structural changes in the cornea of guinea pigs after wearing contact lenses. AMA Arch Ophthalmol 49:335, 1953

181. Spring TF: Reaction to hydrophilic lenses. Med J Aust 1:449, 1974

182. Stark WJ, Martin NF: Extended wear soft contact lenses for myopic correction. Arch Ophthalmol 99:1963, 1981

183. Stenson S: Superior limbic keratoconjunctivitis associated with soft contact lens wear. Arch Ophthalmol 101:402, 1983

184. Stevenson R, Vaja N, Jackson J: Corneal transparency changes resulting from osmotic stress. Ophthal Physiol Opt 3:33, 1983

185. Sweeney DF, Holden BA, Vannas A et al: The clinical significance of corneal endothelial polymegathism. Invest Ophthalmol Vis Sci (Suppl) 26:53, 1985

186. Sweeney DF, Vannas A, Holden BA et al: Evidence for sympathetic neural influence on human corneal epithelial function. Acta Ophthalmol 63:215, 1985

187. Terry JE, Hill RM: Human tear osmotic pressure: Diurnal variation and the closed lid. Arch Ophthalmol 96:120, 1978

188. Thoft RA, Friend J: Corneal epithelial glucose utilization. Arch Ophthalmol 88:58, 1972

189. Thoft RA, Friend J: Biochemical aspects of contact lens wear. Am J Ophthalmol 80:139, 1975

190. Thoft RA, Friend J, Murphy HS: Ocular surface epithelium and corneal vascularization in rabbits; 1. The role of wounding. Invest Ophthalmol Vis Sci 18:85, 1979

191. Tomlinson A, Haas DD: Changes in corneal thickness and circumcorneal vascularization with contact lens wear. Int Contact Lens Clin 7:26, 1980

192. Uniacke CA: Oxygen insufficiency and epithelial swelling with experimental contact lenses. J Am Optom Assoc 42:1274, 1971

193. Uniacke CA, Augsburger A, Hill RM: Epithelial swelling with oxygen insufficiency. Am J Optom Arch Am Acad Optom 48:565, 1971

194. Uniacke CA, Hill RM: The depletion course of epithelial glycogen with corneal anoxia. Arch Ophthalmol 87:56, 1972

195. Uniacke CA, Hill RM, Greenberg M et al: Physiological tests for new contact lens materials. 1. Quantitative effects of selected oxygen atmospheres on glycogen storage, LDH concentration and thickness of the corneal epithelium. Am J Optom Arch Am Acad Optom 49:329, 1972

196. Vannas A, Holden BA, Makitie J: The ultrastructure of contact lens induced changes in the human corneal endothelium. Acta Ophthalmol 62:320, 1984

197. Vannas A, Makitie J, Sulonen J et al: Contact lens induced transient changes in the corneal endothelium. Acta Ophthalmol 59:552, 1981

198. Wechsler S: Striate corneal lines. Am J Optom Physiol Opt 51:852, 1974

199. Weinberg RJ: Deep corneal vascularization caused by aphakic soft contact lens wear. Am J Ophthalmol 83:121, 1977

200. Weissman BA, Fatt I, Rasson J: Diffusion of oxygen in human corneas in vivo. Invest Ophthalmol Vis Sci 20:123, 1981

201. Wilson G, Fatt I: Thickness changes in the epithelium of the excised rabbit cornea. Am J Optom Physiol Opt 51:75, 1974

202. Wilson G, Fatt I: Thickness of the corneal epithelium during anoxia. Am J Optom Physiol Opt 57:409, 1980

203. Wilson G, Fatt I, Freeman RD: Thickness changes in the stroma of an excised rabbit cornea during anoxia. Exp Eye Res 17:165, 1973

204. Wilson G, O'Leary DJ, Vaughan W: Differential swelling in compartments of the corneal stroma. Invest Ophthalmol Vis Sci 25:1105, 1984

205. Wilson RS, Roper-Hall MJ: Effect of age on the endothelial cell count in the normal eye. Br J Ophthalmol 66:513, 1982

206. Yamaguchi T, Asbell PA, Ostrick M et al: Endothelial damage in monkeys after radial keratotomy performed with a diamond blade. Arch Ophthalmol 102:765, 1984

207. Zantos SG, Holden BA: Transient endothelial changes soon after wearing soft contact lenses. Am J Optom Physiol Opt 54:856, 1977

208. Zantos SG, Holden BA: Ocular changes associated with continuous wear of contact lenses. Aust J Optom 61:418, 1978

209. Zantos SG, Holden BA: Guttate endothelial changes with anterior eye inflammation. Br J Ophthalmol 65:101, 1981

210. Zauberman H, Michaelson IC, Bergman F et al: Stimulation of neovascularization of the cornea by biogenic amines. Exp Eye Res 8:72, 1969

CHAPTER TWO

FITTING TECHNIQUES FOR GAS-PERMEABLE RIGID LENSES

JAMES M. GORDON and SIDNEY J. HANISH

Gas-permeable rigid lenses are usually better tolerated, in terms of comfort and wearing time, than conventional hard polymethylmethacrylate (PMMA) lenses. This is a result of the enhanced oxygen transmission of the newer lens materials. Gas-permeable lenses fall into five categories:

1. Cellulose acetate butyrate lenses
2. Siloxanyl/methacrylate lenses
3. Silicone resin and silicone elastomer lenses
4. Fluorocarbon lenses
5. Styrene lenses

The fluorocarbon lenses are not yet available because they are still in investigational studies. The silicone elastomer and silicone resin lenses are no longer available because they have recently been removed from the market by the manufacturer.

Gas permeable lenses have several advantages over soft lenses:

1. Fluorescein can be used to determine the lens–cornea fitting relationship.

2. Visual acuity, especially in the presence of corneal astigmatism, is better.

3. Allergic or toxic reactions are less frequent, because the lenses do not absorb the disinfecting agents. (Soft lenses often absorb the disinfecting agents; their later release causes ocular irritation.)

4. Lens life is longer. Gas-permeable hard lenses are more durable than soft lenses.

DESIGN

These corneal lenses can be lenticular or single cut and have a wide range of parameters. Because of the enhanced oxygen transmission through the lens, it is possible to fit large lenses without inducing corneal edema. A large lens is sometimes advantageous, as it provides for better centration (more surface area of the lens aligned with the cornea) and better vision (larger optical zone). This is especially true when fitting keratoconus patients, post-keratoplasty patients, eyes with significant astigmatism, and patients in whom the interrelationship of the lid anatomy and lens induces a smaller lens to ride high on the cornea.

PARAMETERS

All of the gas-permeable lenses are available in any base curve and diameter one would wish to specify, but most of these lenses are manufactured in certain parameters, as listed in the accompanying tables.

The cellulose acetate butyrate (CAB) lenses were the first gas-permeable rigid lenses. This material has better oxygen transmission than PMMA. Lenses of the siloxanyl/methacrylate type have even better oxygen transmission and are the most common gas-permeable lenses at this time. The search for lens material with improved oxygen transmission has recently led to the development of styrene and fluorocarbon lenses. It is hoped that development of better polymers and improved lens design can continue to improve gas-permeable lens comfort, eventually even realizing an extended-wear gas-permeable lens. It is recognized that optical quality, wetting angle, and material durability are as necessary as oxygen transmission in evaluating gas-permeable lenses.

CELLULOSE ACETATE BUTYRATE LENSES

Parameters for CAB lenses are given in Table 2-1.

Cabcurve Lens

The available diameters range from 8.8 mm to 9.2 mm. The power range is from −8 D to +6 D.

Meso Lens

The available diameters range from 8.8 mm to 9.2 mm. The power range is from −20 D to +20 D.

Rx 56 Lens

The available diameters are 9.2 mm and 9.5 mm. The power range of the 9.2 mm lens is from −6 D to +6 D. The power range of the 9.5 mm lens is from +13 D to +15 D.

TABLE 2-1 Cellulose Acetate Butyrate Lens Parameters*

Lens	Design	Diameter (mm)	OZ (mm)	CPC (mm)	Power (D)
Cabcurve	Lenticular	8.8	7.6	7.18–8.23	−8 to +6
Porofocon B,		9.2	7.6		
Barnes-Hind/Hydrocurve,					
San Diego, Calif.					
Meso	Single cut				−20 to +20
Cabufocon A,	0 to −6 D	8.8		6–9	
Danker Laboratories,	0 to +10 D	8.9			
Tempe, Ariz.	Lenticular	9			
	−7 D and beyond	9.1			
	+11 D and beyond	9.2			
Rx56	Single cut	9.2		6.88–8.44	−6 to +6
Porofocon A,	−7 D to +7 D				
Rynco Laboratories,	Lenticular	9.5		7.35–8.23	+13 to +15
Floral Park, N.Y.	Beyond −7 D or				
	+7 D				

* The parameters are available in the usual inventory set. However, the lenses can be custom ordered from the laboratories in a wider range of parameters.

SILOXANYL/METHACRYLATE COMBINATIONS

Parameters for siloxanyl/methacrylate combination lenses are given in Table 2-2.

Boston Lens II and IV Contact Lens

The Polymer Technology Corporation produces the Boston lens II and IV plastic discs, which are then distributed to authorized contact lens manufacturers. Each company fabricates its lenses in a wide range of parameters. According to the fitting guide of the Polymer Technology Corporation, the suggested diameter for myopic and hyperopic lenses is 9 mm to 9.5 mm; such single-cut lenses are used for refractive error of moderate amount. The suggested diameter for the aphakic lens is 9.5 mm to 10 mm; such lenticular lenses are used for large hyperopic refractive errors. The power range is from −20 D to +30 D.

Optacryl 60 Lens

The Optacryl Company produces only the plastic, which is then distributed to various companies. Each company, in turn, designs lenses in a wide range of parameters.

Paraperm O_2 Lens

The available diameters are 7.5 mm and 9.5 mm. The power range is from −20 D to +20 D.

TABLE 2-2 Siloxanyl/Methacrylate Lens Parameters

Lens	Design	Diameter (mm)	OZ (mm)	CPC (mm)	Power (D)
Boston Lens	Single cut	9–9.5	8	Any base curve	−20 to +10
Itafocon A,					
Polymer Technology,	Lenticular	9.5–10	8	Any base curve	+10 to +30
Wilmington, Mass.					
Optacryl*					
No nonproprietary					
name, Optacryl Co.,					
Denver, Colo.					
Paraperm O$_2$	Lenticular	7.5		Any base curve	−20 to +20
Pasifocon A,	Single cut				
Paragon Laboratories,	Toric	9.5			
Mesa, Ariz.					
Polycon	Lenticular	8.5		7.10–8.35	Plano to −20
Silafocon A,		9		7.20–8.45	−20 to +8
Syntex Laboratories,		9.5		7.20–8.65	−20 to +20
Phoenix, Ariz.		10		7.55–8.65	+8.25 to +20

* The Optacryl Co. produces only the plastic, which is distributed to various companies. Each company, in turn, designs lenses in a wide range of parameters.

Polycon II Lens

The available diameters are 8.5 mm, 9 mm, 9.5 mm, and 10 mm. The power range is from −20 D to +20 D.

STYRENE LENSES

Airlens

The Airlens* is a gas permeable lens that is styrene based (P-butyl styrene). It is available in diameters of 9 mm and 9.5 mm. Powers range from +6 D to −12 D.

FITTING TECHNIQUE

REFRACTION AND KERATOMETRY

Refraction and keratometric measurements are utilized in the same manner as for PMMA lens fitting. When a patient currently wearing PMMA contact lenses is being refitted with gas-permeable lenses, it might be helpful to obtain the original K reading, as well as performing K readings immediately following removal of the lens.

* Wesley-Jessen Co., Chicago, Ill.

SELECTION OF PARAMETERS

Central Posterior Curve

The central posterior curve (CPC), that is, the base curve, is chosen to approximate the cornea. The CPC may be selected so that the lens is fitted on K, or it may be chosen to be slightly steeper than the flattest K if corneal astigmatism is present.

Diameter

The selection of the lens diameter is based on the corneal diameter, the pupillary diameter, and the refractive error.

CORNEAL DIAMETER

The corneal diameter is usually in the 10.5 mm to 12.5 mm range, so most lenses are fitted between 9 mm and 9.5 mm in diameter. If the corneal diameter is less than 10 mm, a lens diameter of 8.5 mm is usually chosen.

PUPILLARY DIAMETER

The pupillary diameter should be measured in a dimly lit room. A millimeter ruler is held adjacent to the eye so that half of the light from a handlight is blocked. Under these circumstances, if the pupillary diameter is greater than 6 mm, consideration should be given to fitting a lens with a diameter larger than 9 mm. If such a person is fitted with a smaller lens, flare may occur, especially from illuminated objects at night. The reason is that in the presence of a large pupil, light rays pass through the junctional area of the optical zone (OZ) of a small lens.

REFRACTIVE ERROR

The power of a contact lens determines its profile, and thus its centering characteristics. To correct a myopic refractive error, a minus power lens is used. Such a lens thickens from the center to the edge. Because of the thick edge, the upper lid can more readily grasp and elevate the lens. High minus lenses (*e.g.,* −8 D or more) may position excessively high. In such an instance, a lens of larger diameter may be used to cover the pupil adequately. Occasionally, when a lens is too high-riding, one must resort to a smaller diameter.

To correct a hyperopic error, a plus power lens is used. Such a lens is thicker in the center than at the edge. In high plus powers, the lens is very thick and heavy. Such a lens in a single-cut design is often low-riding. A lenticular-cut design, incorporating a minus carrier to enhance the capability of upper lid lift, may be necessary.

Power

The power is determined by transposing the spectacle refraction to a minus cylinder, "dropping" the cylinder, and using the remaining spherical power.

Additionally, in high (±4 D) powers, an adjustment must be made for vertex distance. After determining the appropriate power, if the patient is young (and thus able to accommodate readily), it is useful to select an initial trial lens that is slightly overplused.

TRIAL FITTING

Based on the refraction, K readings, corneal diameter, pupillary size, and refractive error, a trial lens is selected. The lens is placed on the cornea, and fluorescein is instilled. The lens is then observed for centration and movement.

Centration

In the usual case of a moderate refractive error, a typical initial trial lens is selected with a diameter of 9 mm and a base curve of 0.5 D to 1 D flatter than the flattest K.

If the initial trial lens positions centrally or slightly high without excessive blink-induced movement,* it is the lens of choice. In this instance, the fluorescein pattern shows a bright green peripheral edge, a diffuse green area centrally, and a slightly darker intermediate area.

If the initial trial lens positions excessively high, visual disturbance will result, because the line of sight is not directed through the center of the lens. In this instance, one should use a larger trial lens, for example, 9 mm to 9.8 mm, so that a sufficient area of OZ will cover the pupil in dim light. To avoid the occurrence of fixed bubbles under the lens, a steep fit should be avoided. The base curve should have a radius that approximates the flattest corneal meridian. The fluorescein pattern should demonstrate minimal apical clearance.

If the initial lens positions excessively low, centration can be improved by using either a larger or a flatter lens. With a larger (9 mm to 9.5 mm) lens with a base curve flatter than K, the increased surface area of the lens allows the upper lid to hold it in a high position throughout the blink cycle. If the initial lens was a single-cut lens, and if the larger lens still positions low, a lenticular lens having a high minus carrier should be evaluated. This design will often enhance the effectiveness of the upper lid in pulling the lens superiorly. If the lens still positions low, one should choose the smallest (8.5 mm) single-cut lens that will remain stable between blinks. Because a smaller lens has less weight, there is less tendency for it to move downward. As with all small lenses, the base curve should be steeper than K. A steep gas-permeable lens is well tolerated because of enhanced oxygen passage through the lens.

---

* Because these lenses permit the passage of atmospheric oxygen, the pumping of tears is not the only source of corneal oxygenation. Thus, blink-induced excursions should be minimized (less than 2 mm) to avoid unnecessary corneal awareness.

Movement

After selecting the diameter, the fit is evaluated in regard to movement. The lens should center well and move approximately 1.5 mm on blinking. Too little movement results in poor tear exchange and poor epithelial oxygenation. Excessive movement causes unnecessary discomfort (because the lid impinges on the lens) and poor vision (because the edge of the OZ crosses the visual axis).

Adequacy of Fit

Once a satisfactory lens is selected, the patient should wear it for about 45 minutes. The fit and the fluorescein pattern then are reevaluated. If the fluorescein pattern is satisfactory, an overrefraction is performed to determine the final power of the lens.

Most patients will fully adapt to the lenses in about 2 weeks. On return office visits, the fluorescein pattern is observed, and the cornea is examined after lens removal. Particular attention is directed to a search for corneal edema (which is best observed using the sclerotic scatter technique) or corneal staining. As with non-gas-permeable hard lenses, peripheral curve modification and fenestration can be done if needed.

The criteria of a successful fit are as follows:

1. *Comfort.* The patient should be able to wear the lenses throughout the day without discomfort.

2. *Clarity of vision.* Normal visual acuity should be obtained. The vision should be crisp and clear.

3. *Appearance.* The patient's conjunctiva should not be hyperemic.

4. *Safety.* The lens should not cause corneal edema, neovascularization, scarring, and so on.

SUMMARY

The fitting technique for gas-permeable hard lenses is only slightly different from that of conventional non-gas-permeable hard lenses. Because gas-permeable lenses permit enhanced oxygen transmission to the cornea, larger diameters can be used. A large diameter is advantageous, because it provides for better centration (more adherence) and clear vision (larger OZ). In contrast to soft lenses, a distinct advantage is that fluorescein can be used to evaluate the fit.

REFERENCES

1. Espy JW: An extended wear contact lens in aphakia. Ann Ophthalmol 3:323, 1979
2. Fatt I, Bieber MT, Pyse SP: Steady state distribution of oxygen and carbon

dioxide in the in vivo cornea of an eye covered by a gas-permeable contact lens. Am J Optom 46:3, 1969
3. Garcia GF: Continuous wear of a gas permeable lens in aphakia. Contact Intraoc Lens Med J 2:29, 1976
4. Gould JG: The management of aphakia with hydrogel, CAB and silicone lenses. Contact Intraoc Lens Med J 4:63, 1978
5. Hartstein J (ed): Introduction to Extended Wear Contact Lenses for Aphakia and Myopia, pp 1–5. St Louis, CV Mosby, 1982
6. Hill RM: In search of a "perfect" polymer. Aust J Optom 61:287, 1978
7. Hill RM, Bailey NJ: Can oxygen pass through PMMA? Int Contact Lens Clin 5:48, 1978
8. Holly FJ: Surface chemistry of contact lens wear. Int Ophthalmol Clin 13:279, 1973
9. Kersley JH: Aphakic prolonged wear lenses brought up-to-date. Contacts 24:17, 1980
10. Lippman JI: Silicone lenses in aphakia: Fact vs. fancy. Contact Intraoc Lens Med J 4:58, 1978
11. Mandell RB: Oxygen permeability of hard contact lenses. Contact Lens Forum 2:35, 1977
12. Polse KA, Mandell RB: Critical oxygen tension at the corneal surface. Arch Ophthalmol 84:505, 1970
13. Roscoe WR, Hill RM: Corneal oxygen demands: A comparison of open and closed eye environments. Am J Optom Physiol Opt 57:67, 1980
14. Ruben M: Fitting hard and soft lenses for aphakia: A review. Aust J Ophthalmol 7:177, 1979
15. Slatt BJ, Stein HA: Complications of prolonged wear hydrogel lenses. Contact Intraoc Lens Med J 5:82, 1979
16. Welsh RC: Continuous use of tiny hard corneal lenses for aphakia (200 cases). Ann Ophthalmol 5:1003, 1973

CHAPTER THREE

HYDROGEL LENSES: APHAKIA

WILLIAM B. ORENBERG
and GULLAPALLI N. RAO

Although nonsurgical approaches to prevent cataract are the subject of intense investigational effort, modern surgical techniques and instrumentation have contributed significantly to enhance the success rate of visual improvement following cataract extraction.

More optimal methods of visual rehabilitation of these patients have added a new dimension to this picture. Contact lenses and intraocular lenses have become standard methods of aphakic correction. Aphakic spectacles are prescribed to a small segment of this population.

The introduction of hydrated polyhydroxyethyl methacrylate (PHEMA) for the production of soft contact lenses by Wichterle and Lim in 1960 ushered in a new chapter in contact lens history.[79] Soft contact lenses manufactured from HEMA, copolymers of HEMA, or other hydrated polymeric materials have been in use in the United States since 1970 when they were first approved by the Food and Drug Administration for therapeutic use in certain painful corneal problems.[26] The FDA approved their use for refractive correction in 1971.

Using Wichterle's methods, Bausch & Lomb pioneered the full-scale production of soft contact lenses in what was to become their Soflens division in the late 1960s. They employed a spin casting method to manufacture the lenses, whereas other companies entering the market used a lathe-cutting process.

Previously, hard lenses were used to correct aphakia.[10,70,78] This modality led to an improvement in the quality of vision as well as the peripheral visual field, and minimized peripheral magnification problems associated with the use of aphakic spectacles.[45] Furthermore, correction of monocular aphakia with contact lenses provided a method for obtaining binocular vision.[20,33,76] The image magnification resulting from aphakic spectacles is on the order of 25% whereas that with aphakic contact lenses is on the order of 7%, the latter differential being within the acceptable range for most patients to attain fusion.[42]

However, a number of aphakic patients were unable to tolerate hard contact lenses either because of problems related to comfort and fit or because of problems resulting from physiologic intolerance.[24] For these patients, the development of hydrophilic daily wear lenses provided a major benefit.[1,3,11,32,50,66,73,77]

The evolution of soft lenses remained an active process with development of new polymers improving the physiologic compatibility with normal corneal metabolic requirements. Higher water contact lenses and thinner lens designs both served to increase the transmission of atmospheric oxygen to the cornea.[60] This led to the concept of extended wear of these lenses.[14,16,28,31,40,43,54,59,64] The first lenses investigated and approved by the FDA for extended wear were for aphakic correction.

This chapter examines the use of soft hydrogel lenses for aphakic correction with specific attention to patient selection, lens selection, and fitting.

SOFT CONTACT LENS MATERIALS AND PROPERTIES

PHEMA is one of the many hydroxylated methacrylates used in the formulation of contact lens materials. There are various other HEMA homopolymers, copolymers of HEMA with other monomers, and non-HEMA polymers that can also be used. The orientation of the macromolecular chains of these polymers is random, that is, an amorphous polymer. A more detailed discussion of contact lenses as biomedical polymers may be found elsewhere.[41,58]

PHEMA contains a polar hydroxyl group that attracts water by means of hydrogen bonding and imbibes about 40% in its crosslinked state, and is used as the construction material of the Soflens contact lens (Polymacon, Bausch & Lomb Soflens Division, Rochester, New York).[62]

PHYSIOLOGY OF THE APHAKIC CORNEA

Optimal oxygen supply to the cornea is a prerequisite for the maintenance of aerobic metabolism, which provides the energy used to maintain the cornea in its normal deturgescent state. Oxygen is made available to the cornea by the atmosphere (*i.e.,* the open eye state) and the bloodstream (*i.e.,* the closed eye state).

Blink-assisted oxygenation or "pumping" of oxygenated tears under the lens is a less important factor with soft lenses, where only about 5% of the tears are exchanged, compared with hard lenses where pumping exchanges about 20% of the tears.[63] Tear pumping, however, is still important with soft lenses because it allows the removal of debris from desquamating epithelial cells and other metabolic waste products. Specifically, an immobile soft lens will lead to corneal edema even if there is high oxygen permeability.

Diffusion of oxygen through oxygen-permeable materials is a more efficient means of meeting the metabolic needs of the cornea than tear pumping.[23] Oxygen and carbon dioxide, the gases of greatest importance with respect to corneal metabolism, are both able to diffuse through hydrogel materials.

In vivo and *in vitro* methods exist for measuring the passage of oxygen through a contact lens. The techniques of measurement have been described elsewhere.[34,35,57,61] The *in vivo* method results in an expression of the equivalent oxygen performance or the equivalent oxygen percent (EOP). Because the oxygen concentration in the atmosphere is 21%, a lens impermeable to oxygen would have an EOP of zero; conversely, a lens completely permeable to oxygen would have an EOP of 21. Thus, hydrogel contact lenses have EOPs between zero and 21. The additional effect of tear pumping is not reflected in this measurement.

The *in vitro* method measures the oxygen flux through a contact lens by means of a laboratory technique. It results in an expression of oxygen permeability, or the DK coefficient, which is a property of a given polymeric material. Oxygen transmissibility refers to the oxygen flux across a lens of given thickness and is expressed as DK/L.

P = Permeability coefficient = DK

D = Diffusion coefficient (which defines how much gas can diffuse through a material)

K = Solubility coefficient (which defines how much gas can be dissolved in a material)

DK is expressed in standard units at a specific temperature, for example, 5.0×10^{-11} cm^3 · cm/cm^2 · s · mmHg at 25°C. The temperature at which this measurement is taken is important because higher temperatures will increase the kinetic energy of a gas, thus increasing its ability to diffuse across a membrane. Therefore, to compare DK values of two different materials, they should be expressed at the same temperature.

DK/L results in an expression of the transmissibility of oxygen across a contact lens of specific thickness, L (L may be taken to mean the central thickness or the average thickness, but should be specified). Therefore, approaches to improving oxygen transmissibility of various contact lenses have concentrated on increasing D (diffusivity) by way of a looser arrangement of polymer chains (as with silicone, for example), increasing K (solubility) by increasing water content, and by decreasing L (lens thickness).[63]

Manufacturers of hydrogel lenses have concentrated on the latter two approaches, resulting in the development of medium and high water content materials into which more atmospheric oxygen can dissolve and thus pass through the lens. Secondly, ultrathin lens designs have been pioneered, decreasing the distance the oxygen must travel to reach the cornea. Oxygen permeability increases exponentially with increases in water content. An increase of 20% in water content doubles the oxygen permeability. To achieve this same goal, the lens thickness should decrease by one half, an arithmetic increase. Increasing water content is thus a more efficient way of improving oxygen transmissibility than is decreasing lens thickness.[63]

Problems with increased hydration are slightly increased lens thickness with more water imbibition and decreased mechanical strength. Problems with decreased lens thickness are difficulty in handling and structural fragility.[63]

Clinical experience suggests that corneal edema develops less frequently in the aphakic cornea compared with the phakic cornea while wearing hydrogel lenses. In a study on the effects of cataract surgery on corneal function, Holden and co-workers noted that the oxygen tensions at the cornea estimated from the oxygen transmissibility values for commonly prescribed aphakic hydrogel lenses are inconsistent with the maintenance of normal corneal transparency.[36,37] The absence of corneal decompensation in these cases clearly suggested that the aphakic cornea has reduced physiologic demands. This has been explained from the observations made by these investigators that corneal epithelial thickness, epithelial oxygen uptake, corneal sensitivity, and endothelial cell density were significantly lower in aphakic eyes.

Under experimental conditions of hypoxia (2 hours with closed eyes) and anoxia (2 hours exposure under goggles to 100% nitrogen), aphakic corneas developed less corneal swelling response, fewer vertical striae, and fewer transient endothelial changes than phakic corneas did. These phenomena were thought to be due to a lower lactate production rate in aphakic corneas. The thinner aphakic epithelium with its lower overall metabolic activity, as correlated with its decreased epithelial oxygen uptake, may explain this. In addition, the surgically induced endothelial changes might increase the endothelial permeability to lactate.

Interestingly, using a differently designed study to measure the corneal oxygen uptake under a soft contact lens in phakic and aphakic eyes, Chaston and Fatt found similar oxygen flux in phakic and aphakic eyes when fitted with soft contact lenses of low power (+1 to −3 D).[13] They concluded that when the oxygen flux is above $1 \ \mu l/cm^2 \cdot h$, the relationship of oxygen flux to contact lens oxygen transmissibility is the same for phakic and aphakic eyes, that is, phakic and aphakic eyes respond similarly to contact lenses if the oxygen tension is above 10 mmHg. They acknowledge that more precise procedures for measuring oxygen flux and oxygen tension under a hydrogel lens are necessary to explore the behavior when flux is less than $1 \ \mu l/cm^2 \cdot h$ or oxygen tension under the lens is less than 10 mmHg. It may be that for the high-plus hydrogel lenses studied in Holden's experiments, the flux is reduced to a level where differences in behavior between phakic and aphakic corneas are manifest.

Corneal functional response, as measured by corneal thickness to high and low water content lenses in aphakic eyes, reveals a statistically significant inverse relationship between lens water content and corneal swelling response. Average lens thickness correlates better with increased corneal thickness than does central lens thickness.[56,60]

MICROBIOLOGY OF THE APHAKIC EYE

Smolin and co-workers studied the microbial flora in eyes fitted with extended-wear soft contact lenses and a matched control group.[68] They found fewer recoverable pathogens in lens wearers than in the control group. Wilson has shown that the presence of a hydrogel lens in the eye does not alter the microbial flora in or around the eye.[12] However, fungal growth within aphakic hydrophilic contact lenses has been reported in uninfected eyes that were experiencing irritation.[7]

PATIENT SELECTION

GENERAL CONSIDERATIONS

Soft hydrogel lenses may be worn on a daily or extended-wear basis. In general, lenses of medium (35% to 50%) water content and standard thickness are worn on a daily-wear basis whereas lenses of higher water content (55% to 80%) or ultrathin design with moderate water content may be worn on an extended-wear basis. The main advantage of daily-wear soft lenses over hard lenses is their improved initial comfort and better physiologic performance.

INDICATIONS

Hard contact lens intolerance. Patients who are uncomfortable with a hard lens because of foreign body sensation may fare much better with a soft lens. Its larger size and semiscleral fit eliminate the contact of the lid with the edge of the lens.

Occupation. Soft lenses may be less easily displaced and lost. Therefore, they are ideally suited for activities such as sports and games.

Ocular surface abnormalities. Eyes with a compromised ocular surface may do better with soft lenses, because hard lenses may aggravate the damage.

Corneal pathology. Conditions like endothelial dystrophy may be more amenable to soft contact lens use compared with hard contact lenses, because of the better physiologic compatibility.

Poor manual dexterity. The introduction of the extended-wear concept was welcomed by the elderly patient with poor manual dexterity.[29] Extended-wear lenses constitute an alternative for patients who are not candidates for intraocular lenses or in whom implantation of an intraocular lens has been aborted.

Postoperative astigmatism. If a patient has been unable to achieve a satisfactory fit with a hard lens because of poor centration secondary to high corneal toricity and if he is willing to wear a spectacle overcorrection, a soft lens may be acceptable. Soft lenses, particularly low or medium water content types, correct a maximum of 1.5 D to 2 D of astigmatism.[17]

The following categories of patients constitute good candidates for extended wear of contact lenses.[19,30]

1. Arthritic or parkinsonian patients who are unable to insert and remove lenses

2. Monocular aphakic patients who are unable to insert and remove lenses

3. Children with monocular aphakia whose parents are unable to remove daily-wear lenses

4. Intraocular lens candidates whose implants were aborted during surgery

5. Monocular pseudophakic patients with aphakia in the fellow eye

CONTRAINDICATIONS

Recognition of contraindications is very important for the successful outcome of extended-wear lenses. The following apply mostly to the situation of extended-wear hydrogel lenses for aphakia.[23,47,55]

Infectious ocular diseases such as chronic blepharitis not responsive to treatment, chronic meibomitis, chronic dacryocystitis, recurrent herpes simplex keratitis, and herpes zoster keratitis are contraindications to the use of extended-wear lenses.

Dry eyes. Borderline dry eye responsive to artificial tears is a relative contraindication, but frank keratitis sicca is an absolute contraindication.

Glaucoma. Cases of glaucoma controlled with nonepinephrine-containing medications are relative contraindications, whereas poorly controlled or advanced glaucoma, especially if filtering blebs are present, constitutes an absolute contraindication.[6]

Chronic or recurrent uveitis. If an eye has been quiescent for 3 to 6 months, an attempt could be made to fit with extended-wear lenses, although with extreme caution. Patients in whom chronic steroid therapy is required should not be fit with extended wear lenses if at all possible.

Endothelial disease. Mild endothelial disease suggests the use of the highest possible water content lens if extended wear is to be considered. Postoperative endothelial damage must be assessed; if severe, extended wear should not be attempted.

Postsurgical lid dysfunction. Patients who have undergone blepharoplasty, facial cosmetic surgery, ptosis repair, or facial reconstructive surgery may have alterations in lid function that may negatively affect the prognosis with extended wear.

Lagophthalmos. Cases of incomplete lid closure during sleep, due to thyroid ophthalmopathy or facial nerve palsy, especially with a poor Bell's phenomenon, are contraindications to extended wear.

Alterations in corneal sensation. Relative contraindications include changes in corneal sensation associated with previous contact lens wear, with the postsurgical state, with drug-induced corneal hypoesthesia (*e.g.,* Timoptic). Stronger contraindications apply to disturbances of sensation associated with neurotrophic keratopathy caused by recurrent herpes simplex keratitis or by herpes zoster keratitis.

Poor motivation is a contraindication because it may lead to lack of desire to adhere to follow-up and lens care regimens.

Poor hygiene leads to increased risk of infection.

Poor compliance and reliability for follow-up care is a contraindication.

Systemic conditions. Diabetes and chronic alcoholism represent higher risk for infection because of corneal alterations as well as altered immune status.

Inability to remove the lens or have someone available to remove the lens in the event of a problem is a contraindication.

Concomitant administration of medications that may decrease tear production (*e.g.,* antihistamines, anticholinergics) is a contraindication.

Other contraindications that are relative to the individual patient's requirements are the following:

1. Employment in certain hazardous industries with exposure to volatile toxic chemicals or particulate matter that may become lodged under the contact lens.

2. Postoperative astigmatism: Soft lenses tend to drape the cornea. Patients with irregular astigmatism will be unhappy with the correction provided by soft lenses. Aphakic patients with regular astigmatism beyond the parameters described above should be willing to wear spectacle overcorrection to achieve best vision.

3. Patients who are already successful hard contact lens wearers and who wish to trade their lenses for the convenience of extended-wear lenses may not be satisfied with the "softness" of the vision provided by the hydrogel lenses.

4. Patients for whom the cost may be prohibitive because of the expense incurred by lens care or by replacement lenses due to lens loss or spoilage.

PREFIT EVALUATION

A thorough ophthalmic evaluation is necessary to rule out the presence of any ocular phenomena that may contraindicate the use of hydrogel lenses.

Particular attention is devoted to an assessment of the integrity of the anterior segment of the eye, as follows: (1) The eyelids are examined for the position, degree of closure, blinking mechanism, and presence of any infective or inflammatory processes. (2) Precorneal tear film is assessed for both qualitative and quantitative changes. (3) Conjunctival status is assessed and documented, paying special attention to upper tarsal conjunctiva. (4) A composite profile of the cornea is obtained. It encompasses fluorescein staining to study epithelial status, biomicroscopic evaluation of endothelium, corneal sensitivity, and thickness, particularly in postsurgical cases and if use of extended-wear lenses is contemplated. (5) In postsurgical patients, particular attention to the location of the cataract incision is also helpful. (6) Additionally, the size and shape of the pupil should be noted to assist in the selection of a lens with an appropriate optical zone.

LENS SELECTION

Once a decision has been made to use an aphakic hydrogel lens, a decision can be made whether to use the lens on a daily or extended-wear basis. Appropriate lens selection for each patient should be made individually and should depend on the anatomic and physiologic status of a given eye. The information obtained at the prefit evaluation should be used as a guideline to select the more appropriate lenses for a given eye. The actual fitting technique is usually on a trial and error basis.

There are many hydrogel lenses on the market for daily wear in aphakia (Table 3-1). Additionally, there are currently three approved lenses for aphakic extended wear (see discussion of Commonly Used Aphakic Hydrogel Lenses for Extended Wear) with an additional three or four lenses being used on an extended-wear basis for aphakia whose approvals are pending.

The selection of a lens is based on several factors such as previous experience and success with a particular lens, quality control of a lens manufacturer, and cost of lenses (*e.g.* cost per lens to the low-volume fitter; volume discounts available to the high-volume fitter). Additionally, specific patient characteristics may help determine the need for a specific lens, for example, a patient with borderline corneal function should receive the highest possible water content lens to enable maximum oxygen transmissibility; alternatively, an ultrathin lens design might also serve this purpose. Another example might be a patient with an eccentric pupil or sector iridectomy who should be fit with a lens with a larger optic zone to eliminate edge flare.

Refer to Table 3-2 for a list of hydrogel lenses for aphakia with various parameters of interest including water content, oxygen permeability, diameter, central thickness, base curve, optical zone, and powers available. A later discussion deals with hydrogel lenses for extended wear in aphakia and includes brief fitting guidelines, evaluation, and experience with particular lenses.

FITTING GUIDELINES

Refer to the fitting guidelines described in the discussion of Commonly Used Aphakic Hydrogel Lenses for Extended Wear for specific criteria; however, some general guidelines for hydrogel lenses are useful.

1. Because these lenses usually are fitted as semiscleral lenses, they should vault the limbus and rest on the corneal apex and paralimbal sclera.

2. The lenses should extend 0.5 mm to 1.5 mm beyond the limbus when centered. Therefore, the lens diameter should be 1 mm to 3 mm larger than the horizontal visible iris diameter (HVID).

3. One general rule of thumb is to fit these lenses flat. The lenses should be fit 3 D to 4 D flatter than the average central corneal curvature (K).

4. The lens should center well.

5. Movement of 0.5 mm to 1.5 mm with the blink is desirable.

6. Slight lag on upgaze (about 1 mm to 2 mm) is also beneficial.

7. Vision should not vary with blinking.

8. Patient comfort is of paramount importance.

A lens is selected and may be placed in the eye by the patient or practitioner. The insertion of the lens should be performed taking all appropriate disinfection precautions. The lens is rinsed with saline and examined to make sure that it is not inverted. The lens is held between thumb and index finger so as to pinch the edges toward the center. Normally, the edges should turn in; otherwise, the lens is inverted. This is called the "taco" test. The right lens is then placed on the fitter's right index finger. While holding the right lower lid down with the right middle finger and the upper lid up with the thumb of the opposite hand, the fitter instructs the patient to look down and then places the lens on the superior bulbar conjunctiva. The patient then looks up and the lens centers on the cornea.

EVALUATION OF FIT

The lens should be allowed to stabilize for at least 15 to 30 minutes, and then should be examined for adequacy of fit.

A *steep fit* is characterized by the following:

1. Poor or absent movement
2. A central air bubble under the lens initially before absorption
3. Paralimbal vessels may appear compressed under the lens edge
4. Pain, discomfort, and photophobia
5. Ciliary injection, epithelial debris, and edema
6. Iritis
7. Variable vision with blinking

A *flat fit* is characterized by the following:

1. Excessive movement, especially with blinking or eye movement
2. Poor centering
3. Peripheral air bubbles
4. Discomfort and tearing
5. Poor visual acuity

FITTING ADJUSTMENTS

Because hydrogel lenses may become steep with time, especially an extended-wear lens, the preferred initial fit should be relatively flat. An important concept in adjusting the lens fit is that of relative sagittal depth

TABLE 3-1 Manufacturing Information for Aphakic Hydrogel Lenses

Lens	Manufacturer	Materials of Construction	Method of Manufacture
Acugel (Droxifilcon A)	Streiter Laboratories	HEMA/VP/MA cross-linked with TEGDMA	Lathe cut
Aquaflex Standard (Tetrafilcon A)	Aquaflex Division of CooperVision	HEMA/VP/MMA	Lathe cut
Cellusoft (Polymacon)	Rynco Scientific Co.	HEMA cross-linked with EGDMA	Lathe cut
CSI High Plus (Crofilcon A)	Syntex Ophthalmics	MMA/glyceryl methacrylate	
CW-79 (Lidofilcon B)	Bausch & Lomb	MMA/VP cross-linked with EGDMA and AMA	Lathe cut
Durasoft (Phemfilcon A)	Wessley-Jessen	HEMA/EOEMA	Lathe cut
Durasoft 2	Wessley-Jessen	HEMA/EOEMA	Lathe cut
Durasoft 3	Wessley-Jessen	HEMA/EOEMA	Lathe cut
Durasoft TT	Wessley-Jessen	HEMA/EOEMA	Lathe cut
Flexlens (Hefilcon A)	Flexlens Inc.	HEMA/VP cross-linked with EGDMA	Lathe cut
Hydracon (Methafilcon A)	Rynco Scientific Co.	HEMA/another monomer (proprietary information)	Lathe cut
Hydrocurve II$_{45}$ (Bufilcon A)	Barnes-Hind/Hydrocurve	HEMA/DAA/MA cross-linked with TMPTMA	Lathe cut
Hydrocurve II$_{55}$ (Bufilcon A)	Barnes-Hind/Hydrocurve	HEMA/DAA/MA cross-linked with TMPTMA	Lathe cut
Hydron (Polymacon)	American Hydron	HEMA cross-linked with EGDMA	Lathe cut
Metrosoft (Deltafilcon A)	Metro Optics	HEMA/BMA cross-linked with TMPTMA	Lathe cut
Permalens (Perfilcon A)	CooperVision	HEMA/VP/MA cross-linked with EGDMA	Lathe cut
Sauflon PW (Lidofilcon B)	American Hospital Supply	MMA/VP cross-linked with EGDMA and AMA	Lathe cut
Sof-Form II (Polymacon)	Salvation Ophth, Inc.	HEMA cross-linked with EGDMA	Lathe cut
Soflens (Polymacon)	Bausch & Lomb	HEMA cross-linked with EGDMA	Spin cast
Softcon (Vifilcon A)	American Optical	PVP/HEMA	Lathe cut
Softcon EW	American Optical	PVP/HEMA	Lathe cut
Softics (Deltafilcon A)	Advanced Soft Optics	HEMA/BMA cross-linked with TEGDMA	Lathe cut
Softics Super Plus	Advanced Soft Optics	HEMA/BMA cross-linked with TEGDMA	Lathe cut
Softsite (Hefilcon A&B)	Softsite Contact Lens Laboratory	Not available	Lathe cut

TABLE 3-1 *(Continued)*

Lens	Manufacturer	Materials of Construction	Method of Manufacture
TC-50 (Daily wear)	Trans Canada Contact Lens	HEMA/MA cross-linked with TEGDMA	Lathe cut
TC-75	Trans Canada Contact Lens	HEMA/MA cross-linked with TEGDMA	Lathe cut
Tresoft (Ocufilcon A)	Alcon Optics	HEMA/MA cross-linked with EGDMA	Lathe cut
Tresoft Thin	Alcon Optics	HEMA/MA cross-linked with EGDMA	Lathe cut
Tripol 43 (Deltafilcon A)	Capital Contact Inc.	HEMA/BMA cross-linked with TEGDMA	Lathe cut
Vistakon Standard (Etafilcon A)	Vistakon, Inc.	Not available	Not available

(RSD), which is calculated by subtracting the base curve from the lens diameter.[46] To loosen a fit, the RSD value must be decreased by using a flatter lens or a smaller lens. To tighten a lens, the RSD value must be increased by using a steeper lens or a larger lens.

Evaluation of the adequacy of lens fit should also include an assessment of visual acuity.[46] Overrefraction will give the spectacle correction necessary to correct such astigmatism. Because it may take approximately 1 week for an extended-wear lens to stabilize in the eye, it is recommended that overrefraction for spectacle overcorrection be delayed until such time.

With an adequate fit, visual acuity should be normal and crisp during blinking. Retinoscopy should give a crisp clear reflex. Keratometry over the lens should show no distortion of the mires and the same amount of astigmatism as without the lens.

With a tightly fitting lens, vision may be poor until blinking, when the lids will compress the lens and prevent the excessive vaulting. Retinoscopy will show a darker reflex centrally with a quicker motion because of the apical vaulting, leading to a plus lens effect. Keratometry will show increased or decreased astigmatism with distortion of the mires.

In a loosely fitting lens, vision will be poor with blinking because of excessive movement. Retinoscopy will show a darker reflex with quicker motion inferiorly because of the plus lens effect inferiorly. Again, keratometry will show increased or decreased cylinder with distortion of the mires.

WHEN TO FIT

An appropriate time to fit an aphakic patient is usually around 8 to 10 weeks following surgery. In cases where cataract extraction is performed through a smaller incision, this period can be reduced to about 4 weeks. However, the

TABLE 3-2 Parameters for Aphakic Hydrogel Lenses[2,23,25,27,47,55,69]

Lens	Water Content	Oxygen Permeability	Diameter (mm)	Thickness (mm)	Base Curve (mm)	Optical Zone (mm)	Power (D)
Acugel (Droxifilcon A)	47%	11×10^{-11} at 25°C	13.5; 14	0.16; 0.07	7.8–9.5 7.8–9.5		−20 to +20 −20 to +20
Aquaflex Standard (Tetrafilcon A)	42.5%	10×10^{-11} at 22°C	13.8	0.42–0.56	8.2; 8.5; 8.8; 9.1; 9.4		+10 to +20
Cellusoft (Polymacon)	38.6%	8×10^{-11} at 24°C	14	0.04–0.12	8.3; 8.5; 8.7; 8.9		−20 to +20
CSI High Plus (Crofilcon A)	40%	Not available	14.8		8.6; 8.9; 9.35		Aphakic range
CW-79 (Lidofilcon B)	79%	48.6×10^{-11} at 32°C	14.4	0.5–0.8	8.1; 8.4; 8.7		+10 to +20
Durasoft (Phemfilcon A)	30%	6.9×10^{-11} at 35°C	13.5	0.09–0.46	8.3; 8.6; 9		−20 to +20
Durasoft 2	38%	9.5×10^{-11} at 35°C	13.5; 14.5	0.07–0.42 0.07–0.42	8.2; 8.5; 8.9 8.2; 8.6; 9		−20 to +20 −20 to +20
Durasoft 3	55%	19×10^{-11} at 35°C	14.5	0.45	8.3; 8.6; 9		−20 to +20
Durasoft TT	30%	6.9×10^{-11} at 35°C	13.5	0.11–0.56	8.6		Spherical −20 to +20 Cylinder −2.75 to −4 Axis: any
Flexlens (Hefilcon A)	45.5%	12×10^{-11} at 35°C	12.6–16.5	0.10–1	6–11		−40 to +40
Hydracon (Methafilcon A)	55%	18.8×10^{-11} at 24°C	15	0.06–0.60	8.3; 8.6; 8.9	8	−20 to +20

Hydrocurve II$_{45}$ (Bufilcon A)	45%	6.5×10^{-1} at 23°C	13.5	0.05	8.3; 8.6		−12 to +20
			14.5	0.05	8.9		−12 to +20
			15.5; 16	0.05	9.2; 9.5; 9.8; 10.1		−12 to +20
Hydrocurve II$_{55}$ (Bufilcon A)	55%	10.5×10^{-11} at 23°C	14	0.05	8.5		−12 to +20
			14.5	0.05	8.8; 9.1		−12 to +20
			15.5; 16	0.24–0.47	9.2; 9.5; 9.8		−12 to +20
Hydron (Polymacon)	38.6%	8×10^{-11} at 24°C	13	0.11–0.45	8.1–8.9; 9.3; 9.7		−20 to +20
			15	0.11–0.45	8.7; 9; 9.3; 9.6		−20 to +20
Metrosoft (Deltafilcon A)	43%	11×10^{-11} at 23°C	13.5	Not available	8.3; 8.6; 8.9		−20 to +20
Permalens (Perfilcon A)	71%	42×10^{-11} at 35°C	14	0.39–0.43	8; 8.3	7.9 for +8 D	+8.50 to +20
			14.5	0.39–0.43	8.3; 8.6; 8.9	6.3 for +20 D	+8.50 to +20
Sauflon PW (Lidofilcon B)	79%	48.6×10^{-11} at 32°C	13.7	0.63–0.96	7.5; 7.8	7	+20 to +35
			14.4	0.23–0.90	8.1; 8.4; 8.7	8	Plano, +25
Sof-Form II (Polymacon)	38.6%	8×10^{-11} at 24°C	14	Not available	8.3; 8.5; 8.7; 8.9	7.4–8.7	−20 to +20
Soflens (Polymacon)	38.6%	10×10^{-11} at 32°C	12.5–14.5	0.035–0.61	Base curve is front surface; varies with series (N, F3, B3, H3, H4)		−20 to +20
Softcon (Vifilcon A)	55%	13×10^{-11} at 20°C	14	0.32–0.64	7.8; 8.1; 8.4; 8.7	7.3	Plano, +18
			14.5	0.32–0.64	8.1; 8.4	7.3	−8 to +18

Continued

TABLE 3-2 (*Continued*)

Lens	Water Content	Oxygen Permeability	Diameter (mm)	Thickness (mm)	Base Curve (mm)	Optical Zone (mm)	Power (D)
Softcon EW	55%	13×10^{-11} at 20°C	14	0.027–0.45	7.8	7.5	+9.5 to +18
			14	0.1–0.45	8.1; 8.4; 8.7	7.5	−6 to +18
			14.5	0.27–0.45	8.1; 8.4	7.5	+9.5 to +18
Softics (Deltafilcon A)	43%	Not available	13.5; 14	Not available	8.3; 8.6; 8.9		−20 to +20
Softics Super Plus	43%	Not available	14	0.1–0.28	8.4		+.25 to +18.5
Softsite (Hefilcon A&B)	45%	Not available	13.5	0.1–0.28	8.3; 8.6		+10 to +20
TC-50 (Daily Wear)	50%	24×10^{-11} at 22°C	13; 13.5;	0.12–0.55	7.8; 8.1;	6–10.3	−20 to +20
			14; 14.5	0.12–0.55	8.4; 8.7; 9	6–10.3	−20 to +20
TC-75	75%	34×10^{-11} at 22°C	13; 13.5;	0.12–0.55	7.8; 8.1;	6–10.3	−20 to +20
			14; 14.5	0.12–0.55	8.4; 8.7; 9	6–10.3	−20 to +20
Tresoft (Ocufilcon A)	46%	5.5×10^{-11} at 24°C	13.5–15	0.1–0.5	8.2; 8.4; 8.6; 8.8	8–11	−20 to +20
Tresoft Thin	44%	10.9×10^{-11} at 24°C	13.7	0.07	8.5		−15 to +15
Tripol 43 (Deltafilcon A)	43%	12×10^{-11} at 24°C	13.5	0.5	8; 8.3; 8.4; 8.6; 8.8		−20 to +20
Vistakon Standard (Etafilcon A)	43%	Not available	14	0.11	8.15–9.05		−20 to +20
			14.5	0.11	8.15–9.05		−20 to +20

ideal criterion is stable keratometric or refractive readings. If any postoperative complications occur, fitting should be delayed for an appropriate length of time.

PATIENT INSTRUCTION

Adequate instruction of the patient is of paramount importance in the successful wear of contact lenses, and should be an integral part of a comprehensive regimen in caring for contact lens patients.

Once an adequate fit has been accomplished, a lens may be dispensed from inventory, or it may be ordered. Upon dispensing, the patient should be instructed in insertion and removal of the lens whether it is to be a daily or extended-wear lens. If the patient is being fitted for extended wear and is unable to handle the lens, someone in the patient's environment (*e.g.,* relative, nurse, optician) should be instructed at least in the removal of the lens. Lens care should be discussed and demonstrated in detail. The patient should be made familiar with potential side-effects of all solutions. Patients should also be made familiar with the danger signs associated with contact lens wear.

FOLLOW UP

Follow-up visits may include evaluations of the lens at 2 to 4 hours after fitting. Daily-wear lenses may be worn for a full waking day starting from day 1. Extended wear lenses may be worn continuously starting from day 1. Lenses should be inspected at 1 day, 1 week, and 1 month.

At the first visit, after 24 hours, a marginally loose fit may be tolerated because the lens may tighten up over time. If the fit has become steeper, it should be flattened. The patient's vision, progress with lens handling (daily wear), and comfort should be assessed.

At the end of the first week, quality of fit and visual acuity are reassessed. Overrefraction and prescription of spectacle overcorrection for astigmatism can be performed.

At the end of 1 month, lens fit should be stabilized. Assessment should be performed with slit lamp, keratometry, and overrefractions. Follow up after this point can be at 6-month intervals for daily-wear patients and at 3-month intervals for extended-wear patients. Patients with potential problems (corneal guttata, low-grade blepharitis, or dry eye) should be seen more frequently and followed more cautiously.

LENS CARE

Patients wearing daily-wear hydrogel lenses must be adept at insertion and removal and must understand the cleaning regimen as well as the importance of compliance.[67]

The daily regimen should consist of cleaning the lens mechanically (rubbing between the fingers) using a surfactant cleaner. This should be followed by rinsing and disinfecting. After disinfection, the lenses should be rinsed with saline before reinsertion: In some cases, an enzyme cleaner is used at least once a week.

Patients on an extended-wear regimen should be instructed in cleaning their lenses similarly, at a frequency to be determined for each patient (*e.g.,* once a week to once every several months). Some extended-wear patients prefer to leave the responsibility of care to the physician. Such patients are instructed in the use of lubricants while the lens is in the eye, to help prevent lipid and proteinaceous deposits on the lens. (Refer to Chapter 10 for a more detailed discussion of solutions for cleaning, disinfection, and storage of lenses.)

Aphakic contact lens wear may lead to several minor problems or major complications.[48] The incidence of morbidity is greater with extended-wear hydrogel lenses. Details on complications are given in Chapter 8.

APHAKIC HYDROGEL LENSES COMMONLY USED FOR EXTENDED WEAR

Contact lens technology is in a state of constant evolution leading to the development of newer lenses and ever-changing indications. This section will review most of the hydrogel lenses currently used for aphakic extended wear.[4,5,15,21,38,39,49,53,69,71]

HIGH WATER CONTENT LENSES

High water content lenses have higher oxygen transmissibility by virtue of their higher water content. Therefore, they are ideal for extended-wear use.

Sauflon PW and CW-79

Sauflon PW and CW-79 both are manufactured from lidofilcon B and are high water content lenses.[8,39,52,65,74] Sauflon PW is made in a 14.4-mm diameter for adult aphakic patients and in a 13.7-mm diameter for pediatric aphakic patients. The optical zone is 8 mm for the adult lens and 7 mm for the pediatric lens. The CW-79 is made in a 14.4-mm diameter only. Thermal or chemical disinfection may be used with either lens. Fitting guidelines suggest that overrefraction over a trial lens closest to the spectacle correction be performed. The lens should be supported by the sclera and the corneal apex. Initial lens selection should be with an 8.4-mm base curve (BC) for adults and a 7.5-mm BC for children. The lens should center well and move 1 mm to 2 mm with blinking.

The Sauflon lens enjoyed 10 years of European experience before receiving Food and Drug Administration approval for aphakic extended wear in the United States. Several authors have reported their experience with an 85% water content Sauflon lens in England.[14,43,59,74] The reports on the 79% water content Sauflon lens available in the United States show for the most part a success rate of 77% to 90%, defined as those patients wearing lenses after 4 weeks on an extended-wear basis.[8,39,52] The rate of deposit formation varied from 11% to 30%.[8,9,39,52] Rates of neovascularization and infection were low. Some practitioners find this lens useful in patients with large pupils or sector iridectomies because of its larger optical zone of 8 mm.

In a national Sauflon study involving 1106 patients, 1427 eyes were fitted with an average wearing time of 15.85 months.[55] Lenses were worn successfully in 71.8%. Best visual acuity without overcorrection was 20/40 or better in 64%, and with overcorrection in 71%. The most common reasons for lens discontinuation were lack of motivation, discomfort, poor acuity, and frequent loss or damage.

Permalens

Permalens is made of perfilcon A and is available in 14-mm and 14.5-mm diameters.[44,47,51,52] Base curves range from 7.8 mm to 8.7 mm with an optical zone of 6.3 mm. It has a water content of 71%. Initial lens selection is recommended to be the 8.6/14.5 lens. If the initial lens is too large, a switch to the 8.3/14.0 lens is recommended; if it is too tight, the 8.9/14.5 should be tried; and if too loose, the 8.3/14.5 should be chosen.

In several different studies, the success rate of this lens is reported to be between 70% and 80%.[12,51,71] In one study, 86% of patients had visual acuities of 20/40 or better without overcorrection and 92% with overcorrection.[71] Most common problems with the lens included tight lens syndrome, mild neovascularization, and conjunctivitis.

TC-75 Lens

The TC-75 lens is available in Canada in 13-mm, 13.5-mm, 14-mm, and 14.5-mm diameters and base curves from 7.8 to 9 mm.[72] The 14-mm diameter is recommended with initial base curve of 3 D to 4 D flatter than K. The material has a 75% water content. Lens thickness is a maximum of 0.49 mm for high plus lenses. The optical zone varies from 6 mm to 10 mm. Visual acuity is reported to be 20/40 or better in 79% of patients without overcorrection and 91% with overcorrection. We found that lenses required removal for cleaning every 1 to 3 months. Corneal neovascularization was not reported to be a problem.

MEDIUM WATER CONTENT LENSES

Softcon EW

The Softcon EW lens is made of vifilcon A in 14-mm and 14.5-mm diameters.[25,66,75] Chemical disinfection is the recommended method of lens care.

In lens selection, the initial lens to be tried is the 8.4/14.0 lens. After a 30-minute stabilization period, the lens should center well with a slight lag on upgaze and slight movement with blinking. If the lens fit is not proper, the base curve or the diameter may be adjusted as necessary.

The Softcon EW is the same 55% water content polymer that was originally studied in the early and mid-1970s for FDA approval as a therapeutic lens.[28,40,66] It is currently made in a thinner design for aphakia with a central thickness from 0.28 mm to 0.45 mm. The 2-year experience with this lens in aphakic patients was reported in a study.[75] Thirty-three patients (44 eyes) were fitted with lenses on an extended-wear basis. Twenty-five patients still wore the lenses after 1 year. Fifty percent were able to go at least 1 month between lens removals for cleaning. Lens replacement was required on the average after 12 to 15 months of extended wear. Forty-eight percent had visual acuity of 20/40 or better without overcorrection. No neovascularization, infection, or microcystic edema was reported. Many practitioners prefer this lens for use in patients with astigmatism up to 2.5 D because of its slightly thicker, more rigid consistency and excellent fitting characteristics.

The Durasoft 3

The Durasoft 3 lens is made of phemfilcon A and is available as a 55% water content lens in one diameter (14.5 mm) and three base curves (8.3 mm, 8.6 mm, and 9 mm). The recommended base curve selection is 8.6 mm, which will fit 80% of patients according to the manufacturer.

ULTRATHIN LENSES

Hydrocurve II

The Hydrocurve II is a lathe-cut lens made from bufilcon-A and is available in four diameters (14 mm, 14.5 mm, 15.5 mm, and 16 mm) with base curves ranging from 8.5 mm to 9.8 mm.[8,23] A 55% water content lens with a flat fit is recommended, as is chemical disinfection. This lens utilizes the thin membrane concept to enable its use for extended wear.

A national study performed to evaluate this lens in support of FDA approval showed visual acuities of 20/30 or better in 79% of aphakic patients. The incidence of corneal edema was less than 0.6% and that of neovascularization was less than 9%. The major problems were soiled, deposit-laden lenses (14%).

CSI Lens

The CSI lens is made of crofilcon A with a 40% water content non-HEMA material.[18,27] A 14.8-mm diameter is available with base curves from 8.6 mm to 9.35 mm. The 8.9-mm base curve is initially recommended and then is adjusted as necessary. The optic zone is 5.2 mm.

In a study by Davis of aphakic patients fitted with this lens on an extended-wear basis, a success rate of 84.5% was reported (defined as continuous wear for 6 months).[18] In a multicenter evaluation of the lens for FDA approval, 179 patients (or 229 eyes) were studied: 78.2% wore their lenses for more than 6 months, 49.1% for more than 1 year, and 16.2% for more than 2 years.[27] Eighty-four percent achieved 20/40 vision or better without overcorrection and 89.9% were 20/40 or better with overcorrection. Adverse reactions included corneal edema (5.75%), staining (15%), and vascularization (1.1%). Additionally, a number of patients reported dryness upon awakening, which was relieved by irrigation with saline. Deposit formation appeared to be an infrequent occurrence with this lens (0.03%).

In addition, there are many other hydrogel lenses used on a daily-wear basis to correct aphakia. There is a paucity of literature about these lenses; therefore, see Table 3-2 for specific lens parameters.

CHOOSING A LENS

The ophthalmologist is often vexed with the problem of which lens to choose for a given patient and which lenses to keep in inventory in a contact lens practice. For those who fit aphakic patients occasionally, familiarity with one of the higher water content lenses and one of the medium water content lenses is probably adequate. The choice of a specific lens from these categories is usually dependent on the experience of the person fitting contact lenses, because no significant difference exists between different lenses on the basis of clinical experience with the various types of lenses available.

For those who deal with a higher volume of contact lens patients, adequate knowledge of the fitting, care, and problems related to different aphakic hydrogel lenses is necessary, because a greater degree of success can be achieved only with the ability to use different lenses. Only a small percentage of the patient population achieves optimal results with one specific lens. In addition to having access to all available lenses, those who have special interest in contact lenses should participate in the clinical studies with newer lenses in the investigational phase.

The variety of lenses available under the different categories makes it possible to achieve desirable results in a large percentage of aphakic patients.

CONCLUSION

Hydrogel contact lenses constitute an excellent modality for the optical correction of aphakia. The success of these lenses is dependent on proper patient selection, lens selection, understanding of contact lens-related corneal physiology, and early recognition and management of complications through proper follow up.

REFERENCES

1. Anderson DP, Lorenzetti DW, Shink R: Aphakic soft contact lens optical considerations. Can J Ophthalmol 9(1):67, 1974
2. Appendix A-3, A-4, A-5, pp A.5–A.13. In Dabezies O (ed): CLAO Book, Contact Lenses. New York, Grune & Stratton, 1984
3. Aquavella JV: New aspects of contact lenses in ophthalmology. Adv Ophthalmol 32:2, 1976
4. Aquavella JV, Rao GN: Which lens: Contact lenses currently available for extended wear in aphakia. Ophthalmology 87(2):151, 1980
5. Barner S, Marner K, Fahmy JA: Clinical experience with continuous wear hydrophilic contact lenses in aphakia. Acta Ophthalmol (Copenh) 58(1):83, 1980
6. Bellows AR, McCully JP: Endophthalmitis in aphakic patients with unplanned filtering blebs wearing contact lenses. Ophthalmology 88(8):839, 1981
7. Berger RO, Streeten BW: Fungal growth in aphakic soft contact lenses. Am J Ophthalmol 91(5):630, 1981
8. Binder PS, Woodward C: Extended wear Hydrocurve and Sauflon contact lenses. Am J Ophthalmol 90(3):309, 1980
9. Boyd BF: Extended wear contact lenses in 525 aphakic eyes. Am J Ophthalmol 88:351, 1979
10. Boyd HH: Hard contact lens corrections in aphakia. Ophthalmology 86(3):399, 1979
11. Carter DB, Brucker D: Hydrophilic contact lenses for aphakia. Am J Optom 50(4):316, 1973
12. Cavanagh HD, Bodner BI, Wilson LA: Extended wear hydrogel lenses. Ophthalmology 87(9):871, 1980
13. Chaston J, Fatt I: Corneal oxygen uptake under a soft contact lens in phakic and aphakic eyes. Invest Ophthalmol Vis Sci 23(2):234, 1982
14. Clement DB: Continuous wear soft lenses in the treatment of aphakia. Trans Ophthalmol Soc UK 97(1):145, 1977
15. Contact Lenses. Vol XVII, 6:47, 1984
16. Coon LJ, Miller JP, Meier RF: Overview of extended wear contact lenses. J Am Optom Assoc 50(6):745, 1979
17. Dabezies O, Farris RL, Rosenthal P: Correction of aphakia. In Dabezies O (ed): CLAO Book, Contact Lenses. 56:56.12, 1984
18. Davis HE: The CSI-TM Crofilcon A, a membrane lens for aphakic extended wear. J Am Optom Assoc 51(3):217, 1980
19. Durham DG, Kuhwald EP: Extended wear of hydrophilic contact lenses in aphakia: An alternative to intraocular lens implantation. Trans Am Ophthalmol Soc 77:355, 1979
20. Enoch JM: Restoration of binocularity in unilateral aphakia by non-surgical means. Int Ophthalmol Clin 18(2):273, 1978
21. Extended wear lenses. Symposium CLAO Meeting, 28 January 1982. CLAO J 8(4):71, 1982
22. Fatt I, Lin D: Oxygen tension under a soft or hard gas permeable contact lens in the presence of tear pumping. Am J Optom Physiol Opt 53:104, 1976
23. Feldman G: Hydrocurve soft contact lenses for extended wear in Hartstein J (ed): Extended Wear Contact Lenses for Aphakia 5:103, 1982

24. Ferris RL: Complications associated with aphakic contact lenses. Ophthalmology 86(6):1120, 1979
25. Freeman MI: The Softcon (Vifilcon A) hydrophilic contact lens for extended wear in ocular disease and aphakia. In Hartstein J (ed): Extended Wear Contact Lenses for Aphakia 7:161, 1982
26. Gasset AR, Kaufman HE: The therapeutic uses of hydrophilic contact lenses. Am J Ophthalmol 69:252, 1970
27. Gordon JM, Korb DR: The use of CSI (Crofilcon A) contact lenses in aphakic extended wear. In Hartstein J (ed): Extended Wear Contact Lenses for Aphakia 6:138–160, 1982.
28. Gould HL: Aphakia: Continuous wearing of soft contact lenses NY State J Med 77(6):913, 1977
29. Hakkinen L, Salminen L: Hydrophilic contact lenses in aphakia: Experience with geriatric patients intolerant to spectacle correction. CLAO J 9(2):141, 1983
30. Hartstein J: Extended wear contact lenses for aphakia and myopia. In Hartstein J (ed): Extended wear contact lenses for aphakia 1:1, 1982.
31. Hartstein J: Prolonged wearing of contact lenses and preliminary results. Ophthalmology 86(3):409, 1979
32. Highman VN: Correction of aphakia with contact lenses. Doc Ophthalmol 43(1):155, 1977
33. Highman VN: Stereopsis and aniseikonia in uniocular aphakia. Br J Ophthalmol 61(1):30, 1977
34. Hill RM, Mauger TF: Oxygen uptake: Hydrophilics. Int Contact Lens Clin 7:224, 1980
35. Holly FJ, Refojo MF: Oxygen permeability of hydrogel contact lenses. J Am Optom Assoc 43:1173, 1972
36. Holden BA, Mertz GW, Guillon M: Corneal swelling response of the aphakic eye. Invest Ophthalmol Vis Sci 19(11):1394, 1980
37. Holden BA, Polse KA, Fonn D et al: Effects of cataract surgery on corneal function. Invest Ophthalmol Vis Sci 22(3): 343, 1982
38. Houde WL, Rubin ML: Extended wear lenses: An update. Surv Ophthalmol 26(2):103, 1981
39. Ing MR: Experience with extended wear hydrogel lenses for aphakia. Ann Ophthalmol 13(2):181, 1981
40. Jackson GK, Aquavella JV: Clinical experience with hydrophilic lenses in monocular aphakia. Ann Ophthalmol 8(2):156, 1976
41. Kastl P, Refojo M, Dabezies O: Review of polymerization for the contact lens fitter. In Dabezies O (ed): CLAO Book, Contact Lenses 6:6.1, 1984
42. Kersley HJ: Contact lenses in aphakia. Trans Ophthalmol Soc UK 97:142, 1977
43. Kersley HJ, Kerr C, Pierse D: Hydrophilic lenses for continuous wear in aphakia: Definitive fitting and problems that occur. Br J Ophthalmol 61(1):38, 1977
44. Kracher GP, Stark WJ, Hirst LW: Extended wear contact lenses for aphakia. Am J Optom Physiol Opt 58(6):467, 1981
45. Krohn DL: Enhancement of the sensitivity of the peripheral visual field of aphakic eyes by a soft contact lens correction. Trans Am Ophthalmol Soc 77:308, 1979
46. Lembach RG: Fitting techniques of soft lenses. In Dabezies O (ed): CLAO Book, Contact Lenses 38:38.1, 1984

47. Lembach RG, Keates RH: Permalens extended wear contact lenses. In Hartstein J (ed): Extended Wear Contact Lenses for Aphakia 3:44, 1982
48. Lembach RG, Wilson LA: Extended wear contact lenses. In Dabezies O (ed): CLAO Book, Contact Lenses 61:61.1, 1984
49. Lenses and lens care, PDR for Ophthalmology 8:135, 1985
50. Lobascher D, Chaston J, Morris J et al: Soft contact lenses in cases of aphakia. Br J Ophthalmol 58(12):1009, 1974
51. Manchester PT Jr: Extended wear contact lenses for aphakic correction: Experience with the Cooper Permalens, A Preliminary Report. Trans Am Ophthalmol Soc 78:47, 1980
52. Martin NF, Kracher GP, Stark WJ et al: Extended wear soft contact lenses for aphakic correction. Arch Ophthalmol 101(1):39, 1983
53. Mobilia EF, Foster CS: A comparison of various extended wear lenses for use in aphakia. CLAO J 8(1):12, 1982
54. Nesburn AB: Prolonged-wear contact lenses in aphakia. Ophthalmology 85(1):73, 1978
55. Nesburn AB, Maguen E: Sauflon contact lenses for extended wear. In Hartstein J (ed): Extended Wear Contact Lenses for Aphakia 4:78, 1982
56. Nilsson SE, Morris JA: Corneal thickness response to high and low water content lenses in aphakic eyes. Br J Ophthalmol 67(5):317, 1983
57. Novicky NN, Hill RM: Oxygen measurements: Dk's and EOP's. Int Contact Lens Clin 8:41, 1981
58. Peppas N: Contact lenses as biomedical polymers. In Hartstein J (ed): Extended Wear Contact Lenses in Aphakia 2:6, 1982
59. Pierse D, Kersey HJ: Hydrophilic lenses for "continuous" wear in aphakia: Fitting at operation. Br J Ophthalmol 61(1):34, 1977
60. Polse KA, Sarver MD, Harris ME: Corneal effects of high plus hydrogel lenses. Am J Optom Physiol Opt 55(4):234, 1978
61. Rasson JE, Fatt I: Oxygen flux through a soft contact lens on the eye. Am J Optom Physiol Opt 59:203, 1982
62. Refojo M: Water imbibition. In Dabezies O (ed): The CLAO Book, Contact Lenses 9:9.1, 1984
63. Refojo M, Farris RL, Dabezies O: Gas transmission. In Dabezies O (ed): The CLAO Book, Contact Lenses 10:10.1, 1984
64. Salz JJ, Schlanger JL: Prolonged wear soft contact lenses. J Am Intraocul Implant Soc 6(3):246, 1980
65. Schonder AA, Conklin TR, Angelini EA: Clinical evaluation of extended wear Lidofilcon B contact lenses in aphakia. Ann Ophthalmol 14(10):935, 1982
66. Shaw EL, Gassett AR: Experience in the use of soft contact lenses for the correction of monocular and binocular aphakia. Ann Ophthalmol 5(9):937, 1973
67. Sibley MJ, Dabezies O: Soft lens hygiene. In Dabezies O (ed): The CLAO Book, Contact Lenses 40:40.1, 1984
68. Smolin G, Okumoto M, Nozik R: The microbial flora in extended wear soft contact lens wearers. Am J Ophthalmol 88(3):543, 1979
69. Soft contact lenses. (Section 6) Table 35, pp 29–35; Table 37, p 38. In PDR for Ophthalmology, 1985.
70. Soper JW: Contact lens correction of aphakia. Int Ophthalmol Clin 18(2):247, 1978

71. Stark WJ, Kracher GP, Cowan CL et al: Extended wear contact lenses and intraocular lenses for aphakic correction. Am J Ophthalmol 88:535, 1979

72. Stein HA, Harrison KW: Canadian experience with the TC-75 lens for extended wear. In Hartstein J (ed): Extended Wear Contact Lenses for Aphakia and Myopia 8:124–196, 1982

73. Stein HA, Slatt B: Contact lenses after cataract surgery: A review of 200 aphakic patients fitted with soft lenses. Can J Ophthalmol 9(1):79, 1974

74. Tandon MK, Davies MS, Wishart D et al: Extended wear soft contact lenses in the correction of aphakia. Trans Ophthalmol Soc UK 101(1):65, 1981

75. Traykovski A, Freudenerg C, Janoff L: Extended wear of Softcon Vifilcon A lenses by aphakic patients: A 2 year study. CLAO J 9(4):327, 1983

76. Vannas S, Vannas A, Blowater R et al: Binocular vision in monocular aphakia correctable with contact lenses. Acta Ophthalmol 50(4):589, 1972

77. Wakelin DL, Shirley SY: Soft contact lenses in aphakia. Can J Ophthalmol 9(1):56, 1974

78. Weis DR: Long term results wearing hard contact lenses in monocular aphakia. Ophthalmology 89(9):1003, 1982

79. Wichterle O, Lim D: Hydrophilic gels for biological use. Nature 185:117, 1960

CHAPTER FOUR

HYDROGEL LENSES: COSMETIC

THOMAS JOHN

HISTORY

Wichterle and Lim described the first soft contact lenses in 1960.[61,62] These lenses were made of a cross-linked polymer of 2-hydroxyethyl methacrylate (poly HEMA) and had a water content of about 30%. Wichterle's soft hydrophilic lenses and the spin casting and xerogel lathing techniques were later acquired by Bausch & Lomb. It was not until 1965 that soft contact lenses were introduced on a trial basis into the United States by the National Patent Company. One year later, Bausch & Lomb introduced the spin-cast soft lens followed by the advent of the first lathe-cut Griffin lens, which later became the American Optical Softcon lens.

In the evolution of soft contact lenses, the "second generation" lenses had greater water content of 30% to 50%. With the advent of "third generation" soft contact lenses with a higher water content, the Food and Drug Administration in January 1981 cleared the Hydrocurve II (Barnes-Hind Hydrocurve) 55% hydrated lens and the Permalens (Cooper-Vision, Inc.) 71% hydrated lens for myopic extended wear. Presently, FDA-approved cosmetic soft contact lenses with a high water content of up to 79% for hyperopia (*e.g.,* Sauflon PW; American Medical Optics) are available for extended wear.

CLASSIFICATION OF SOFT CONTACT LENSES

Soft contact lenses may be considered under different categories either on the basis of the water content of the lens or the thickness of the lens, with these two factors bearing an inverse relationship. The different categories have been alluded to in another chapter.

MANUFACTURE OF HYDROGEL CONTACT LENSES

Hydrogel contact lenses are made by either a spin-casting or a lathe-cutting process.

SPIN CASTING

In this method, liquid plastic is injected into a concave spherical spinning mold (Fig. 4-1*A*). The vertical axis of rotation passes through the center of curvature of the mold (Fig. 4-1*B*). The inner concave curvature of the mold matches the front surface of the lens. Thus, the shape of the mold determines the sagittal depth, cord diameter, and the anterior surface of the lens. The back surface of the lens forms a shape that is dependent on the rate of speed. A faster speed would result in less plastic in the central region, with more plastic being displaced to the periphery due to the greater centrifugal force, giving rise to a greater amount of minus power.

Lens parameters are governed by the shape of the mold, amount of injected material, surface tension, and spin speed of the mold.[3,15] Having chosen the mold design and the monomer mixture, the variables left to alter the refractive power of the contact lens are the volume of monomer injected and the spin speed. Once the injected monomer mixture attains equilibrium, the polymerization process is initiated. Finally the lens is hydrated, removed from its mold, and placed in distilled water at 190°F to remove any unreacted monomer or other water soluble substances. The lens is then inspected, its power is checked, and it is bottled in 0.9% saline and sterilized in an autoclave.

In this process, both the anterior and posterior surfaces of the lens can be altered independently of each other. Hence, it is possible to produce a variety of lens features.

Advantages of Spin Casting

Spin casting is an automated process with computer controlled spin speed, which produces lenses that are accurate and reproducible. The lenses manufactured by this method have a superior optical surface compared to the lathe-cut lenses, and the plastic is durable. Unlike lathe-cut lenses, spin-cast lenses do not have the tool marks or peripheral grooves that may occur in lathe cutting.

LATHE CUTTING

Polymeric material in a dehydrated state is cast in the form of buttons (Fig. 4-2*A*), which are then cut using the lathe (Fig. 4-2*B*), similar to hard

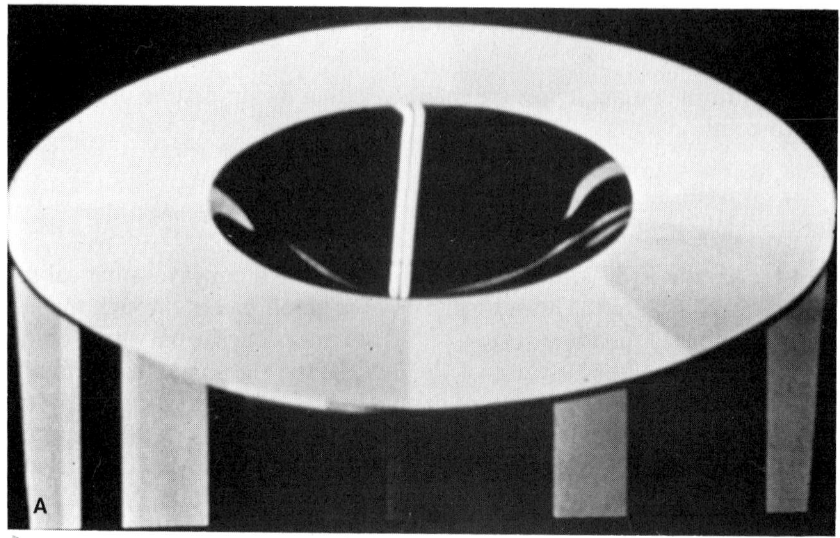

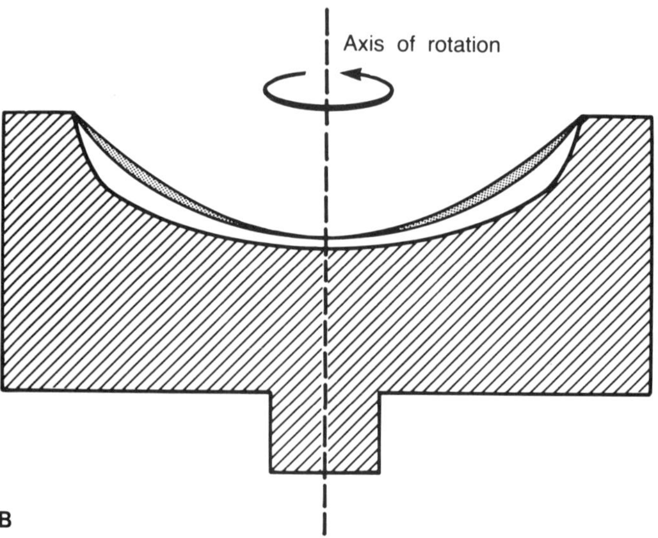

Figure 4-1 (*A*) Mold used for spin casting soft contact lens (Courtesy Bausch & Lomb, Inc.). (*B*) Diagrammatic representation of spin-cast molding process.

lenses.[45,46,49] The button is cut to the desired diameter and the back surface is cut on the lathe to the required curvature (Fig. 4-2*C*). The back surface is then polished using the polishing machine (Fig. 4-2*D*). This process is repeated on the front surface of the lens (Figs. 4-2*E, F*). The peripheral curves are added and the edges are polished (Fig. 4-2*G*). Next the lens is hydrated for several hours in a water bath. Following inspection, lenses are bottled, autoclaved, and ready for dispatch.

Advantages of Lathe Cutting

In lathe cutting, the parameters of the lens can be changed. Any anterior or posterior curve can be cut on the lathe. The power of the lens is changed by changing the anterior curve of the lens. Identification of the lens is simplified by engraving on the lens. High-quality surfaces can be achieved in the lathe-cutting process.

Some of the differences between the spin-cast and lathe-cut processes in the manufacture of soft contact lenses are shown in Table 4-1.

TORIC SOFT LENSES

Aspheric hydrophilic lenses are manufactured in a similar way to hard lenses using the lathe.[23] Cylinders are added by crimping. The amount of "cylinder bend" can be varied by changing the degree of crimping. Methods used to prevent lens rotation on the eye include prism ballast, truncation, and thin circular peripheries.

LENS DESIGN

The two basic lens designs are the single-cut (Fig. 4-3) and lenticular-cut (Fig. 4-4) designs.[26] The single-cut design is used in spin casting of low minus lenses. The lenticular-cut design is used in spin casting for high minus power lenses and most plus power contact lenses. The lenticular-cut design is also used for most lathe-cut lenses, of plus and minus powers.

CONTACT LENS PARAMETERS

Some of the parameters of a contact lens are described below.

Base curve: The base curve or posterior central curve of a contact lens is the radius of curvature of the cental posterior optical portion in millimeters.

Power is the dioptric power of the contact lens, specified to the nearest 0.12 D. The power in a spin-cast lens depends on the curvature of the back surface of the lens, whereas the power in a lathe-cut lens is determined by the curvature of the front surface.

Diameter is the overall linear, chord dimension of the lens from edge to edge, in millimeters. Truncated contact lenses have two diameters placed at right angles to each other.

Thickness: Central thickness of a lens is indicated in millimeters.

Optical zones: There are two optical zones, namely, an anterior optical zone (AOZ) on the front surface of the lens (see Figs. 4-3, 4-4) and a posterior optical zone (POZ) on the back surface of the lens (see Figs. 4-3, 4-4). The chord length, or diameter, of the anterior central curve represents the AOZ whereas that of the central posterior curve is the POZ, specified to the nearest 0.1 mm.

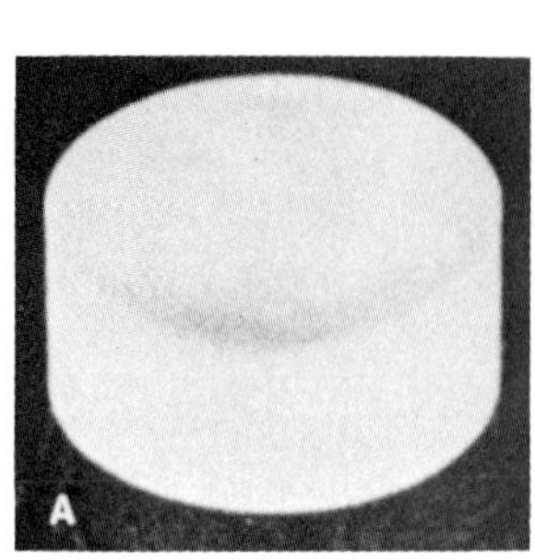

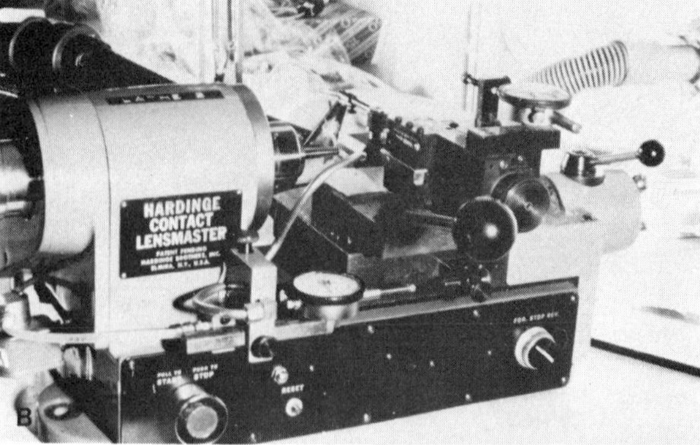

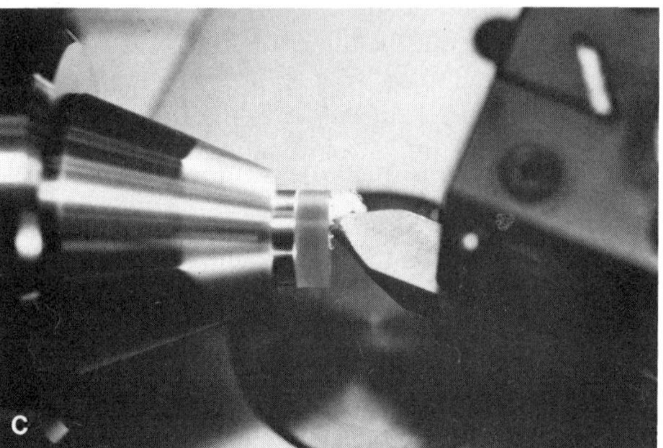

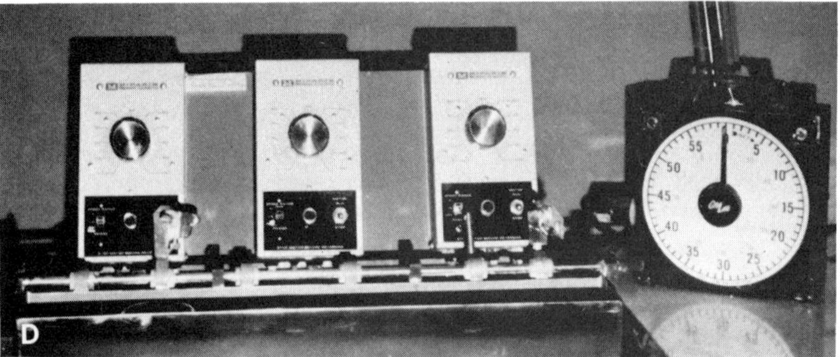

Figure 4-2 (*A*) Button of soft lens material in the dehydrated state used in manufacturing lathe-cut lens (Courtesy American Hydron, Inc.). (*B*) Lathe. (*C*) Using the lathe, the base curve is cut. (*D*) Polishing machine. (*E*) In lathe-cut lens, power is ground on the front surface of the lens. (*F*) The front surface of the lens is polished. (*G*) The edges of the lens are polished while the lens is still mounted (*B–G*, Courtesy Bausch & Lomb, Inc.).

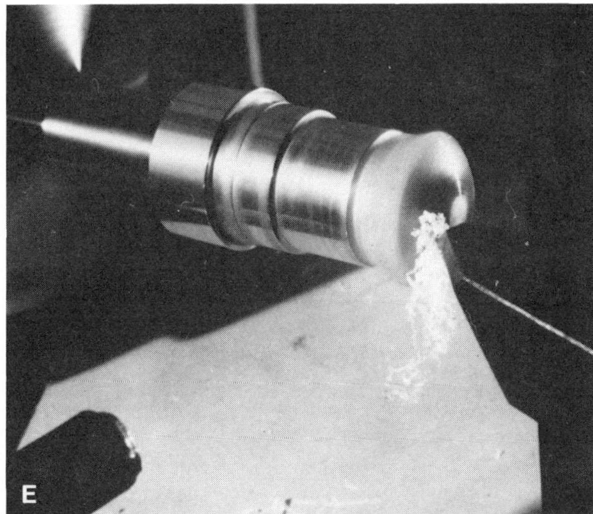

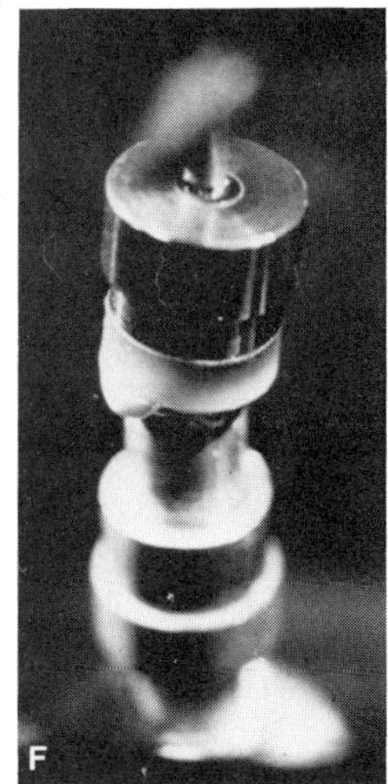

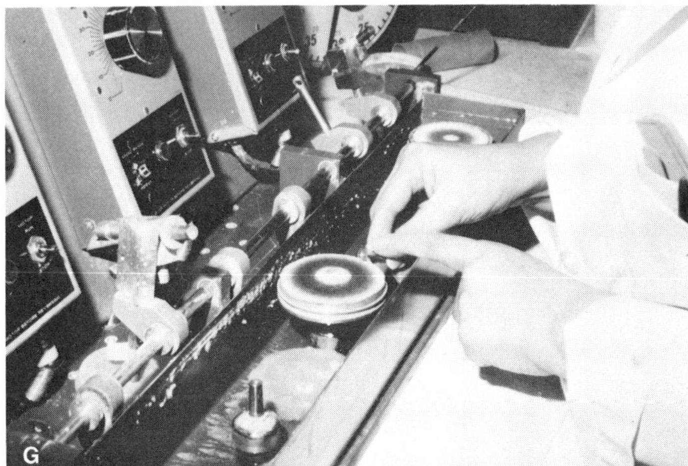

Figure 4-2 (*Continued*)

Peripheral curves: At the periphery of spin-cast lenses, there is a bevel on the anterior surface called the anterior peripheral curve (APC) (see Fig. 4-3), whereas in lathe-cut lenses, the peripheral bevel is on the posterior surface and is called the posterior peripheral curve (PPC) (see Fig. 4-4). The bevel usually varies from 0.8 mm to 1 mm.

Blend is the point of transition between the radii of curvature from one curve to another.

Tint refers to the coloring in a lens. For the most part, soft lenses are clear. Recently, tinted soft lenses have been introduced for cosmetic use.

Sagittal depth is the distance between a flat surface and the back surface of the central portion of a lens.

TABLE 4-1 Comparison of Spin Casting and Lathe-Cutting Processes for Soft Contact Lenses

	Spin Casting	Lathe Cutting
Manufacture	Liquid plastic is injected into spinning molds, polymerized, and hydrated	Unhydrated polymeric material is cut into buttons, lathe cut, polished, and hydrated
Lens Power Governed by Peripheral Construction	Posterior lens curvature Bevel is present on anterior surface (Fig. 4-3)	Anterior lens curvature Bevel is present on posterior surface (Fig. 4-4)
Anterior Optical Zone (AOZ)	Corresponds to front surface of the lens minus the anterior peripheral curve	Corresponds to the optical portion of the lens (i.e., front surface minus carrier portion of the lens)
Posterior Optical Zone (POZ)	Includes the entire diameter of the back surface of the lens (Fig. 4-3)	Is the back surface of the lens, less the posterior peripheral curve (Fig. 4-4)

ADVANTAGES AND DISADVANTAGES OF SOFT CONTACT LENSES

Advantages

Initial comfort and easy adaptation

Option of intermittent usage

Little or no spectacle blur

Easy to fit

Foreign bodies do not get lodged under the lens

Eyes may be rubbed with lenses in place

Less corneal physiologic change

Usually does not fall out of the eye (useful in athletics)

Cosmetically excellent

Iris color can be changed with tinted lenses

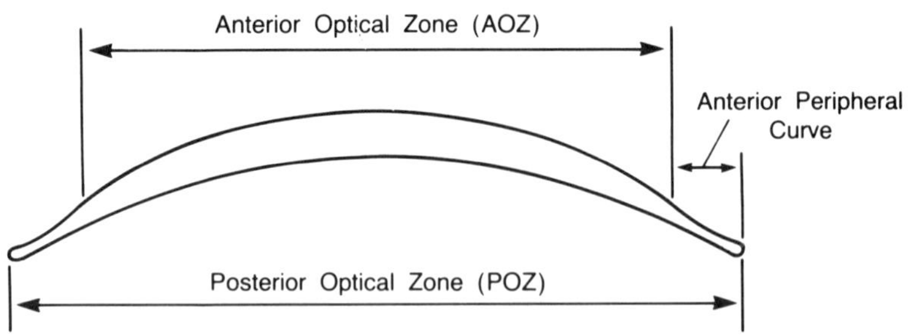

Figure 4-3 Spin-cast soft contact lens construction with a single-cut lens design.

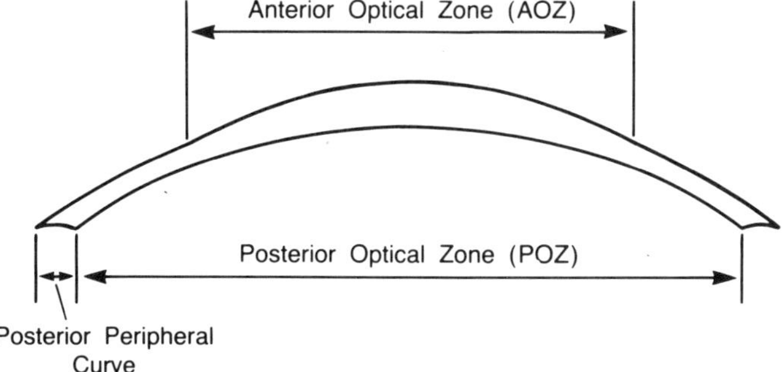

Figure 4-4 Lathe-cut soft lens construction with a lenticular-cut design.

Corneal or anterior segment pathology can be masked with certain soft lenses

Disadvantages

Visual acuity may be reduced

Costs more than hard contact lens

Requires meticulous care

Spherical lens does not correct astigmatism

Lenses may tear easily

Drying of the lens can cause blurred vision

Lens replacement more frequent

Storage and cleaning may be difficult while travelling

FITTING SOFT LENSES

Objectives

A successful contact lens fit should provide a good, steady visual acuity comparable to that obtained with spectacles, without any discomfort or any major alterations in corneal physiology.

Choice of Soft Lens

A soft contact lens is preferred when rapid adaptation to the lens is required. A soft lens is more comfortable compared with a hard lens, and hence it is useful in patients with a low threshold for discomfort. A soft lens is chosen in persons unable to wear hard lenses. Because a soft lens is more stable on the eye than a hard lens, it is preferred for athletes, especially those involved in body contact sports such as hockey, football, and basketball. Unlike hard lenses, soft lenses do not drop to a great extent inferiorly when the eyes are raised, and thus are preferred in games such as tennis. Because of the relative stability of the soft lens on the eye, it is also useful for pilots, machinists working with heavy, dangerous machinery, swimmers, and in patients with nystagmus. It offers an attractive alternative to some who prefer to wear contact lenses intermittently.

Avoidance of Contact Lenses

Contact lenses should be discouraged in patients who lack self-motivation and in those with poor hygiene habits. Contact lenses should not be used for cosmesis in the presence of corneal or conjunctival inflammation or infection.

Prefitting Evaluation

The prefitting evaluation should start with thorough information taken about the medical history of the patient. The history should include information about any previous use of contact lenses, hard or soft, daily or extended-wear lenses, and whether there were any adverse reactions in the past while using a contact lens. Detailed information about the method of lens care should also be obtained. If the person was a hard lens wearer, he or she should have discontinued wearing the lens for at least 7 days, to allow the cornea to resume its near normal contour. Following the assessment of visual acuity, refraction and keratometer readings of the central cornea should be obtained followed by thorough slit lamp biomicroscopy.

In the evaluation of the eyelids, the position of the eyelid should be checked. The size of the palpebral fissures should be examined to see if they are normal or excessively narrow. A smaller lens may be helpful in patients with narrow palpebral fissures. The eyelashes are to be scrutinized for any anterior or posterior blepharitis. The upper tarsal conjunctiva should be specifically examined for any papillary changes. The evaluation of the tear film and tear meniscus is of paramount importance. The height of the lower tear meniscus and the presence of debris in the tears should be noted. The qualitative and quantitative integrity of tear film is vital for proper performance of soft contact lenses. Conjunctiva and conjunctival vessels are then evaluated with special attention paid to check for pinguecula, pterygium, filtering bleb, and cysts. Detailed corneal evaluation is the next step. This includes observations about any neovascularization, sensitivity, and thickness, as well as the status of epithelium and endothelium.

Methods of Fitting

Soft contact lenses may be fitted using the diagnostic lens method or the inventory lens method.[32]

DIAGNOSTIC LENS METHOD

Lathe-cut lenses are usually fitted using the diagnostic lens method. A set of diagnostic trial lenses with standard diameter and base curves are utilized to obtain adequate fit. The lenses have differing base curves and diameters but only one power. At least 15 minutes should be allowed for the trial lens to "settle" on the cornea before evaluating the fit of the lens. This allows the lens to adjust to the ocular environment. Once a good lens fit is attained, the power of the lens is ascertained by manifest refraction over the lens. If there is a large change in the power of the lens (greater than 2 D to 3 D), this may entail using a new lens with different fitting characteristics than the initial trial lens. This problem can be overcome if one uses an inventory set with all the available powers. However, a complete inventory of lathe-cut lenses is rather expensive.

INVENTORY LENS METHOD

The inventory lens method is usually used to fit spin-cast lenses. A complete inventory of lenses of different series is used for fitting. The curvatures of the anterior and posterior peripheral portion of the lens are constant within each series of lenses. Only the curvature of the posterior surface of the central portion of the lenses, which determines the lens power, varies within each series of lenses. This enables one to obtain both an adequate lens fit and proper lens power in the initial fitting session. Hence, the lens can be dispensed at the initial visit, which is advantageous to both the practitioner and the patient.

Technique of Fitting

To understand the basis of fitting a soft contact lens, it is important to review the lens–eye relationship. A normal fitting soft lens should have a three-point touch, namely, at the corneal apex and at the superior and inferior limbi.[32,53] This ideal fit will keep the lens well centered and will allow for slight motion with eye movement, which will provide adequate tear flow beneath the lens. The lens fit can be altered by varying the sagittal depth. To obtain a tighter fit, the sagittal depth is increased by using a steeper base curve or a larger contact lens. Conversely, a looser fit may be attained by using a flatter lens or a smaller lens.

EVALUATION OF LENS FIT

When fitting a soft contact lens, the type of fit and the lens–eye relationship should be evaluated (Table 4-2).[14,32,53,59] The fitting is initiated by using a lens that is 2 D to 3 D flatter than the central K reading. The fit of the lens should be evaluated after 20 to 30 minutes of wearing time to allow the lens to stabilize on the eye. An optimum fit results in a well-centered lens that moves slightly with ocular movement (1 mm to 2 mm). Good centration will provide a good optical result and the slight movement will allow oxygenated tears to flow under the lens. A well-fit lens will be comfortable with stable vision (see Table 4-2).

TABLE 4-2 Effect of Soft-Lens Fit

Parameter	Type of Fit		
	GOOD	FLAT/LOOSE	STEEP/TIGHT
Comfort	Good	Increased lens awareness	Comfortable initially, becomes uncomfortable later during the day
Vision	Stable	Variable; clear initially, poor after blinking	Variable; clears momentarily after blinking
Centration	Good or slight lag in primary position	Poor (Fig. 4-5)	Good (Fig. 4-5)
Movement	Slight (Fig. 4-5)	Excessive (Fig. 4-5)	Poor or absent (Fig. 4-5)
Slit-lamp examination	No compression of peripheral limbal tissues	Bubble under lens edge or edge standoff (Fig. 4-5)	Vascular blanching at lens edge; later, circumcorneal injection; central air bubble may be present (Fig. 4-5)
Keratometry	Clear mires (Fig. 4-6)	Clear mires, blurs after blink (Fig. 4-6)	Distorted mires, clears immediately after blink (Fig. 4-6)
Retinoscopic reflex	Clear (Fig. 4-7)	Clear at first, blurs after blinking (Fig. 4-7)	Blurred reflex, clears momentarily after blink (Fig. 4-7)

Movement

Good fit: A lens with an optimum fit will display good centration in primary position and would lag behind about 0.5 mm to 1.5 mm when the patient looks in an upward direction (Fig. 4-5). If the patient blinks while he or she continues to look up, the lens would elevate about 1 mm and then return down 1 mm to recenter on the cornea.

Flat/loose fit: With a flat-fitting lens, there is excessive movement of the lens with both eye movement and blinking. This may even result in the lens sliding off the cornea. In primary gaze, the lens would show poor centration and may have air bubbles beneath the periphery of the lens (see Fig. 4-5).

Steep/tight fit: A steep-fitting lens may have an air bubble in the center and may blanch conjunctival vessels at the lens periphery or result in engorgement of more peripheral vessels with wear. There is little or no lens movement when the patient moves his eye or blinks (see Fig. 4-5). In some instances, this can lead to the extreme manifestation of tight lens syndrome with its characteristic clinical features.

Keratometry

Keratometry over the lens also assists in evaluating the lens fit.

Good fit: With a good lens fit, no distortion of the mires is seen (Fig. 4-6), and the keratometric readings show the same amount of astigmatism that was present before insertion of the lens.

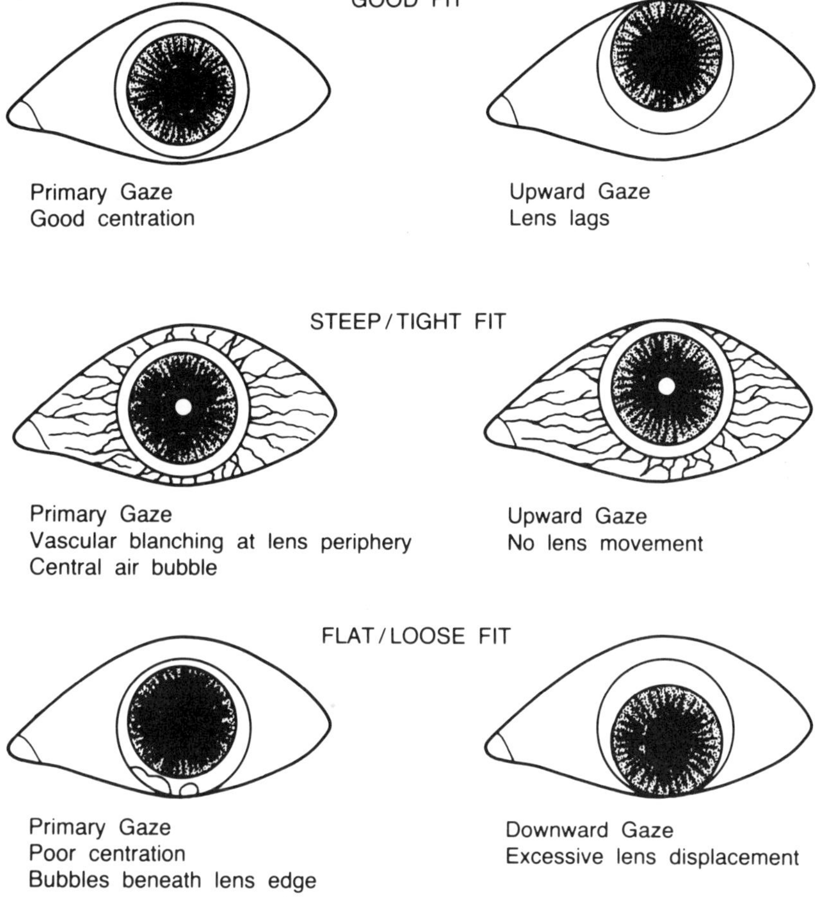

Figure 4-5 Evaluation of soft contact lens fit based on centration and movement of the lens.

Flat/loose fit: The central portion of a lens that has a flat fit will rest intermittently on the cornea. The mires that are clear will then get distorted just after a blink (see Fig. 4-6).

Steep/tight fit: On the other hand, the central part of a steep-fitting lens vaults the cornea. Thus, initially blurred mires become more regular when the tight lens is flattened by a blink (see Fig. 4-6). Also, with both a tight and loose-fitting lens, the keratometric readings will show a change in astigmatism.

Retinoscopy

Retinoscopy over the lens can be used to assess the adequacy of lens fit. With a good fit, the retinoscopic reflex is clear and crisp, as if no lens were in

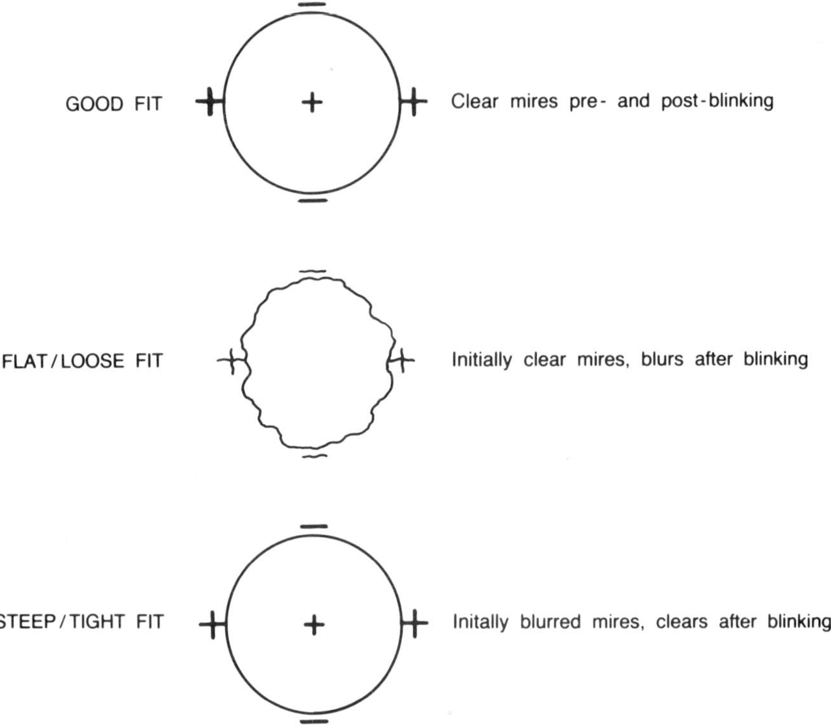

Figure 4-6 Checking the adequacy of a soft lens fit after blinking using a keratometer.

place. In a flat fit, the retinoscopic shadow may be blurred immediately after a blink. If the lens is steep, prior to blinking there will be a spreading of the streak centrally, which will clear following a blink due to ironing out of the apical vault of the lens (Fig. 4-7).

Refraction Over the Lens

Overrefraction can help in evaluating the adequacy of fit. If this results in more than −0.5 D than would be anticipated based on refraction and K reading, then the lens is fit steep. The tear lens beneath the vault of a steep lens would induce a plus power effect, which accounts for the requirement of minus power. However, in a flat fit, the tear lens induces a minus power effect, which would result in the patient accepting more than +0.5 D.

Thus, various subjective and objective modalities may be used to help the practitioner in attaining the optimum lens fit for the patient (see Table 4-2).

FITTING DAILY-WEAR SOFT LENSES

A large number of soft lenses that are approved by the FDA are currently available for the correction of myopia, hyperopia, and astigmatism. These

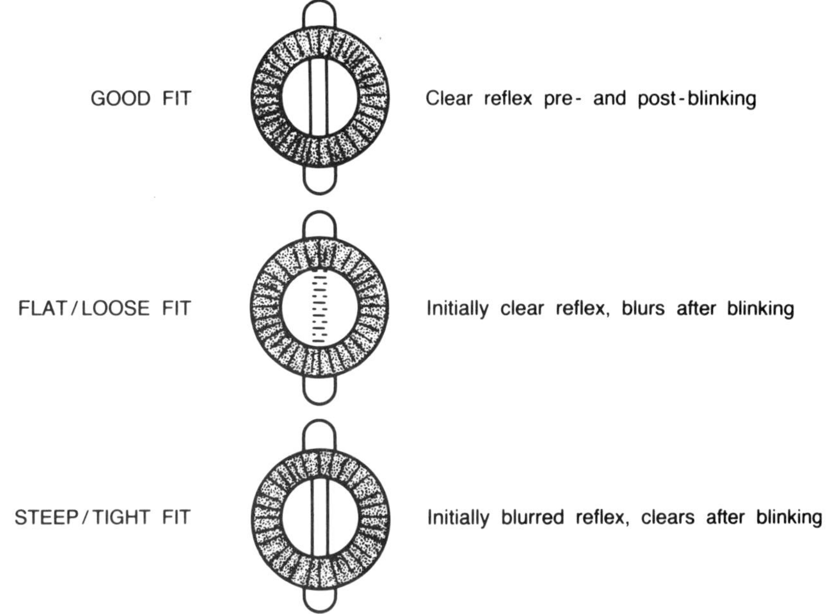

Figure 4-7 *Changes in retinoscopic reflexes after a blink, in soft contact lens that has a good, loose, or tight lens fit.*

lenses vary in the type of polymer, water content, diameter, base curve, central thickness, oxygen transmission, and edge shape. Some lenses are spin cast or molded, whereas others are lathe cut. Lens design varies with different manufacturers. Each contact lens manufacturer produces lenses with differing lens design, with a choice of base curve, diameter, and central thickness. This gives the practitioner a wide range of parameters from which to choose an appropriate lens to suit the need of the patient.

Myopia

A large variety of daily wear soft lenses are available for the correction of myopia. Consequently, there is no "single method" or "best method" of lens fitting. The practitioner has to choose a lens that is best suited for each patient. The fitting procedures for a few of the lenses are described later. Table 4-3 lists some of these lenses.

MYOPIA UP TO −20 D WITH AVERAGE OR LARGE DIAMETER CORNEAS

DuraSoft 3 The DuraSoft 3 lens has a water content of 55% and a tensile strength of 4 kg/cm^2, which contributes to its durability. Oxygen transmission is high ($Dk/L \times 10^{-9} = 22.3$). Phemfilcon A is said to provide resistance to protein deposits. It provides good optical properties and has a large optical zone.

TABLE 4-3 Partial List of Daily-Wear Contact Lenses for Myopia

Lens/Manufacturer	Polymer	Water Content (%)	Power Range (D)
Softcon; American Optical Corp.	Vifilcon A	55	−0.25 to −8
Hydrocurve II; Barnes-Hind/Hydrocurve	Bufilcon A	45	Plano to −20
CSI; Syntex Ophthalmics	Crofilcon A	38.5	Plano to −20
Soflens; Bausch & Lomb	Polymacon	38.6	−0.25 to −20
Aquaflex; CooperVision	Tetrafilcon A	42.5	Plano to −20
DuraSoft; Wesley-Jessen	Phemfilcon A	30, 38, 55	Plano to −20
Hydron; American Hydron	Polymacon	38	Plano to −20
Cibasoft Minus; Ciba Vision Care	Tefilcon	37.5	Plano to −10

The lens has a diameter of 14.5 mm. The fitting should be started with an 8.6-mm base curve (flattest central $K = 41.5$ to 44.5) and the fit evaluated after about 20 minutes. According to the manufacturer, this base curve provides adequate fit to about 80% of the patients. If the fit is loose, one should switch to a lens with a base curve of 8.3 mm; if the lens is tight, a 9-mm base curve lens should be tried.

Having obtained the base curve, the lens power required should be determined. The spectacle correction is expressed in minus cylinder and only the spherical component has to be considered. The vertex distance is compensated for, if the power is greater than ±4 D. A lens with a power as close as possible to the patient's requirements is then fitted. The final power of the lens is determined by overrefraction. If spherical power alone provides good vision, a DuraSoft spherical lens is dispensed. When the overrefraction sphere power exceeds ±4 D, compensation has to be provided for vertex distance. (Diagnostic lens power + overrefraction = final lens power.)

If cylinder power is necessary to provide good vision, a toric lens has to be fitted. When a lens is to be ordered, the base curve, diameter, and power have to be specified.

MYOPIA UP TO −12 D WITH AVERAGE DIAMETER CORNEAS

Hydrocurve II A 13.5-mm diameter lens with a base curve of 8.6 mm has to be selected as the initial lens, if the cornea is not especially steep. The fit is evaluated after 20 minutes. If the fit is too tight, a larger diameter Hydrocurve II lens of 14.5 mm, 15.5 mm, or 16 mm is tried with an appropriate base curve based on the flattest K. If the fit is too loose, then a lens with an 8.3-mm base curve with the same diameter as the initial lens is tried.

Initial Lens

8.3 mm   _{too loose} ←   8.6 mm   _{too tight} → try larger
(13.5-mm diameter)   (13.5-mm diameter)   diameter lens
with appropriate
base curve

Hydrocurve II is made of Bufilcon A polymer. It is a lathe-cut lens with a 45% water content. It has a spherical posterior (concave) surface, minimum central thickness, and a flattened posterior peripheral curve.

MYOPIA UP TO −10 D WITH AVERAGE OR LARGE DIAMETER CORNEAS

Cibasoft Minus Cibasoft Minus has a 14.5-mm diameter and comes in three different base curves. An 8.9-mm base curve is to be used for corneas from 7.5 mm to 8.1 mm. For corneas flatter than 8.1 mm, a base curve of 9.2 mm is recommended. If the cornea is steeper than 7.5 mm, an 8.6-mm base curve lens is the first lens to be tried. This lens has a water content of 37.5%, provides good visual results, and is easy to handle.

MYOPIA UP TO −6 D WITH AVERAGE DIAMETER CORNEAS

Hydron Zero 6 The Hydron Zero 6 lens has a diameter of 14 mm, with a central thickness of 0.06 mm, and a water content of 38%. It is comfortable, easy to handle, and affords good vision.

For corneas ranging from 7.6 mm to 8.1 mm, an 8.7-mm base curve lens is to be selected, with an 8.4-mm base curve lens for corneas of 7.5 mm or steeper. For corneas 8.15 mm and flatter, a 9-mm base curve lens is tried first.

MYOPIA UP TO −8 D WITH VERY SENSITIVE LIDS
OR HANDLING DIFFICULTIES

Softcon An 8.1-mm base curve lens is to be tried for corneas of 7.2 mm to 7.5 mm. For corneas 7.5 mm and flatter, an 8.4-mm base curve lens is to be tried. For corneas 7.1 mm and steeper, a 7.8-mm base curve lens is used. The lens comes in 14 mm and 14.5 mm diameters, with the former having base curves of 7.8 mm and 8.1 mm, and the latter 8.1 mm and 8.4 mm. This lens has 55% water content and an excellent edge design, which makes it very comfortable.

MYOPIA FROM −8 D TO −20 D WITH AVERAGE
CORNEAL DIAMETER AND SENSITIVE LIDS

B & L HO-4 Lens The B & L HO-4 lens has a central thickness of 0.035 mm with edges that are thin and comfortable. It has a diameter of 14.5 mm and a single base curve.

MYOPIA UP TO −20 D WITH LARGE CORNEAL DIAMETER

Hydrocurve II Use a 15.5-mm or 16-mm diameter Hydrocurve II lens, each of which comes in four different base curves (9.2 mm, 9.5 mm, 9.8

mm, and 10.1 mm). Choose the appropriate base curve based on the flattest *K*. For flattest *K* reading of 45.25 D to 47 D, use 9.2-mm base curve; for a reading of 44 D to 45 D, use 9.5 mm; for a reading of 41.25 D to 43.75 D, use 9.8 mm; and for a reading of 40 D to 41 D, select a 10.1-mm base curve.

CSI Lens Most patients can be fitted successfully with the 8.9-mm base curve CSI lens. This should be the initial lens of choice, except on flat corneas of 41.75 D and less, where the 9.35-mm base curve is used first. For steep corneas, use the 8.6-mm lens. This lens is comfortable to use.

MYOPIA UP TO −20 D WITH SMALL DIAMETER CORNEAS

Aquaflex Superthin Minus Lens The Aquaflex Superthin Minus lens is made of Tetrafilcon A polymer and has a water content of 42.5%. The diameter is 13.8 mm, with four different base curves (Vault I, 9.1 mm; Vault II, 8.8 mm; Vault III, 8.5 mm; and Vault IV, 8.2 mm). The central thickness is 0.06 mm. Although thin, the lens has good handling characteristics. From Vaults I to IV, the lens becomes progressively steeper.

Hydron Mini Lens The Hydron (polymacon) lathed mini lens is a hydrophilic lens of 38% water and a central thickness of 0.52 mm to 0.12 mm, depending on the power. The lens has a wider range of base curves in 0.2-mm increments, which gives the practitioner control over fitting. It has good mechanical strength and returns to original shape after deformation.

The diameter is 13 mm and base curves are available in 8.1 mm, 8.3 mm, 8.5 mm, 8.7 mm, and 8.9 mm. To select a base curve, convert the *K* reading to millimeters and add 0.9 mm to the flat *K*.

8.1	8.3	8.5	8.7	8.9

steep ⎯⎯⎯⎯⎯⎯⎯⎯⎯⎯⎯⎯→ flat

In the majority of cases, 8.7 mm will give the best fit.

MYOPIA UP TO −10 D WITH SMALL DIAMETER CORNEAS

Aquaflex Standard Minus Lenses The Aquaflex Standard Minus lens is made of Tetrafilcon A with a water content of 42.5%. It has a 13-mm diameter and has five different base curves (Vault 0, 9 mm; Vault I, 8.7 mm; Vault II, 8.4 mm; Vault III, 8.1 mm; and Vault IV, 7.8 mm). The base curves vary from flat in Vault 0 to steep in Vault IV. The lens is easy to handle, and it provides excellent vision.

MYOPIA UP TO −12 D WITH SMALL CORNEAL DIAMETER

Hydrocurve II Daily Wear Spherical The Hydrocurve II Daily Wear Spherical lens, with a diameter of 13.5 mm, may be used on small corneas. It has a single base curve of 8.6 mm. It is made of Bufilcon A, with a 45% water content.

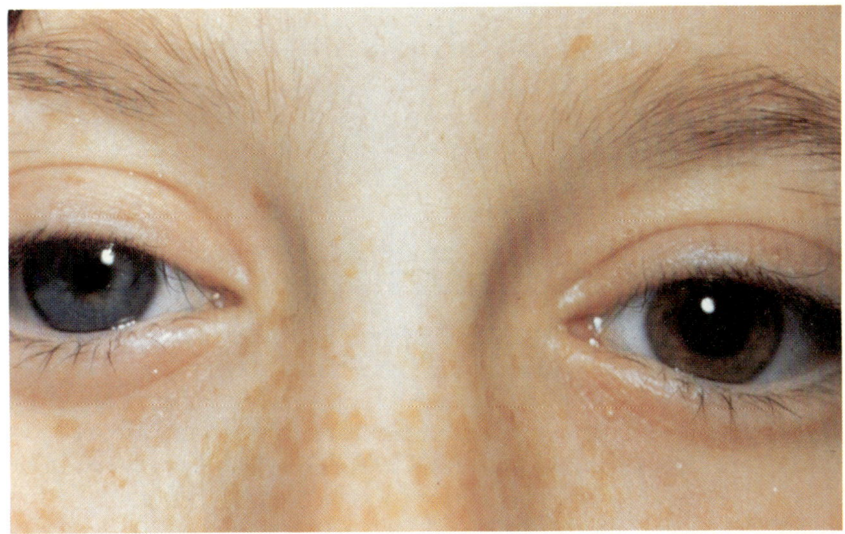

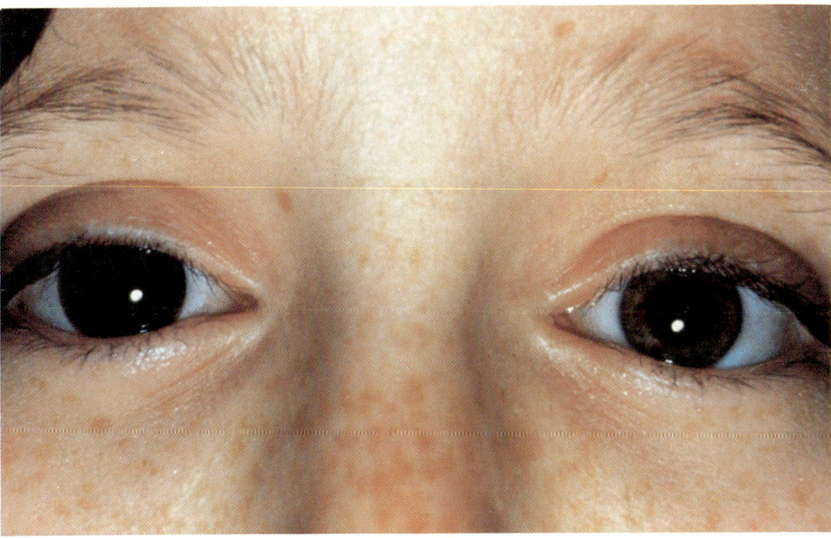

Color Figure 4-1 Cosmetic correction of heterochromia iridis (*A*) with a tinted soft contact lens (*B*). (Courtesy Narcissus Medical Foundation)

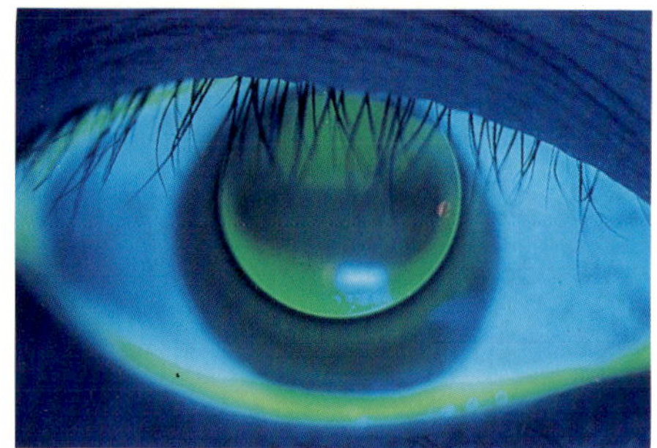

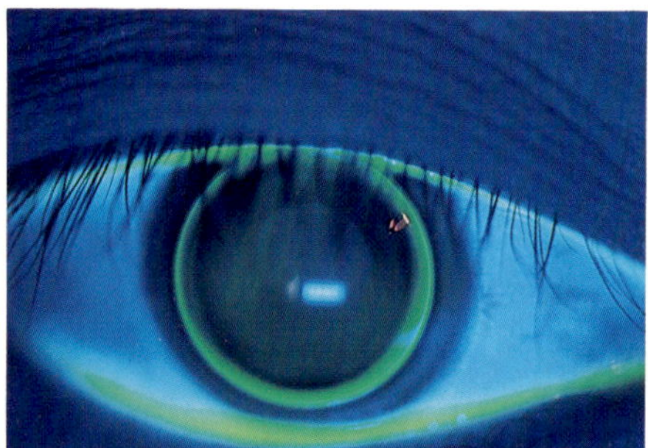

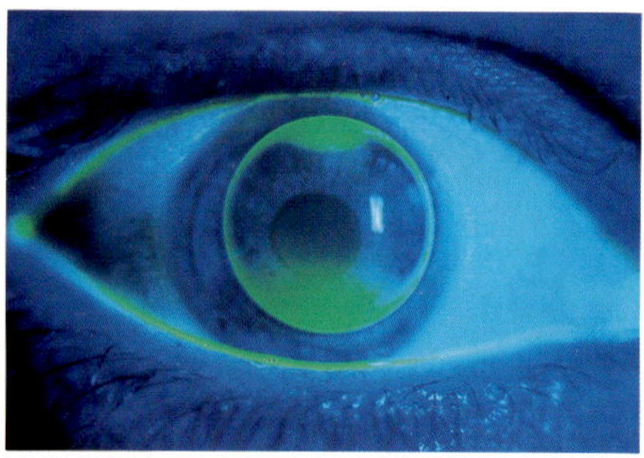

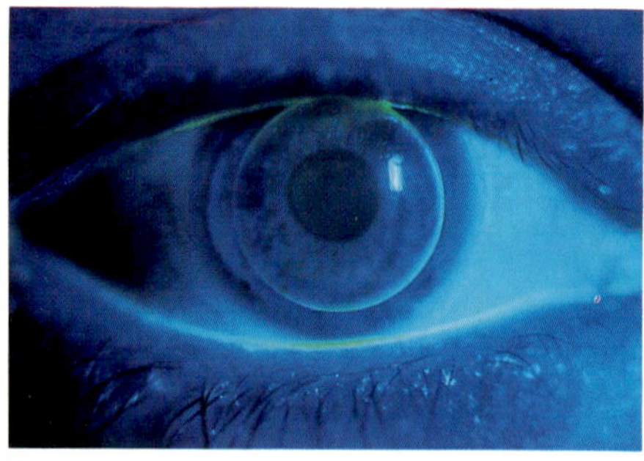

Color Figure 7-1 (*A*) Fluorescein pattern of a spherical lens fitted to a highly toric cornea. The lens rides high, and there is horizontal band touch with superior and inferior pooling (with-the-rule toric fluorescein pattern). (*B*) The same cornea as in *A* fitted with a toric base curve lens. The lens now centers well and has an even distribution of fluorescein underneath. (*C*) Fluorescein pattern of a spherical lens fitted to a highly toric cornea. In this case, the lens decenters in, and there is a with-the-rule pattern of superior and inferior pooling with horizontal bearing. (*D*) The same cornea as in *C* fitted with a toric base lens. The lens centers well and has an even distribution of fluorescein under it.

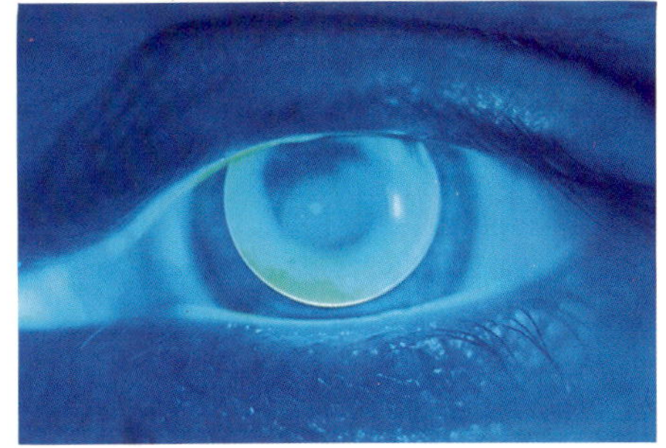

A

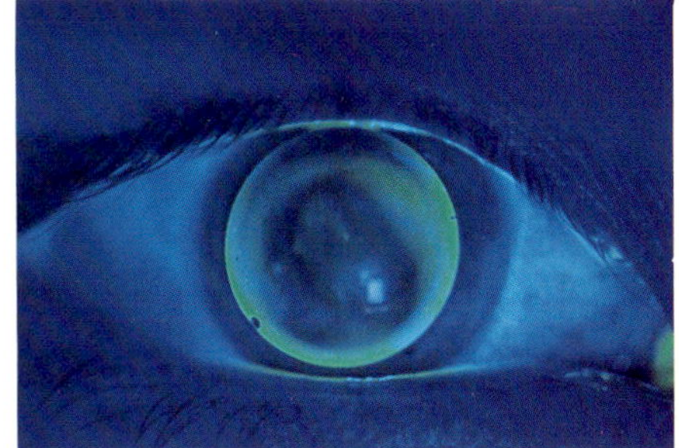

B

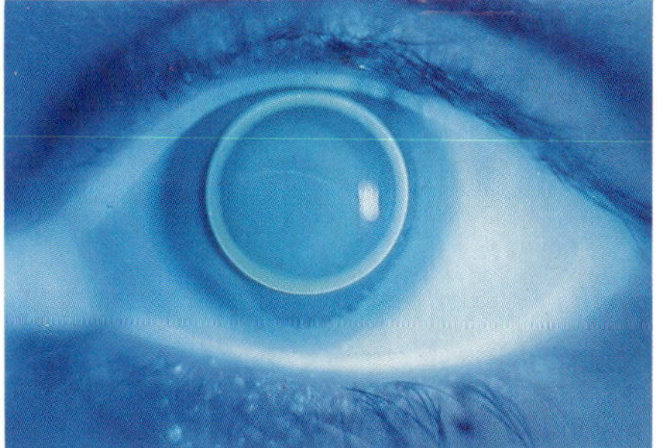

C

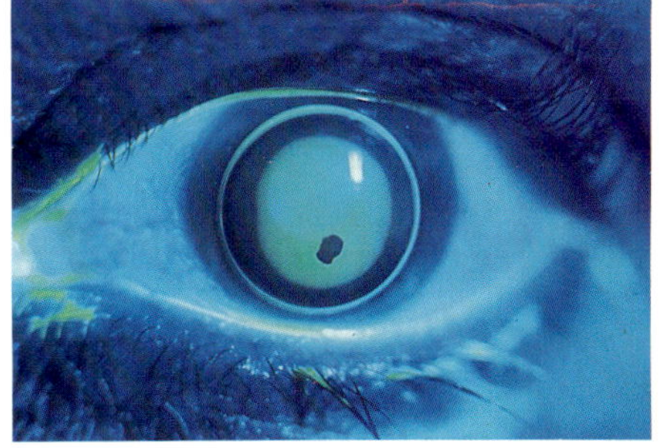

D

Color Figure 7-2 *(A)* Fluorescein pattern of keratoconic cornea fitted with a flat base curve. Heavy central touch is accompanied by wide, dark green peripheral pattern. This lens may be uncomfortable, will tend to decenter, and may lead to corneal scarring. *(B)* Fluorescein pattern of keratoconic cornea fitted slightly flat with overly flat peripheral system. Pressure is distributed over a wider area than in *A*, but there is still too much apical bearing. Bubble under peripheral curve indicates that it is too flat. *(C)* Ideal fitting lens on a keratoconic cornea. Very faint central touch avoids excessive pressure on the cone, and the lens is supported by mid-peripheral bearing. Pooling in the pericentral area is due to bridging of the spherical base curve over the cone-shaped corneal topography. Peripheral system shows an adequate but not excessive tear reservoir. *(D)* Fluorescein pattern of a steep fit to a keratoconic cornea. Central pooling is accompanied by a bubble to the side of the cone. In addition, the peripheral system is too narrow, as evidenced by the thin green band surrounding the heavy mid-peripheral bearing. This lens does not move well on the cornea and may cause pressure rings (corneal indentation).

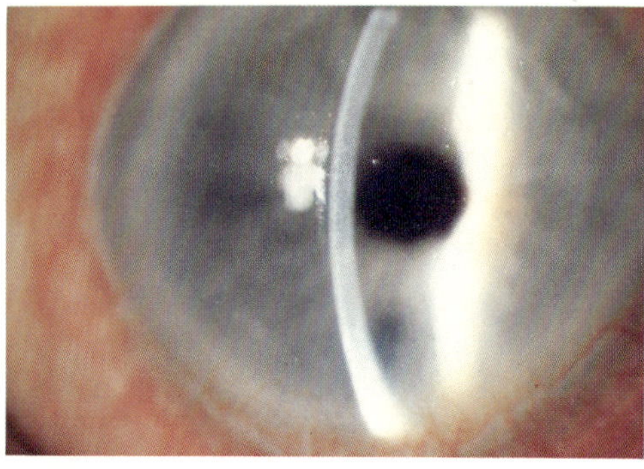

Color Figure 9-1 Tight lens syndrome demonstrates marked ciliary injection and corneal edema with evidence of iritis in a 73-year-old aphakic patient who had been using extended-wear hydrophilic contact lenses.

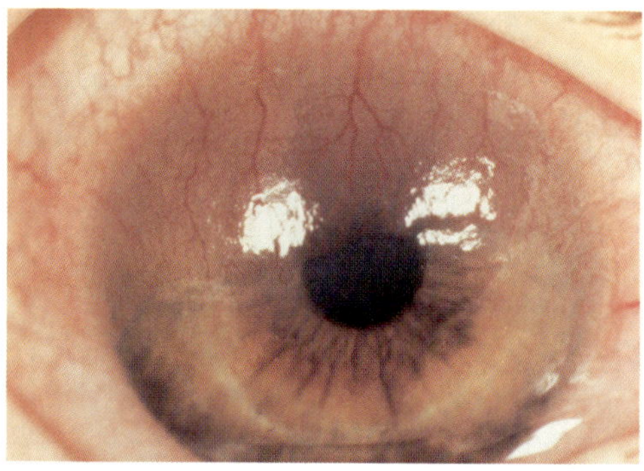

Color Figure 9-2 Superior limbic keratoconjunctivitis with the upper part of the cornea demonstrating infiltration and vascularization. The adjacent limbal area demonstrated considerable hyperemia.

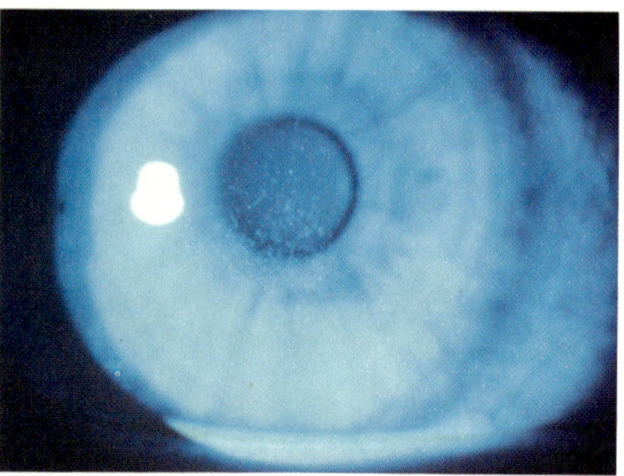

Color Figure 9-3 Superficial punctate keratopathy confined to the apex of the cornea in a patient fitted with a Polycon contact lens. This was secondary to fitting problems. (Courtesy of Dr. Jeffrey K. Harris)

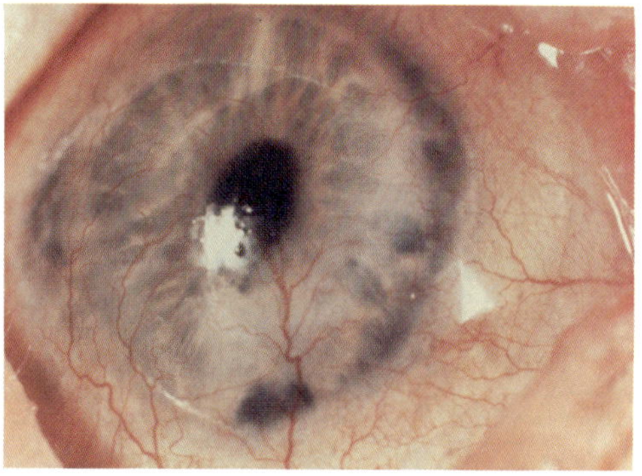

Color Figure 9-4 Cornea demonstrating deep stromal vascularization with lipid deposition at the edge of the vascularization in the cornea.

"FIRST FIT" METHOD OF BAUSCH & LOMB SOFLENS (POLYMACON) CONTACT LENSES FOR MYOPIA

The "first fit" method of Bausch & Lomb for myopia utilizes lens diameter, central thickness, and power as the three variables for obtaining an optimal lens fit for Soflens (Fig. 4-8). The lens power is determined by taking the patient's spherical equivalent refractive error, corrected for vertex distance. Next, the horizontal visible iris diameter (HVID) is measured. This will help in making the initial lens selection.

HVID	*Diameter*	*Series*
Small, < 11.5 mm	12.5 mm	U or F
Medium, 11.5 mm to 12 mm	13.5 mm	O_3, U_3, or B_3
Large, > 12 mm	14.5 mm	O_4, U_4, or B_4

The next step is to select the lens thickness. The lens with the least mass that provides full corneal coverage is best, keeping in mind patient comfort, patient's dexterity, and overall corneal oxygen requirements. Finally, the fit is to be evaluated. If the initial lens fails to cover the cornea, the next larger diameter lens in the same thickness has to be tried (*e.g.,* from a U_3 go to a U_4, and from an O_3 go to an O_4). If the initially chosen lens is a B_4, one can try a lens of U_4 series next, followed by one from an O_4 series. If there is excessive lens awareness, lag, or visual fluctuations and if the initial lens is a standard series, an ultra-thin lens of the same diameter should be tried. If the initial lens is an ultra-thin series, then an O_3 or O_4 lens of the same diameter may be suitable. If handling or damage is a problem, a lens of greater thickness has to be tried.

Hyperopia

Some of the daily-wear soft lenses that are available for the correction of hyperopia (Table 4-4) are discussed below.

HYPEROPIA UP TO +20 D WITH AVERAGE OR LARGE DIAMETER CORNEAS

Hydromarc Standard The Hydromarc lens is a lathe-cut, soft hydrophilic lens with a large spherical posterior optical zone and flattened peripheral curve. It has a water content of 43%. It is very comfortable for daily wear and has excellent longevity. The lens is available in two diameters, 14 mm and 14.5 mm. It is manufactured with various base curves: 8.15 mm, 8.3 mm, 8.45 mm, 8.6 mm, 8.75 mm, 8.9 mm, and 9.05 mm. The base curves and diameters of the standard diagnostic set are in 0.15-mm and 0.5-mm steps, respectively. The initial lens diameter should be 2 mm larger than the corneal diameter. The flattest keratometer reading is converted to millimeters of radius to which 1 mm is added, and the base curve closest to that number is selected. The power is determined from spectacle refraction in

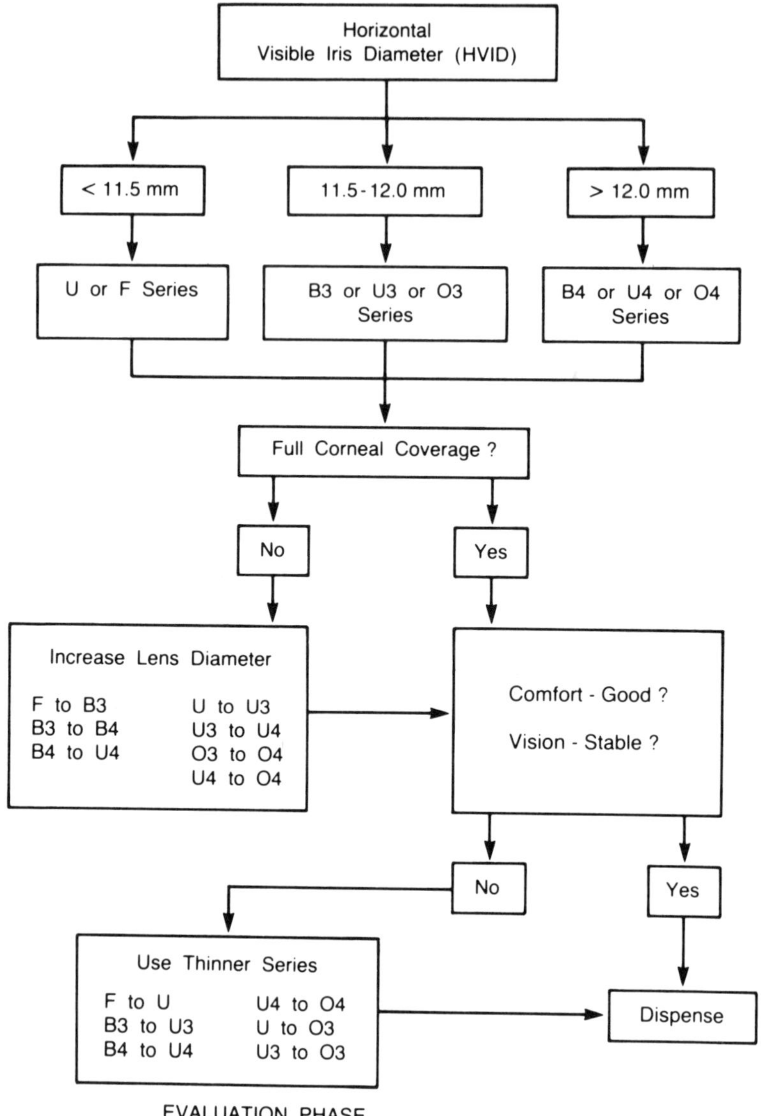

Figure 4-8 *"First fit" method for Bausch & Lomb Soflens (Polymacon). Initial selection phase for minus lenses.*

minus cylinder form corrected for vertex distance, if needed. The cylinder is dropped and +0.25 D is added to compensate for the tear lens. Due to different corneal and scleral eccentricities, more than one trial lens may be required. The proper diameter is determined first, followed by varying the base curve of the lens.

TABLE 4-4 Partial List of Daily-Wear Contact Lenses for Hyperopia

Lens/Manufacturer	Polymer	Water Content (%)	Power Range (D)
Softcon; American Optical Corp.	Vifilcon A	55	Plano to +18
Hydrocurve II; Barnes-Hind/Hydrocurve	Bufilcon A	45	Plano to +7
CSI; Syntex Ophthalmics	Crofilcon A	38.5	+0.25 to +8
Soflens; Bausch & Lomb	Polymacon	38.6	+0.25 to +20
Aquaflex; CooperVision	Tetrafilcon A	42.5	Plano to +20
DuraSoft; Wesley-Jessen	Phemfilcon A	30, 38, 55	Plano to +20
Hydron; American Hydron	Polymacon	38	Plano to +20

DuraSoft 2 DuraSoft 2 is a lathe-cut hydrophilic soft lens with optimized thin design. The water content of the lens is 38%. The D2-T4 lens has a diameter of 14.5 mm. The three base curves for this lens are 8.3 mm, 8.6 mm, and 9 mm. The median base curve of 8.6 mm is tried first. If the fit is loose, an 8.3-mm base curve is to be used. If the lens has a tight fit, then a lens of 9-mm base curve is to be tried.

HYPEROPIA UP TO +7 D WITH AVERAGE OR LARGE CORNEAL DIAMETER

Vistamarc The Vistamarc lens is a lathe-cut, soft lens with a water content of 58%. The lens diameters and base curves are as follows: 14 mm/8 mm, 8.4 mm, 8.9 mm; 14.5 mm/8.7 mm, 9 mm. The 14-mm lens will fit most corneas and the initial base curve selected is determined by the K reading: for a reading steeper than 46, an 8-mm base curve lens is used; for 46 and 42, an 8.4-mm base curve is used; and for flatter than 42, an 8.9-mm base curve is used. For larger corneas, or for better centration with K readings between 46 and 42, an 8.7/14.5-mm lens is to be used. For corneas flatter than 42 where better centration may be required, a 9/14.5-mm lens is to be selected.

HYPEROPIA UP TO +4.5 D WITH AVERAGE CORNEAL DIAMETER

Hydromarc Ultra-thin The Hydromarc Ultra-thin is a lathe-cut soft lens with optimum draping qualities. The lens contains 43% water by weight. One base curve and one diameter will fit a wide range of corneal curvatures. The lens is available in one diameter, 14 mm, and two base curves, 8.4 mm and 8.8 mm. The 14 mm diameter has excellent centering qualities and allows good movement in 90% of the patients. The initial lens selection is based on the keratometric reading. For corneas measuring 43 or steeper, the 8.4-mm base curve is chosen; for corneas flatter than 43, the 8.8-mm base curve is used.

HYPEROPIA UP TO +18 D WITH VERY SENSITIVE LIDS OR HANDLING DIFFICULTIES

Softcon The Softcon lens is a lathe-cut, soft, hydrophilic lens with a water content of 55% by weight. The higher water content combined with the excellent edge design provides superior corneal compatibility and all-day comfort. The refractive power is cut on the anterior surface, making power relatively independent of fit. This lens is very easy to handle. The available diameters are 14 mm and 14.5 mm, and the base curves are 7.8 mm, 8.1 mm, 8.4 mm, and 8.7 mm. The trial fit has to be started using the 8.4/14 mm lens with a power close to the patient's prescription for corneas measuring 7.3 mm to 7.9 mm, an 8.1-mm base curve for corneas steeper than 7.3 mm, and an 8.7-mm base curve for corneas flatter than 7.9 mm. Once a proper fit is established, overrefraction has to be done. No adaptation period is necessary, and the patient is asked to wear the lenses 8 to 16 hours the day they are dispensed.

HYPEROPIA UP TO +20 D WITH SMALL CORNEAS

Hydron Mini Lens The Hydron Mini soft lens is a small, thin lens of 13 mm that is easy to handle. It is a monocurve with a full 13-mm fitting zone, strong centering capabilities, and a unique edge design that provides a smooth transition from eye to lens with minimum lid movement resistance. It is available in base curves from 8.1 mm to 9.1 mm in 0.2-mm steps. An 8.3-mm base curve lens is used for corneas measuring 7.4 mm and steeper; for corneas measuring 7.5 mm to 8.1 mm, an 8.5-mm base curve lens is used; and for corneas measuring flatter than 8.2 mm, an 8.7-mm base curve lens is used.

"FIRST FIT" METHOD OF BAUSCH & LOMB SOFLENS (POLYMACON) CONTACT LENSES FOR HYPEROPIA

In the "first fit" method of Bausch & Lomb Soflens for hyperopia, the lens power is determined by taking the patient's spherical equivalent refractive error, corrected for vertex distance. Because of lens flexure on the eye, there is a need to add power to the spherical equivalent refractive error before selecting the initial lens. The greater the power, the greater the adjustment required. Next, the horizontal visible iris diameter (HVID) is measured. These parameters will aid in the initial lens choice (Fig. 4-9).

HVID	*Low + Series*	*High + Series*
Small, < 11.5 mm	+N (12.5 mm)	+H3 (13.5 mm)
Medium, 11.5 mm to 12 mm	+B3 (13.5 mm)	+H3 (13.5 mm)
Large, > 12 mm	+B4 (14.5 mm)	+H4 (14.5 mm)

If the initial lens fails to cover the cornea, the next larger diameter is tried. For most patients, the +B3 or +H3 lens will be suitable.

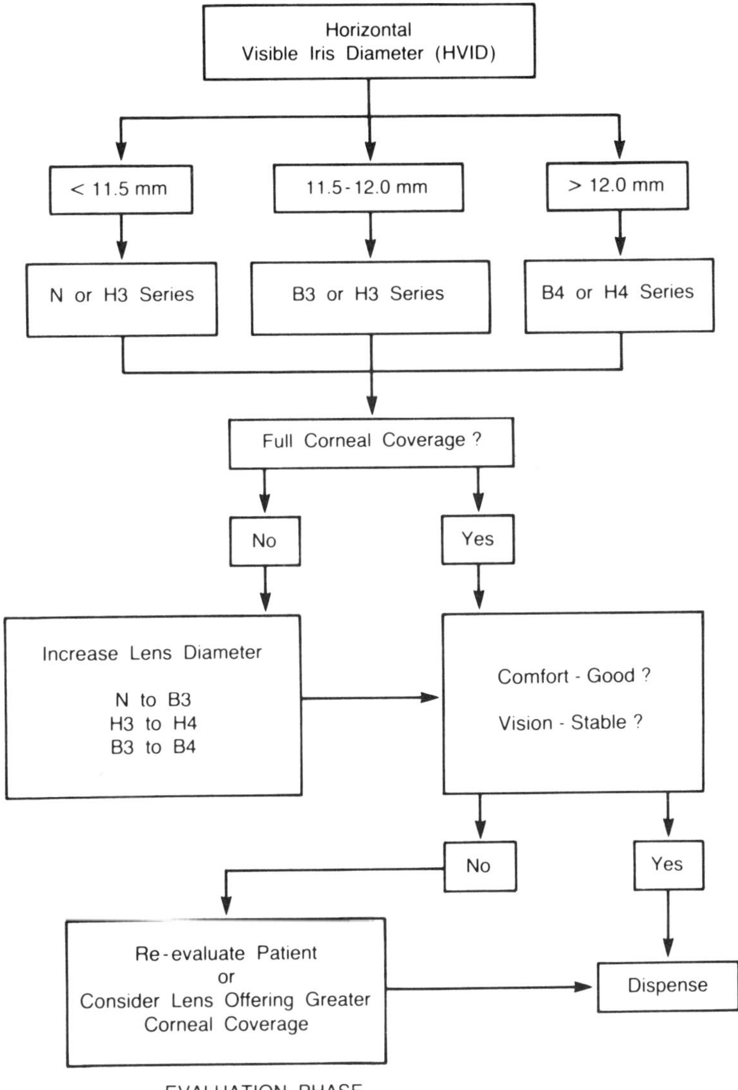

Figure 4-9 *"First fit" method for Bausch & Lomb Soflens (Polymacon). Initial selection phase for plus lenses.*

Toric Soft Contact Lenses for Astigmatism

Of all lens prescriptions, 80% contain a cylinder and of these only 2% to 3% exceed 3 D.[39] Many of these patients may wish to use contact lenses for correcting their refractive error. Spherical soft lenses should be tried initially if the astimgatism is less than 1 D or one-fourth the total refractive error, especially if there is significant myopia (*i.e.,* greater than 8 D). The amount of corneal astigmatism can be determined by using the keratometer.

Recently available are the toric soft lenses (Table 4-5). They are designed for patients with astigmatic error in the range of -1 D to -3 D who do not wish to use hard or gas-permeable lenses. The best visual results are obtained in patients whose spectacle prescription cylinders are located at or near 180° or 90° with both eyes correctable to 20/20 visual acuity. There are two types of flexible toric lenses, front and back surface toric designs. There appears to be no optical or fitting advantage to either front or back surface toric designs. Both are single toric lenses and assume bitoric characteristics and configuration when placed on a toric cornea.[42]

To ensure optimum vision, the axis of the trial lens should be within 10° of the spectacle prescription axis. The axis markings on the toric lenses are either at 6 o'clock position or at the 180° line. To compensate for rotating axis, the following procedure should be observed:

If the lens rotates in a clockwise direction, the amount of rotation has to be added to the cylinder axis.

On the other hand, if the lens rotates counterclockwise, the amount of rotation has to be subtracted from the cylinder axis.

TABLE 4-5 Toric Daily-Wear Contact Lenses for Astigmatism

Lens/Manufacturer	Polymer	Water Content (%)	Diameter (mm)	Base Curve (mm)
Torisoft; Ciba Vision Care	Tefilcon	37.5	14.5	8.6; 8.9; 9.2
DuraSoft 2 Toric Standard; Wesley-Jessen	Phemfilcon A	38	13.5 14.5	8.2; 8.5 8.3; 8.6
DuraSoft 2 Custom; Wesley-Jessen	Phemfilcon A	38	13.5 14.5	7.9; 8.2; 8.5; 8.9 8.3; 8.6; 9
Hydron Zero T; American Hydron	Polymacon	38	14.3 (horizontal); 13.0 (vertical)	8.3
Hydromarc Toric; Vistakon	Etafilcon A	43	14.5	Series 1 (8.3); Series 2 (8.75); Series 3 (9.1)
Hydrocurve II; Barnes-Hind/Hydrocurve	Bufilcon A	45, 55	13.5; 14.5	8.6; 8.8; 8.9
Bausch & Lomb Toric; Bausch & Lomb	Hefilcon B	45	14	8.3; 8.6

Patients should be advised that visual acuity may fluctuate because of drying and lens rotation. The major design features that try to minimize lens rotation include double truncation, prism ballast, and prism ballast with inferior edge truncation and thin zones. Little has been done with double truncation of soft lenses, other than the clinical study reported by Bayshore.[6,7] In lenses with prism ballast, gravity causes the heavier, thicker part of the lens to rotate with prism base in the down (vertical) position and maintain rotation stability. Lenses with prism ballast and inferior edge truncation may enhance the meridional stability of the lens in some designs.[56] The lower truncation would conform to the lower lid margin, or in large diameter lenses would tend to "lock" into the lower conjunctiva. Lenses with thin zones have the superior and inferior portions of the lens bevelled or "slabbed off" to decrease the lens thickness at these areas. The resultant thicker central area aligns horizontally within the palpebral fissure. This lens design is used by European and Canadian manufacturers.[13] American contact lens manufacturers dealing with soft toric lenses are using prism ballast with or without a lower edge truncation and special edge-thinning features. This lens construction, aided by the stabilizing effect of a toric lens surface in apposition with a similarly toroidal cornea, has resulted in fairly effective nonrotating lenses.[43]

Front (F) or Back (B) Surface Toric	Ballast Plan	Sphere Power Range (D)	Cylinder Power Range (D)
F	"Thin zone" (double slab-off)	Plano to −6	−1, −1.75; Axes: 10°, 20°, 70°, 80°, 90°, 100°, 110°, 160°, 170°. 180°
F	Prism and truncation	+20 to −20	−0.75 to −3 in 0.25-D steps
F	Prism and truncation	+20 to −20	−0.75 to −4 in 0.25-D steps
F	Prism and truncation	Plano to −6	−0.75 to −2 in −0.25-D steps; Axes: 180° ± 20° and 90° ± 20° both in 5° steps
F	Prism with slab-off	+0.25 to +4; plano to −5	−0.75 to −2 in 0.25-D steps; Axes: 180° ± 20°; 90° ± 20° in 5°-steps
B	Prism	+0.25 to +3; plano to −6	−1.25, −2; Axes: ±25° from 90° and 180° in 5°-steps
F	Prism	−6 to +4	−0.75, −1.25, −1.75; Axes: 90° ± 20°, 180° ± 20° in 10°-steps

FITTING SOFT ASTIGMATIC LENSES

The flattest fitting soft toric lens that will remain centered and meridionally stable on the cornea without compromising comfort or visual consistency has to be used. Thick or tight-fitting lenses have to be avoided, because "steep fitting" lenses also reduce the effectiveness of the lens ballasting or locating system.[18,28,37]

ASTIGMATIC MYOPIA AND HYPEROPIA UP TO ±20 D SPHERICAL POWER WITH AVERAGE TO LARGE CORNEAS

DuraSoft 2 Toric Standard The DuraSoft 2 Toric Standard lens is a lathe-cut hydrophilic lens with an effective truncated, prism ballast design. It contains 38% water by weight and is available in two diameters, 14.5 mm and 13.5 mm. The diagnostic lens with cylinder power and axis as close as possible to the patient's spectacle refraction is selected. The adequacy of fit is evaluated after about 20 minutes. The lens must move freely with the blink and then center promptly and reasonably well. If the truncation is horizontal, overrefraction has to be done to obtain the best visual acuity. Only spheres have to be used. The power of the lens to be ordered is equal to the power of the diagnostic lens plus the overrefraction. For example:

Diagnostic lens power	$-3 - 1.25 \times 10$
Over-refraction	$+2$
Lens required	$-1 - 1.25 \times 10$

If the truncation is not in a horizontal position, then the cylinder axis is not properly oriented. Because the lens position cannot be changed, it is necessary to compensate by changing the cylinder axis.

The angle of truncation has to be measured. To do this, a trial frame with a cylinder lens of lower power is to be used. The axis markings on the trial frame have to be aligned with the truncation of the contact lens, and the angle shown on the trial frame scale is to be noted. *If the angle shown is less than 90°*, no further calculation is required. Truncation angle equals that shown on the trial frame. *If the angle is greater than 90°*, this has to be subtracted from 180°. For example:

	180°
Trial frame reading	−170°
Truncation angle	10°

The axis now has to be compensated as follows:

If the truncation position has rotated clockwise, then the rotation angle has to be added to the axis of spectacle refraction.

If the truncation position has rotated counterclockwise, then the rotation angle has to be subtracted from the axis of spectacle refraction.

If the fit is unacceptable, then the DuraSoft TT Custom lenses have to be tried.

ASTIGMATIC MYOPIA UP TO −6 D SPHERICAL POWER
WITH AVERAGE TO LARGE CORNEAS

Torisoft Lens The Torisoft is a lathe-cut, soft contact lens with a water content of 37.5% by weight. The lens has a diameter of 14.5 mm with an excellent edge design for comfort and a thin zone for stable orientation. The available cylinders are shown in Table 4-5. For corneas ranging from 7.5 mm to 8.2 mm, an 8.9-mm base curve lens is to be tried; for corneas steeper than 7.4 mm, use an 8.6-mm base curve lens; and for corneas flatter than 8.2 mm, use a 9.2-mm base curve lens.

ASTIGMATIC MYOPES UP TO −6 D WITH SMALL TO AVERAGE CORNEAS

Hydron Zero T The Hydron Zero T lens provides excellent comfort. It has only one base curve of 8.3 mm, and the diameter is 14.3 mm (horizontal) and 13 mm (vertical). At 0.06-mm central thickness, it offers optimum oxygen transmissibility. The cylinder is on the front surface and both prism ballast and truncation are provided for maximum stability. Cylinders available are from −0.75 D to −2 D in 0.25-D increments. Axes available are 180° ± 20° and 90° ± 20° (both in 5° increments).

ASTIGMATIC HYPEROPES FROM +0.25 D TO +4 D AND ASTIGMATIC
MYOPES UP TO −5 D WITH AVERAGE TO LARGE CORNEAS

Hydromarc Toric The Hydromarc Toric is a lathe-cut, soft lens with the cylindrical correction ground on the front surface of the lens. The axis is stabilized with 1.5-D prism ballast. For orientation, the lens has a dot at the 6 o'clock position. It has only one diameter, 14.5 mm, and three base curves: series 1 (8.3 mm), series 2 (8.7 mm), and series 3 (9.1 mm). Available cylinder powers are −0.75 D to −2 D in 0.25-D steps, with axes of 180° ± 20° and 90° ± 20° in 5° increments. The lens is circular with prism ballast and slab-off to control rotation.

ASTIGMATIC HYPEROPES FROM +0.25 D TO +3 D AND MYOPES
UP TO −6 D WITH SMALL TO LARGE CORNEAS

Hydrocurve II The Hydrocurve II is a lathe-cut, soft hydrophilic lens with a toric back surface. It is stabilized by one prism diopter to minimize lens rotation. It is available in 45% and 55% water by weight. The available diameters are 13.5 mm and 14.5 mm, with base curves of 8.6 mm, 8.8 mm, and 8.9 mm. Cylinder powers are −1.25 D and −2 D with axes of ±25° from 90° and 180° in 5° increments.

ASTIGMATIC HYPEROPES UP TO +4 D AND MYOPES UP TO −6 D WITH
SMALL OR AVERAGE CORNEAS OR LENS HANDLING DIFFICULTIES

Bausch & Lomb Toric The Bausch & Lomb Toric hydrophilic lens has a spherical posterior and a spherocylindrical anterior surface in the optic zone to accommodate the required astigmatic power. The lens contains 45% water by weight. The diameter is 14 mm, and the base curves are 8.3 mm and 8.6 mm. A base curve of 8.3 mm is used for corneas 7.6 mm or steeper, and an 8.6-mm base curve is used for corneas 7.7 mm and flatter. The available spherical powers are from -6 D to $+4$ D. The lens is easy to handle. Three micro-thin guide marks at the 5, 6, and 7 o'clock positions aid in determining lens stability.

EXTENDED-WEAR SOFT CONTACT LENSES

Extended-wear lenses are a recent addition to the contact lenses used to correct myopia, hyperopia, and astigmatism (Tables 4-6 to 4-8). Extended-wear contact lenses can be worn during the day and night (during sleep), and are removed at regular intervals for cleaning and disinfecting.[16]

Extended-wear contact lenses are very comfortable and have excellent gas

TABLE 4-6 Extended-Wear Contact Lens for Myopia

Lens/Manufacturer	Polymer	Water Content (%)	Diameter (mm)	Base Curve (mm)	Central Thickness (mm)	Power Range (D)
Hydrocurve II; Barnes-Hind/Hydrocurve	Bufilcon A	55 45	14 14.5	8.5 8.8; 9.1	0.05	Plano to -12
Permalens; CooperVision	Perfilcon A	71	13.5 14.2	7.7; 8; 8.3 8.6	1 to 0.24	Plano to -20
Permaflex; CooperVision	Surfilcon A	74	14.4	8.7	0.22 to 0.08	-0.5 to -10
Softcon; American Optical Corp.	Vifilcon A	55	14 14.5	8.1 8.4; 8.7	0.43 to 0.10	-0.5 to -8
CSI T; Syntex Ophthalmics	Crofilcon A	38.5	13.5 14.8	8.3; 8.6 8.9; 9.35	0.035	Plano to -7
O₃ Lens; Bausch & Lomb	Polymacon	38.6	13.5	Variable	0.035	-1 to -9
O₄ Lens; Bausch & Lomb	Polymacon	38.6	14.5	Variable	0.035	-1 to -9
B & L 70; Bausch & Lomb	Lidofilcon A	70	14.3	8.4; 8.7; 9	0.14	Plano to -6
Genesis-4; Channel Laboratories	Lidofilcon A	70	14.3	8.4; 8.7; 9	0.14	-0.25 to -6
DuraSoft 3; Wesley-Jessen	Phemfilcon A	55	14.5	8.3; 8.6; 8.9	0.06	-0.25 to -20
Hydromarc; Vistakon	Etafilcon A	58	14 14.5	8; 8.4; 8.9 8.7	0.06	-0.25 to -7
PDC-70; Products Development Consortium	Lidofilcon A	38	14.3	8.4; 8.7; 9	0.06	-0.25 to -8
Q & E 70; Breger-Mueller Welt Corp.	Lidofilcon A	70	14.3	8.4; 8.7; 9	0.14	-0.25 to -8
Sauflon-70; American Medical Optics	Lidofilcon B	70	14.3	8.4; 8.7; 9	0.17 to 0.39	Plano to -12

TABLE 4-7 Extended-Wear Contact Lens for Hyperopia

Lens/Manufacturer	Polymer	Water Content (%)	Diameter (mm)	Base Curve (mm)	Central Thickness (mm)	Power Range (D)
Hydrocurve II; Barnes-Hind/Hydrocurve	Bufilcon A	55	14 14.5	8.5 8.8; 9.1	0.1 to 0.18	+0.25 to +7
Softcon; American Optical Corp.	Vifilcon A	55	14.0	8.1; 8.4; 8.7	0.1 to 0.43	Plano to +18
PDC-70; Products Development Consortium	Lidofilcon A	38	14.3	8.4; 8.7; 9	0.06	+0.25 to +6
Sauflon; American Medical Optics	Lidofilcon B	79	14.4	8.1; 8.4; 8.7	0.25 to 0.45	Plano to +20
Vistamarc; Vistakon	Etafilcon A	58	14 14.5	8; 8.4; 8.9 8.7	0.06	+0.25 to +4
DuraSoft 3; Wesley-Jessen	Phemfilcon A	55	14.5	8.3; 8.6; 9	0.06	+0.25 to +20
Permalens; CooperVision	Perfilcon A	71	14	8; 8.3; 8.6	0.35	+0.25 to +8

transmission; thus, they can be worn continuously for more than 24 hours. Oxygen transmission is essential for maintaining the aerobic metabolism of the cornea. Oxygen transmission is usually expressed as Dk/L. Corneal oxygen requirements and the O_2 permeability of various lens materials have been discussed previously.[19,25,41] Oxygen transmission is critical when the eyes are closed during sleep, when environmental O_2 pressure drops from 155 mmHg (at sea level) to approximately 50 mmHg.[33] The O_2 transmission is directly proportional to the water content of the hydrogel lens and inversely proportional to its thickness.[33] The higher the water content, the higher the oxygen transmission. Lens thickness is also important. By dividing the percent of water content of a lens (hydration) by its thickness (center thickness in millimeters), the hydration/thickness (H/T) index of any lens can be determined.[33] The higher the index, the greater the amount of oxygen transmission by the lens. As a general rule, the oxygen permeability is doubled by increasing water content by 20% or by reducing the thickness by one half.[27] Fatt and Lin have shown that it is more efficient for the cornea to obtain oxygen through the contact lens rather than from beneath the lens (by a pumping mechanism).[20]

A prospective candidate for extended-wear contact lenses should be made aware of all the risks and benefits of their use. Recently, several reports have emphasized the incidence of vision-threatening bacterial keratitis and ulceration (including *Pseudomonas aeruginosa*) associated with extended-wear soft contact lenses. This has dampened the initial enthusiasm for cosmetic extended-wear soft lenses in many centers. The ideal patients are those who have used either hard or soft daily-wear lenses. The patient should also be

TABLE 4-8 Toric Extended-Wear Contact Lenses for Astigmatism

Lens/Manufacturer	Polymer	Water Content (%)	Diameter (mm)	Base Curve (mm)
Hydrocurve II; Barnes Hind/Hydrocurve	Bufilcon A	55	14.5	8.8
DuraSoft 3; Wesley-Jessen	Phemfilcon A	55	14.5	8.3; 8.6

informed of the necessity of frequent lens replacement. Some of the advantages and disadvantages of extended-wear lens are mentioned in the following list.

Advantages

Convenience

Comfort

Instant vision on awakening

Useful in patients with physical or mental handicaps

Reduced lens care

Disadvantages

Frequent replacement increases overall cost of the lens

Corneal vascularization may occur

During sleep, lens may be lost due to drying

Visual acuity may fluctuate

Lens deposits

Lens replacement required approximately every 6 to 9 months

History taking and prefitting evaluation for extended-wear contact lenses is similar to that described for daily-wear soft lenses. The cardinal fitting rule is to use the largest and flattest lens that will remain stable on the eye and provide good visual acuity and a healthy cornea.[27] It is best to obtain a flatter fit for extended-wear lenses because there is a definite tendency for soft lenses to tighten with duration of wear.[35] It is essential to obtain an optimum fit before dispensing extended-wear lenses. Patients should also be taught to remove the lens so that they can discontinue wearing it at the earliest onset of symptoms, and to seek an ocular examination and therapy if indicated.

Extended-Wear Soft Lens for Myopia

Since the FDA's first approval of extended-wear soft contact lenses to correct myopia in January 1981, many studies have been published.[8–10,24,29,31,34,40,50–52,55] Currently, several FDA-approved soft contact lenses are available (see Table 4-6). The water content of these lenses varies

Front (F) or Back (B) Surface Toric	Ballast Plan	Sphere Range (D)	Cylinder Power Range (D)
B	Prism	Plano to −8; +0.25 to +3	−1.25, −2; Axes: 90°, 180°/−25
F	Truncated	−12 to +8	−0.75 to −3 in 0.25 D steps; any axis

from 38% to more than 70%. Some of these lenses are described below. Extended-wear soft contact lenses may be an alternative for patients considering keratorefractive procedures for the correction of myopia.[5,21,30,48,57]

MYOPIA UP TO −12 D WITH AVERAGE TO LARGE CORNEAS

Hydrocurve II The Hydrocurve II was one of the first two lenses to be approved by the FDA for myopic extended wear. It is a lathe-cut soft lens that has minimal interference with corneal metabolism. The thin design aids in centration and stability. The central thickness is only 0.5 mm at −3 D. It is soft and pliable and provides excellent comfort. The relatively large optical zone aids in reducing or eliminating the problems of glare. This lens is available with 45% or 55% water by weight. It is available in 14 mm and 14.5 mm diameters and in base curves of 8.5 mm, 8.8 mm, and 9.1 mm. It is easy to handle, and because of its lower water content, is more durable. The initial lens selection should be 8.8 mm/14.5 mm. If adequate lens movement is not obtained, an 8.5 mm/14 mm lens has to be tried.

In 1983, Binder published the results of 1099 patients who were fitted with Hydrocurve II_{55} soft contact lens for extended wear by 42 investigators.[9] The motivation for obtaining extended-wear lenses was cosmetic in 97% and occupation/sports in 3% of the patients in this group. Fifty-five percent of the patients previously had been successful daily wearers of hard or soft contact lenses. Of these patients, 98% achieved a corrected acuity of 20/30 or better and 84% obtained an acuity of 20/20 or better. There was no permanent change in visual acuity in any patient during this study. The study concluded that myopic extended wear is highly successful.

MYOPIA UP TO −20 D WITH AVERAGE OR SMALL CORNEAS

Permalens The Permalens is a lathe-cut or molded soft lens. It has the same water content (71%) as the aphakic lens, and is available in base curves of 7.7 mm, 8 mm, and 8.3 mm in a single 13.5-mm diameter. Also available is an 8.6-mm base curve lens with a 14.2-mm diameter. If the smaller diameter lens is chosen, an 8-mm base curve lens is chosen for corneas ranging from 7.5 mm to 8 mm. To steepen the fit, a 7.7-mm lens is tried; to loosen the fit, an 8.3-mm lens is tried. The 8.6 mm/14.2 mm lens is said to be a "one size fits all" lens. Because it is easy to fit, it may be the initial lens of choice.

Stark and Martin evaluated the long-term effects of Permalens as an extended-wear soft contact lens for myopia in 106 patients who had worn the lens successfully for 4 to 8 years.[52] The visual acuity with the contact lens alone was 20/40 or better in 95% of eyes; this figure increased to 97% when eyes with amblyopia, macular degneration, or astigmatism greater than 1 D were excluded. There were no cases of infectious corneal ulcer, scarring, or permanent visual loss from the use of this lens. Mild neovascularization was noted in 8.7% of patients without any significant effect on their vision.

MYOPIA FROM −1 D TO −12 D WITH SMALL TO AVERAGE CORNEAS

Sauflon-70 Sauflon-70 contains 9% to 10% less water than Sauflon PW lenses, although both are made from the same polymer. A reduction in water content from 79% to 70% results in an increase in the tensile property of the lens.[24] The tensile strength of Lidofilcon B in 70% hydration compares favorably with PHEMA; hence, it is durable.[24] It is manufactured with a single diameter of 14.3 mm and three base curves, 8.4 mm, 8.7 mm, and 9 mm. Hartstein studied Sauflon-70 soft lens for extended wear in 64 myopic patients and found the lens to be safe, easy to handle, and effective for extended wear in myopia.[24]

MYOPIA FROM −1 D TO −6 D WITH SMALL TO LARGE CORNEAS

O_3/O_4 Soflens The Bausch & Lomb O_3/O_4 lenses are membrane-type, spin-cast, low water content (38.6%) hydrophilic polymer lenses. They are available in two diameters, 13.5 mm (O_3) and 14.5 mm (O_4). They are comfortable and provide adequate oxygen transmission because of their center thinness of 0.035 mm. However, they are difficult to handle.

The initial lens selection is based on HVID, with the O_3 lens being used at 12 mm or less and the O_4 lens at greater than 12 mm. Generally, most patients wearing the O_3 series can be fit with the O_4 series, but not vice versa.

Solomon and co-workers studied Bausch & Lomb "O" series lenses that were fit on 245 myopic eyes.[50] They reported that the lenses are safe, provide excellent comfort, and have a low rate of lens replacement (0.9 lenses per eye per year).

MYOPIA UP TO −8 D WITH AVERAGE TO LARGE CORNEAS

Softcon The Softcon lens is similar to the aphakic lens both in its water content (55%) and the polymer (Vifilcon A) used. It is available in base curves of 8.1 mm, 8.4 mm, and 8.7 mm with two diameters, 14 mm and 14.5 mm. The initial lens may be either 8.1 mm/14 mm or 8.7 mm/14.5 mm, with the diameter or base curve changed to obtain optimum lens fit. The refractive power is cut on the anterior surface, making the power relatively independent of the fit. It is aproved for therapeutic and myopic extended wear.

MYOPIA UP TO −7 D WITH AVERAGE TO VERY LARGE CORNEAS

CSI T The CSI T hydrophilic, membrane-type, lathe-cut extended-wear lens is not a HEMA lens, and thus differs from other hydrogel lenses. It is a copolymer of glyceryl methacrylate (GMA) and methyl methacrylate (MMA). The lens is made ultra thin (0.035 mm) to compensate for its low water content of 38.5%. It is available in base curves of 8.3 mm and 8.6 mm in 13.8-mm diameter, and base curves of 8.6 mm, 8.9 mm, and 9.35 mm in 14.8-mm diameter. When using the 14.8-mm diameter lens for corneas ranging from 7.5 mm to 8 mm, an 8.9-mm base curve is used to obtain a steeper fit, and a base curve of 8.6 mm or 9.35 mm is used to obtain a flatter fit. For an ultra-thin lens, it has good handling properties, is durable, and resists hard deposit formation.

Extended-Wear Lenses for Myopia Compared with Lenses for Aphakia

Myopic patients and extended-wear lenses for myopia have certain advantages over aphakic patients and extended-wear lenses for aphakia. The lenses for myopia permit more oxygen transmission, and myopic patients have healthier eyes. Because they are nearsighted, myopic patients can examine the lenses and leave them out if necessary until examined by a practitioner. Because younger myopic patients are also manually dexterous, they can remove the lenses at the first sign of ocular infection, discomfort, or pain. Also, the younger, healthier myopic eyes have better tear function than aphakic eyes; therefore, the likelihood of successful wear is increased. On the other hand, the lens for aphakia is thicker, and it transmits less oxygen to the corneal epithelium, which probably is altered following surgery and is not as healthy compared with the young myopic eye. Because aphakic patients may not be able to remove the lens by themselves, they may present late for management of corneal infection associated with contact lens wear. However, there is a need for extended-wear lenses for aphakic patients, because they are unable to insert and remove contact lenses on a daily basis.

Extended-Wear Lenses for Myopia Compared with Keratorefractive Procedures

Extended-wear contact lenses are an alternative correction for myopic patients because they offer the potential for excellent vision while avoiding the inconveniences associated with spectacles or daily-wear contact lenses and the risks of keratorefractive surgery.[47] Radial keratotomy has continued to gain acceptance, and more corneal and anterior segment surgeons are performing the procedure.[1,2,11,12,17,21,22,44,48,58] Radial keratotomy is effective in reducing myopic refractive error, but the amount of reduction is unpredictable, and postoperative regression may occur.[47] Extended-wear contact lenses for myopia carry less risk of serious complications than does radial keratotomy, because they can be removed promptly if problems arise. However, to minimize potential complications (*e.g.,* corneal ulceration) related to extended-wear soft contact lenses, proper patient selection, adequate patient and fitter education, and removal of the lens at least twice weekly is recommended. Myopic keratomileusis and epikeratophakia have problems related to predictability.[4,5,36,54,60] In addition, the long-term effects of surgical correction of myopia on the cornea and vision are yet to be studied.

Extended-Wear Soft Contact Lenses for Hyperopia

HYPEROPIA UP TO +20 D WITH AVERAGE CORNEAS

Sauflon Sauflon PW lenses are lathe-cut lenses with a water content of 79%. This lens has high oxygen permeability. Use an 8.4-mm base curve for corneas ranging from 7.5 mm to 8 mm. Use an 8.1-mm base curve for corneas 7.4 mm and steeper, and an 8.7-mm base curve for corneas 8.1 mm and flatter. The lens has a single diameter of 14.4 mm.

HYPEROPIA UP TO +8 D WITH SMALL CORNEAS

Permalens The cosmetic Permalens for correction of hyperopia is available in three base curves (8 mm, 8.3 mm, and 8.6 mm) and a single diameter of 14 mm. This lens has a water content of 71%. Although compared to the minus lens, it is thicker centrally by 0.15 mm, and it has an oxygen flux adequate for extended wear. The initial lens to be tried is the 8.3 mm/14 mm lens. If the lens has a loose or a tight fit, the 8 mm/14 mm or the 8.6 mm/14 mm lenses, respectively, have to be tried. Use an 8-mm base curve for corneas measuring 7.5 mm and steeper. The 8.6-mm base curve is recommended for corneas 8.2 mm and flatter.

HYPEROPIA UP TO +7 D WITH SMALL TO LARGE CORNEAS

Hydrocurve II The lathe-cut hydrophilic Hydrocurve II soft lens has the same water content as the extended-wear lens for myopia. It is available from +0.25 D to +5 D in 0.25-D steps, and from +5.5 D to +8 D in 0.5-D steps. Depending on the power of the lens, the central thickness varies from 0.1 mm to 0.18 mm. The fitting process is initiated by selecting the flattest base curve that provides full corneal coverage. Allow the lens to stay on the eye to achieve equilibrium, and then evaluate the size and base curvature relationship. The lens often chosen for cosmetic correction of hyperopia is the 8.5 mm/14 mm lens.

HYPEROPIA UP TO +18 D WITH SMALL CORNEAS

Softcon The Softcon extended-wear lens is a lathe-cut hydrophilic lens that provides good comfort and acuity. This lens has the same amount of water content as the myopic extended-wear contact lens (see Tables 4-6 and 4-7). The lens diameter is 14 mm and it has three base curves in 0.3-mm steps (see Table 4-7). Optimum fit is achieved by varying the base curve. The initial lens to be tried should be close in power to the patient's refraction, and should be of the 8.4 mm/14 mm geometry. The fit has to be evaluated after 30 minutes. For a flatter fit, the 8.7 mm/14 mm lens is to be used; for a steeper fit, an 8.1 mm/14 mm lens is to be used.

EXTENDED-WEAR SOFT CONTACT LENSES FOR ASTIGMATISM

Hydrocurve II The first toric lens approved by the FDA for extended wear is the Hydrocurve II. The lens has a base curve of 8.8 mm and a diameter of

14.5 mm and is available in powers ranging from plano to -8 D and from $+0.25$ D to $+3$ D. The available cylindrical powers are -1.25 D and -2 D with the axis set at 90° or 180°, or 25° to either side in 5° steps. It is fit similar to any of the standard prism ballast, back toric soft lenses. The inferior prism ballast stabilizes the lens on the eye.

The DuraSoft 3 (see Table 4-8) lens manufactured by Wesley-Jessen was recently FDA-approved as a toric extended-wear contact lens.

APPLICATION AND REMOVAL OF SOFT LENSES

The patient should be instructed in the proper method of application and removal of the soft lens. The practitioner should spend adequate time with the patient until he or she is comfortable with these maneuvers.

INSERTION BY THE PRACTITIONER

It is helpful to keep the fingernails short on the fingers being used for lens application and removal. Having washed the hands with soap and rinsed well, it is advisable to use a lint-free towel to dry them. The right lens is then removed from its container and rinsed thoroughly with saline solution. Avoid touching the inside surface of the lens after rinsing. The lens is then placed on the tip of the index finger with the convex side down.

The practitioner now positions himself on the right side of the patient, and retracts the lower eyelid using the middle finger of the hand holding the lens. The upper lid is retracted using the finger(s) of the other hand (Fig. 4-10). During this time, the patient holds the head erect and looks straight ahead, fixing on some object in front. The lens is placed directly on the cornea, and both eyelids are gently released. The patient closes the eye and the practitioner gently massages the upper lid to express any air bubbles that may be trapped beneath the lens. The patient should also blink or squeeze the eye as necessary to eliminate all air bubbles. The same procedure is repeated for the opposite lens. If the patient has discomfort following insertion of the lens, then the lens is displaced to the conjunctiva to allow increased tear flow beneath the lens, and the lens is recentered.

The other methods of insertion include placing the lens on the inferior conjunctiva while the patient is looking up, placing it on the superior conjunctiva with the patient looking down, or placing it on the temporal conjunctiva with the patient looking nasally.

REMOVAL BY THE PRACTITIONER

When removing the lens, the practitioner's hands should be clean and dry. The patient should hold the head erect and look up. The practitioner retracts the lower eyelid with the middle finger, touches the peripheral portion of the lens with the index finger, and slides the lens down to the inferior conjunctiva. The practitioner places his thumb adjacent to his index finger, presses the lens gently between the two fingers, and removes the lens (Fig. 4-11).

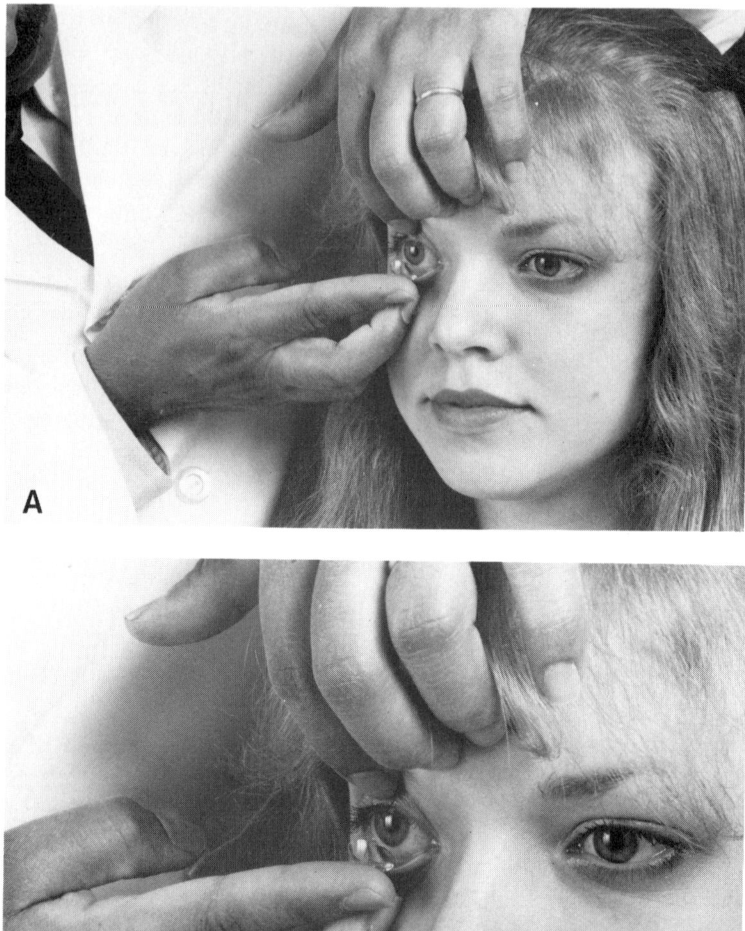

Figure 4-10 *(A, B)* Contact lens insertion by practitioner.

APPLICATION BY THE PATIENT

Good personal hygienic habits are a basic requisite for the successful use of soft contact lenses. The patient should keep the fingernails short. The hands have to be washed well with soap, rinsed, and dried. The right lens is removed from the vial by emptying the contents into the palm of the hand. The excess fluid is removed and the right lens is placed on the right index finger with the concave side facing up. The lower lid is retracted with the middle finger of the right hand while the upper eyelid is retracted with the

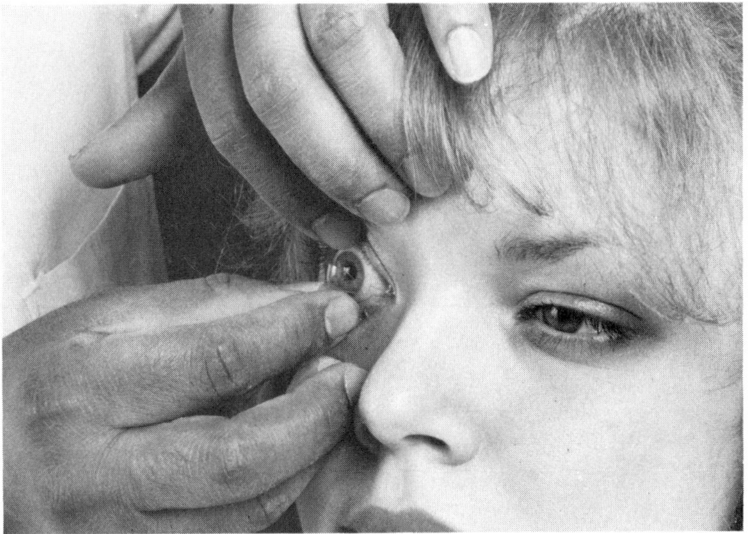

Figure 4-11   Removal of contact lens by practitioner.

left hand. The patient then stares straight ahead into a mirror and gently places the lens onto the corneal surface (Fig. 4-12). Any air bubbles are expressed by gentle pressure, and then the index finger is removed. Next, the lower eyelid is gently released followed by the upper eyelid. To center the lens, the patient can also close the eyes and gently massage the lids (Fig. 4-13). The vision has to be checked to make sure that the lens is centered.

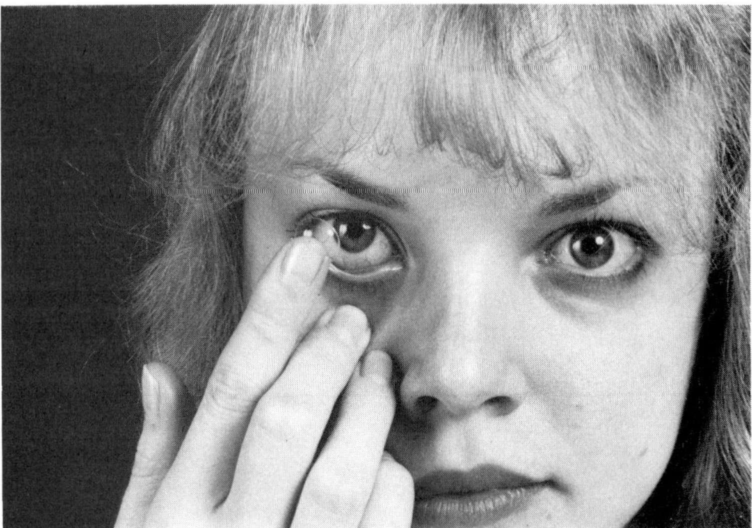

Figure 4-12   Application of contact lens by patient.

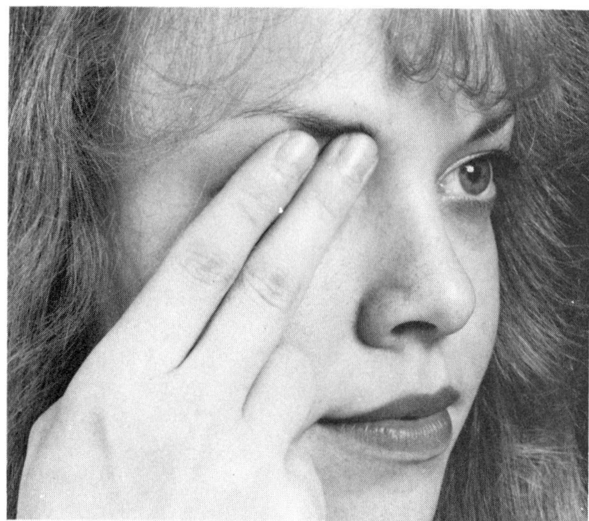

Figure 4-13 Patient centers the lens through closed eyelid.

The same procedure is repeated for the left lens. If the patient is comfortable, the procedure can be performed with the aid of a mirror. The patient fixates straight ahead on any object.

Another method is for the patient to look up and fixate on any object above. While doing so, the lower eyelid is retracted with the middle finger and the lens is placed on the inferior conjunctiva (Fig. 4-14). The lens is then gently moved to center it on the cornea.

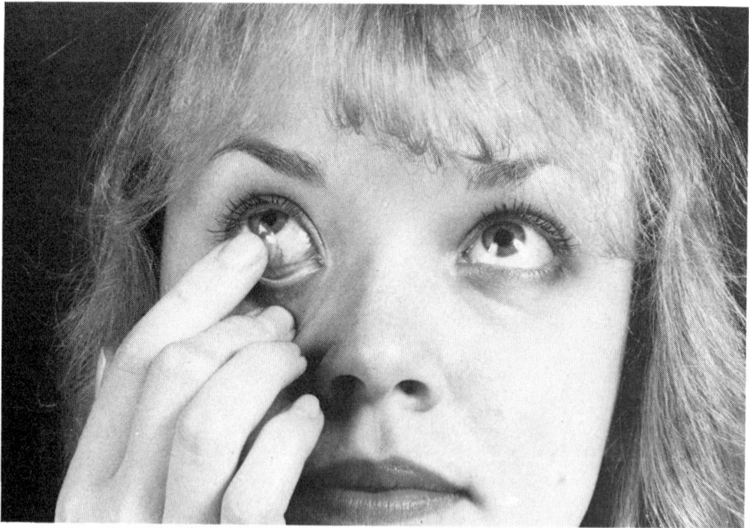

Figure 4-14 Patient places the contact lens on the inferior conjunctiva while looking in an upward direction.

Sometimes the thin edge of a high plus lens may fold over while the patient is attempting to place it on the cornea. This difficulty can be minimized if the lens is held on the finger for about 50 to 60 seconds prior to placement. This permits drying, which decreases lens flexibility.

REMOVAL BY THE PATIENT

Before removing the lens, the patient confirms the presence of the lens on the cornea by checking the vision of each eye separately. The hands are washed thoroughly and dried. While looking upwards, the lower lid is retracted with the middle finger and the index finger is placed on the inferior portion of the lens. The lens is slid down and compressed between the thumb and the index finger, and then is removed (Fig. 4-15).

Another method of removal involves looking into a mirror that is placed slightly above the eyes. The superior gaze displaces the lens inferiorly. Using the thumb and index finger, the lens is gently grasped and removed. The lens can also be removed by looking nasally, sliding the lens to the temporal part of the eye (Fig. 4-16), and then folding it off using the thumb and index finger. The lens can also be removed without using a mirror, with the patient fixating straight ahead on some object with both eyes. Yet another method is to use the right index finger or thumb to press the lower lid up while the left index finger is used to hold the upper lid edge. Squeezing and blinking then causes the lens to fall out, and it can be grasped by the thumb and forefinger.

Taco Test

The "taco" test is used to ensure that the lens is not inverted. Fold the lens gently between the thumb and forefinger. The lens edges should be directed

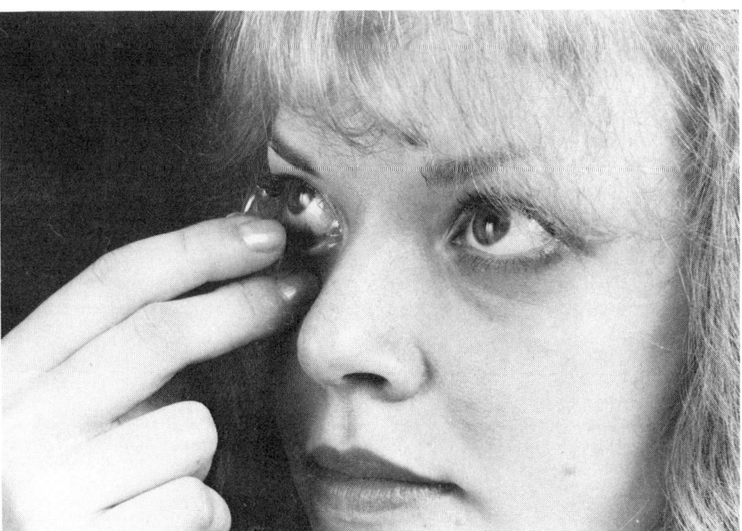

Figure 4-15 Lens removal by patient.

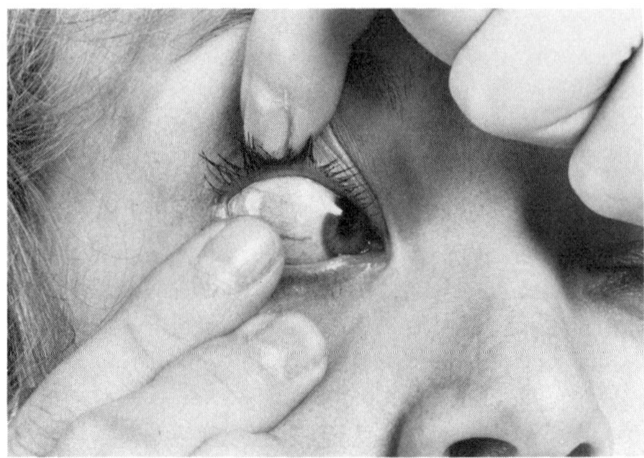

Figure 4-16 Patient slides the lens to the temporal part of the globe prior to removal.

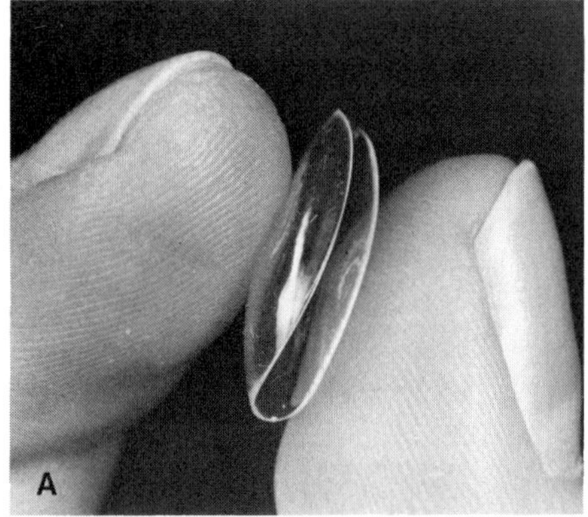

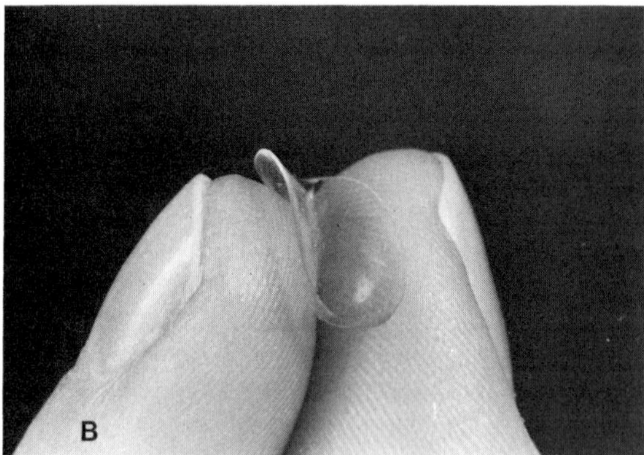

Figure 4-17 (A) Taco test to check the correct side of the lens. On gently compressing the lens between the thumb and index finger, the edges point inward when the lens has the correct side. (B) When the lens is inside out, the edges fold back on the fingers.

inward until they look like a Mexican taco with the edges touching (Fig. 4-17*A*). When the edges evert rather than turn in (Fig. 4-17*B*), the lens is inverted and must be reversed prior to application on the cornea. To minimize false results, the lens should be grasped and folded near the apex rather than at the edges.

TINTED SOFT CONTACT LENSES

Tinted soft lenses can provide significant cosmetic improvement for patients with disfigured eyes.[38] Meshel and Gregory have developed a technique for tinting HEMA lenses. They are able to imprint any image on any portion of the lens. They state that the colors are stable and nontoxic. The images incorporated into the soft lens can be either translucent or opaque. Translucent images are modified by whatever color is behind them. Hence, it is not possible to create a lighter image than what is behind the lens. A blue or hazel iris can be made to look dark, but a dark iris cannot be made to look lighter (see Color Fig. 4-1). Translucent lenses can also be used to treat photophobia. A lens with a translucent dark pupil can be used to hide an inoperable cataract. If a dark iris is to be changed to a lighter-looking iris, then an opaque lens should be used. For a scarred nonseeing eye, an opaque lens can completely recreate a pupil and iris (Figs. 4-18 and 4-19), and offers excellent cosmesis. Pseudo-iris lenses for albino and aniridic patients not only improve their appearance but also provide visual comfort by cutting

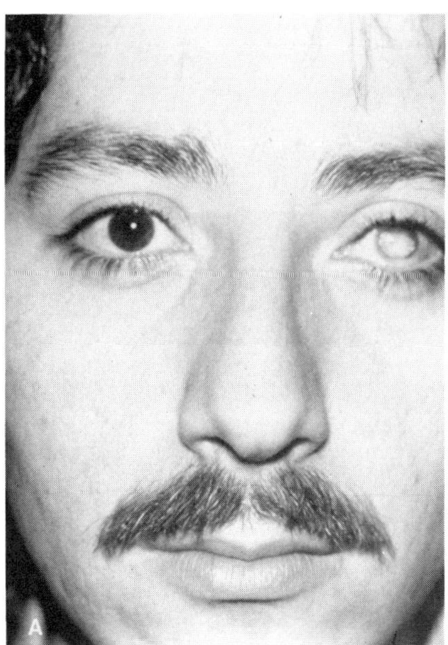
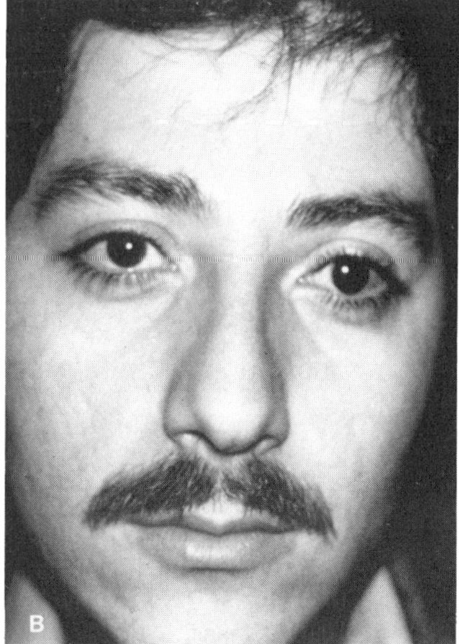

Figure 4-18 Scarred, nonseeing eye (*A*) is transformed to a normal-looking eye (*B*) using an opaque tinted soft lens. (*Courtesy Narcissus Medical Foundation*)

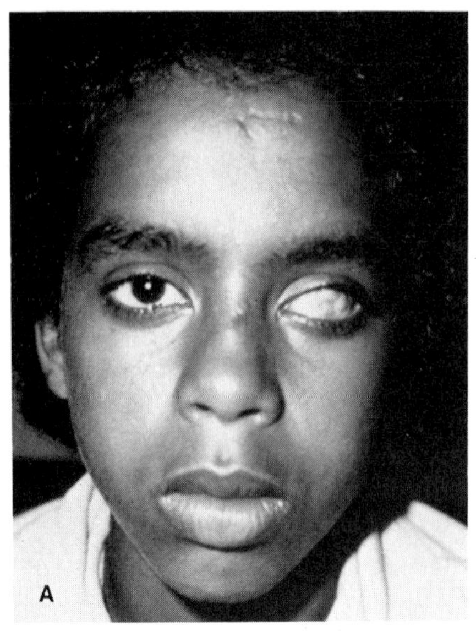

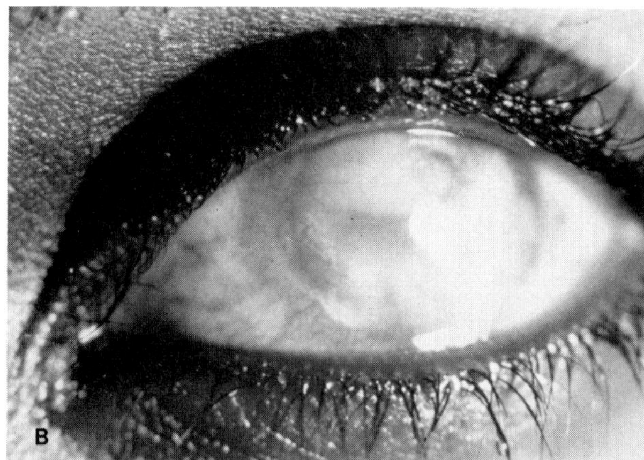

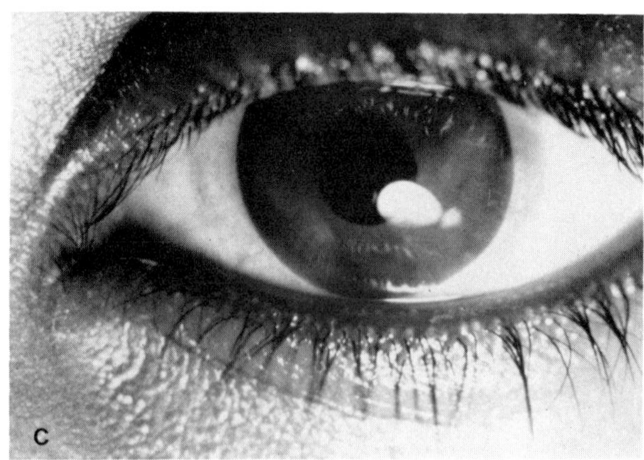

Figure 4-19 Scarred, nonseeing eye (*A, B*) is transformed to a normal-looking eye (*C*) using an opaque tinted soft lens. (Courtesy Narcissus Medical Foundation)

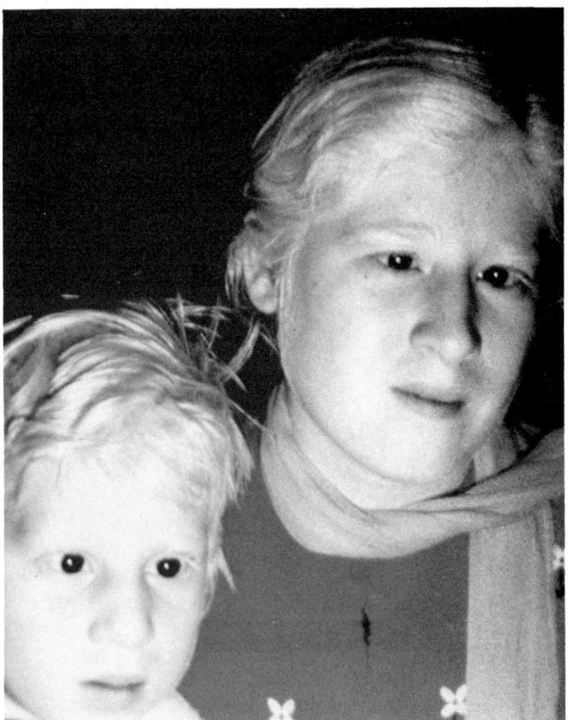

Figure 4-20 Albino brother and sister wearing tinted soft lenses. (Courtesy Narcissus Medical Foundation)

down on the amount of light transmission (Fig. 4-20). In patients with surgical or congenital colobomas, portions of the iris can be created to hide the iris defect. To make a nonseeing eye appear straight, weighted lenses with decentered images are used. An opaque lens can also be used for diplopia or amblyopia therapy. Every lens is custom-tinted to match the patient's healthy eye, and can be obtained from the Narcissus Medical Foundation (a nonprofit organization) in San Francisco. The manufacturers claim that the tinting process does not alter the lens. They recommend cold chemical sterilization for these contact lenses.

Cosmetically tinted soft lenses, either with tinted iris and a clear pupil and a clear periphery, or with tint covering both the iris and pupil leaving a clear periphery, are available from different manufacturers, for example, Narcissus Medical Foundation, Bausch & Lomb, and CibaVision Care. These lenses can alter the color of a lighter iris but offer no significant color change on dark-eyed patients.

REFERENCES

1. Arrowsmith PN, Marks RG: Visual, refractive, and keratometric results of radial keratotomy; one-year follow-up. Arch Ophthalmol 102:1612, 1984

2. Arrowsmith PN, Sanders DR, Marks RG: Visual, refractive, and keratometric results of radial keratotomy. Arch Ophthalmol 101:873, 1983
3. Banko PE: Production of contact lenses by spin-casting. Aust J Optom 59:286, 1976
4. Barraquer JI: Keratomileusis for myopia and aphakia. Ophthalmology 88:701, 1981
5. Barraquer JI: Queratomileusis y Quertofaquia. Bogota, Colombia, Instituto Barraquer de America, 1980
6. Bayshore CA: Astigmatic soft contact lenses. A report of 88 patients. Int Contact Lens Clin 2:69, 1975
7. Bayshore CA: Astigmatic soft contact lenses: A report of 140 patients. Int Contact Lens Clin 4:56, 1977
8. Benson C: Continuous use of contact lenses. Aust J Ophthalmol 4:99, 1976
9. Binder PS: Myopic extended wear with the Hydrocurve II soft contact lens. Ophthalmology 90:623, 1983
10. Binder PS, Woodard C: Extended wear Hydrocurve and Sauflon contact lenses. Am J Ophthalmol 90:306, 1980
11. Bores LD: Historical review and clinical results of radial keratotomy. Int Ophthalmol Clin 23:93, 1983
12. Bores LD, Meyers W, Cowden J: Radial keratotomy: An analysis of the American experience. Ann Ophthalmol 13:941, 1981
13. Callendar M, Egan DJ: A clinical evaluation of the Weicon-T and Durasoft-TT toric soft contact lenses. Int Contact Lens Clin 5:209, 1978
14. Cogger SK: Fitting daily wear soft lenses. In Fitting Contact Lenses, pp 49–59. New York, Raven Press, 1985
15. Coombs WF: Spin casting of HEMA lenses. Int Contact Lens Clin 9:169, 1982
16. Coon LJ, Miller JP, Meier RF: Overview of extended wear contact lenses. J Am Optom Assoc 50:745, 1979
17. Cowden JW, Bores LD: A clinical investigation of the surgical correction of myopia by the method of Fyodorov. Ophthalmology 88:737, 1981
18. Ewell DG: Clinical application of toric soft lenses. Contact Lens Forum 5:23, 1980
19. Fatt I, Freeman RD, Lin D: Oxygen tension distribution in the cornea: A re-examination. Exp Eye Res 18:357, 1974
20. Fatt I, Lin D: Oxygen tension under a soft or hard gas permeable contact lens in the presence of tear pumping. Am J Optom Physiol Opt 53:104, 1976
21. Fyodorov SN, Durnev VV: Operation of dosaged dissection of corneal circular ligaments in cases of myopia of mild degree. Ann Ophthalmol 11:1885, 1979
22. Gelender H, Flynn HW, Mandelbaum SH: Endophthalmitis from radial keratotomy. Am J Ophthalmol 93:323, 1982
23. Hales RH: Manufacturing of contact lenses. In Contact Lenses: A Clinical Approach to Fitting, 2nd ed, pp 71–76. Baltimore, Williams & Wilkins, 1982
24. Hartstein J: Experience with the Sauflon 70 (Lidofilcon A) soft contact lenses for extended wear in myopia. Ann Ophthalmol 16:422, 1984
25. Hill RM: Oxygen permeable contact lenses: How convinced is the cornea? Int Contact Lens Clin 4:34, 1977
26. Hoefle FB, Dabezies OH: Nomenclature, parameters, and design of soft lenses. In Dabezies OH (ed): Contact Lenses, Vol 2, pp 37.1–37.7. New York, Grune & Stratton, 1984
27. Houde WL, Rubin ML: Extended wear lenses. An update. Surv Ophthalmol 26:103, 1981

28. Jurkus J, Tomlinson A, Gilbault DC et al: The effect of fit and parameter changes on soft lens rotation. Am J Optom Physiol Opt 56:734, 1979

29. Koetting RA: A retrospective study of patients fitted with extended wear lenses. Contacto 27:7, 1983

30. Krwawicz T: Lamellar corneal stromectomy for the operative treatment of myopia: A preliminary report. Am J Ophthalmol 57:828, 1964

31. Lamer L: Extended wear contact lenses for myopes: A follow-up study of 400 cases. Ophthalmology 90:156, 1983

32. Lembach RG: Fitting techniques of soft lenses. In Dabezies OH (ed): Contact Lenses, Vol 2, pp 38.1–38.9. New York, Grune & Stratton, 1984

33. Lembach RG, Wilson LA: Extended wear contact lenses. In Dabezies OH (ed): Contact Lenses, Vol 2, pp 61.1–61.19. New York, Grune & Stratton, 1984

34. Maguen E, Nesburn AB, Verity SM et al: Myopic extended wear contact lenses in 100 patients. A retrospective study. Contact Lenses 10:335, 1984

35. Mandell RB: Contact lens practice, 2nd ed, p 490. Springfield, IL, Charles C Thomas, 1974

36. McDonald MB: The current state of epikeratophakia. In Jakobiec FA (ed): Advanced Techniques in Ocular Surgery, pp 1–23. Philadelphia, WB Saunders, 1984

37. McMonnies CW, Parker DP: Predicting the rotational performance of toric soft lenses. Austr J Optom 60:130, 1977

38. Meshel LG: Interview: Tinted lenses: New "life" for dead eyes. Contact Lens Forum, p 13, March 1978

39. Michaels DD: Ametropia. In Visual Optics and Refraction: A Clinical Approach, 2nd ed, p 524. St Louis, CV Mosby, 1980

40. Miller JP, Coon LJ, Meier RF: Extended wear of Hydrocurve II_{55} soft contact lenses. J Am Optom Assoc 51:225, 1980

41. Polse KA, Mandell RB: Critical oxygen tension at the corneal surface. Arch Ophthalmol 84:505, 1970

42. Remba MJ: Clinical evaluation of FDA approved toric hydrophilic soft contact lenses (Part 1). J Am Optom Assoc 50:289, 1979

43. Remba MJ: Clinical evaluation of toric hydrophilic contact lenses (Part II). J Am Optom Assoc 52:211, 1981

44. Rowsey JJ, Balyeat HD, Rabinovitch B et al: Predicting the results of radial keratotomy. Ophthalmology 90:642, 1983

45. Salvatori AL: Manufacturing HEMA soft lenses by lathe: Part 1. Contact Lens Forum p 27, November 1981

46. Salvatori AL: Manufacturing HEMA soft lenses by lathe: Part 2. Contact Lens Forum p 32, December 1981

47. Sarno EM, Smith RE, Schanzlin DJ: Comparison of clinical results following radial keratotomy, extended wear contact lenses, and myopic keratomileusis. Int Ophthalmol Clin 23:167, 1983

48. Sato T, Akiyamo K, Shibata H: A new surgical approach to myopia. Am J Ophthalmol 36:823, 1953

49. Skudder CD: Lathe-cut hydron lenses. In Montague R (ed): Soft Contact Lenses: Clinical and Applied Technology, pp 427–432. London, Bailliere Tindall, 1978

50. Solomon OD, Sholiton DB, Slonim C et al: Bausch and Lomb "O" lenses for extended wear. Contact Lenses 9:137, 1983

51. Stark WJ, Kracher G, Martin NF: Extended wear soft contact lenses for aphakia and myopia. In Koch DD, Park II DW, Paton D (eds): Current Management in Ophthalmology, pp 87–114. New York, Churchill Livingstone, 1983

52. Stark WJ, Martin NF: Extended wear contact lenses for myopic correction. Arch Ophthalmol 99:1963, 1981
53. Stein HA, Slatt BJ: How to fit soft lenses. In Fitting Guide for Hard and Soft Contact Lenses: A Practical Approach, pp 62–70. St Louis, CV Mosby, 1977
54. Swinger CA, Barker BA: Prospective evaluation of myopic keratomileusis. Ophthalmology 91:785, 1984
55. Temprano J: Our experience with extended wear contact lenses: Permalens. Contact Lens 17:18, 1979
56. Tomlinson A, Jurkus J, Bibby MM: Evaluation and control of Durasoft lens rotation. Am J Optom Physiol Opt 55:365, 1978
57. Tucker DN, Barraquer JI: Refractive keratoplasty. Clinical results in 67 cases. Ann Ophthalmol 5:335, 1973
58. Waring GO, Lynn MJ, Gelender H et al: Results of the prospective evaluation of radial keratotomy (PERK) study, one year after surgery. Ophthalmology 92:177, 1985
59. Weismann BA: Soft lenses for myopia and hypermetropia. In Contact Lens Primer: A Manual, pp 31–36. Philadelphia, Lea & Febiger, 1984
60. Werblin TP, Klyce SD: Epikeratophakia: The surgical correction of myopia. I. Lathing of corneal tissue. Curr Eye Res 1:591, 1981/1982
61. Wichterle O: Interview: Birthplace of the soft lens: Czechoslovakia. Contact Lens Forum p 33, May 1982
62. Wichterle O, Lim D: Hydrophilic lenses for biological use. Nature 185:117, 1960

CHAPTER FIVE

CONTACT LENS CORRECTION OF PRESBYOPIA

ALAN TOMLINSON

The demand for contact lens correction of presbyopia is likely to grow dramatically as the average age of the American population increases. Between 1980 and 1995 it is anticipated that the population in the age range 40 years to 59 years, the prime candidates for such correction, will increase by over one third from 46.2 million to 62.3 million.[52] The reasons for this increase include the "creation" of an aging population by modern medicine and the entry into the presbyopic ranks of the "baby boom" generation. Contact lens practitioners are thus faced with a large group of potential patients who, in many cases, wear single vision contact lenses and whose interest in presbyopic correction is fueled by televised consumer advertising. To meet this demand, several contact lens modalities have been developed for the correction of presbyopia.

CORRECTION OF PRESBYOPIA WITH SINGLE VISION CONTACT LENSES

In early presbyopia the prescription of distance single vision contact lenses may delay the need for actual correction of the presbyopia. Single vision contact lenses for incipient presbyopes will postpone the need for a reading addition in the case of hyperopes, but will advance the time at which a myope will need correction for presbyopia. The myope has to accommodate more with contact lenses than with spectacles, whereas the opposite is the case for the hyperope.[15] Slight overcorrection of hyperopia or undercorrection of myopia with single vision contact lenses may also postpone the need for a reading correction in the younger presbyopic age groups.[6] However, this technique cannot be adopted when the reading addition exceeds 1 D. In other cases, single vision lenses may be prescribed to compensate fully for the loss of accommodation in middle age. This technique is known as monovision correction of presbyopia.

MONOVISION LENSES

The correction of presbyopia with single vision contact lenses where one eye is corrected for distance and the other eye for near has been advocated by many clinicians.[6,16,17,21,25,36] The basis most frequently cited for this technique is the case of the presbyope who is myopic in one eye and emmetropic or hyperopic in the other eye.[6,36] Such a patient has no problems in reading or performing distance vision tasks well after reaching the presbyopic age.

The advantage of monovision correction of presbyopia over the use of bifocal contact lenses is that the technique of fitting is simple and similar to that with single vision correction of ametropia. In addition, the patient has a wide field of view at both distance and near. The time involvement and consequent expense for patients and practitioners is somewhat less than required for most bifocal contact lens fittings. For these reasons the technique has remained popular even despite the development of rigid and hydrogel bifocal contact lenses.[4]

However, there are disadvantages to the technique. These include the loss of binocularity.[36] Surprisingly, however, this does not seem to reduce stereopsis to the extent that might be anticipated. Indeed, with additions of less than 1 D, very little loss of stereopsis is found.[36] The loss with monovision contact lenses is considerably less than that found with similar reading additions made in spectacle lens form.[44] Another and often more significant problem is the flare, blur, or haze in vision at distance and near reported by many patients.[6,36] In some cases this reduces with adaptation. The adaptation period to monovision may take several weeks.[6,21,36] During adaptation the development of the ability to fuse two dissimilar images without vision problems, or the suppression of one image effectively makes the patient monocular at distance and near.[15] Only in such cases is the patient able to accept monovision. In other instances patients can fuse the dissimilar images only with difficulty, resulting in discomfort and inefficient single vision or diplopia. In these cases the patient requires some other form of correction.

Fitting Monovision Lenses

Fitting a patient with monovision correction for presbyopia is similar to fitting single vision rigid or hydrogel contact lenses. The only difference lies in the determination of the correction for near. Some authorities suggest that patients be given both distance and near vision corrections in contact lens form. The patient is given the option of choosing one eye for distance and one eye for near after wearing the pairs of contact lenses in different combinations.[21] However, most fitters adopt a technique in which the dominant eye is corrected for distance and the nondominant eye for near.[6,36] This technique is not universally applied, however. In certain occupational situations it is necessary to correct the dominant eye for near. For example, in the case of a left eye dominant patient requiring near vision on the left side because of the organization of his work station, the left eye is corrected for near. In other instances where patients have concentrated distance vision tasks such as driving, cinema, or the theatre, a third lens corrected for distance is prescribed for the eye normally corrected for near vision.[6,36]

Monovision contact lenses for correction of presbyopia are most effective when fitted to previous contact lens patients. For this reason it is often advocated that distance vision correction is offered to patients first so that they may adapt to contact lens wear, before having to adapt to monovision.[36]

PINHOLE LENSES

Alternative forms of single vision contact lenses for presbyopia have been suggested. These have included the pinhole lens and the multirange or cosmetic bifocal.[37,55] Both of these lenses work on the principle of the pinhole camera in which only a small, clear aperture in the center of the lens allows rays of light to enter the eye. Because of the great depth of focus of such a system, both distance and near vision rays are in focus at the retina at the same time.[36] The disadvantage of this system is that it reduces the field of view and the brightness of the retinal image, making it difficult for patients to read in many situations. The multirange lens uses a system in which the central pinhole is surrounded by several radial lines. This improves the field of view, but still leads to reductions in retinal image brightness. These lenses have not been widely accepted.

MODIFIED MONOVISION CORRECTION OF PRESBYOPIA

Two forms of modified monovision correction have been suggested. In one, overcorrection of plus power in one eye is combined with the use of a bifocal contact lens.[17] This gives binocular vision at near when the patient's principal requirement is for near vision, together with distance vision monocularly in the eye wearing the bifocal contact lens. Obviously, in situations where the patient's principal requirement is for binocular distance vision, the single vision lens incorporates the distance vision correction.

Alternative forms of modified monovision have developed with the fitting of hydrogel bifocal contact lenses. In the first, the Bausch & Lomb hydrogel bifocal contact lenses, which give maximum addition of 0.75 D to 1.25 D, have been prescribed for both eyes.[33] The nondominant eye is overplussed to maximize near vision in this eye, and the other eye is optimally corrected for distance. With this technique good distance vision is obtained with one eye and near vision with the second eye, while binocularity is maintained with a minimum amount of anisometropia. The technique offers some of the benefits of monovision correction with the binocularity offered by bifocal contact lenses.

Experience with current simultaneous hydrogel bifocal contact lenses suggests that good distance vision is provided by the Bausch & Lomb PA1 lens, whereas the Ciba Bi-Soft lens provides better near vision. Accordingly, some practitioners have adopted a second approach in which the Bausch & Lomb and Ciba lenses are fitted to the same patient to give a modified monovision correction in which the distance vision is provided by the Bausch and Lomb bifocal and the near vision by the Ciba Bi-Soft.

CORRECTION OF PRESBYOPIA WITH BIFOCAL CONTACT LENSES

In addition to the correction of presbyopia by single vision contact lenses, several designs of hard and soft bifocal contact lenses have been developed.

Two basic forms of bifocal contact lenses have been described: simultaneous vision lenses and alternating vision lenses. The general principles of these types of lenses will be discussed first.

SIMULTANEOUS VISION BIFOCAL LENSES

The patient is fitted with a relatively stable, well-centered lens that has two distinct optical zones. The central zone of the lens is corrected for distance and an annular peripheral zone is corrected for near. The diameter of the distance optical zone must be smaller than that of the patient's pupil to allow rays from both the distance and near vision zones of the lens to enter the pupil. In this lens design, rays of light from both distant and near objects fall on the retina simultaneously (Fig. 5-1).

The advantage of a properly fitted simultaneous vision lens is that it provides constant distance and near vision without the need for lens movement, a requirement with the alternating bifocal design. Because the simultaneous vision lens has a concentric reading zone, there is no real need for movement or translation on the eye. In reality, however, slight movements

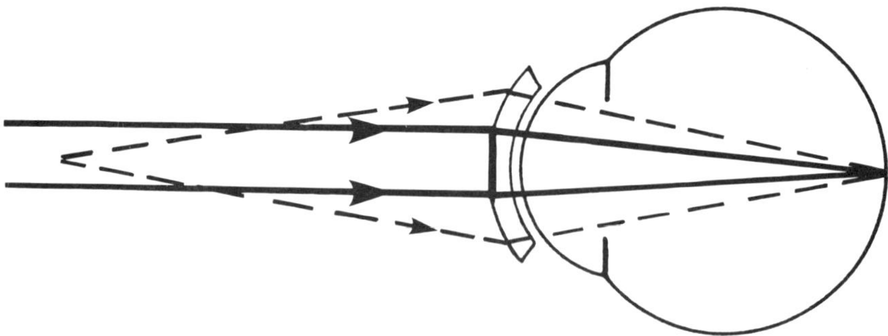

Figure 5-1 Simultaneous vision bifocal contact lenses. Rays of light from distant (*complete lines*) and near (*dotted lines*) enter the eye through a simultaneous bifocal contact lens. Images of distant and near objects are focused at the retina.

of "simultaneous" bifocal lenses on the eye may aid changes in focus from distance to near by shifting the near vision zone into the pupil area in the same way as occurs with an alternating bifocal. Most bifocal contact lenses probably work by a combining the simultaneous and alternating vision techniques.

The simultaneous bifocal is usually made as a completely round lens, which gives good comfort and allows any size lens to be fitted. The absence of a need for the stabilization mechanisms required in alternating lenses allows the simultaneous lens to be made thinner, giving better physiological tolerance.[8]

However, the disadvantage of this lens design lies in the dependence of its performance on good centration and the size of the patient's pupil. Pupils of less than 2 mm in diameter (Fig. 5-2) preclude fitting this type of lens, because most simultaneous bifocal lenses have distance optical zones of 2 mm to 4 mm.[58]

A period of patient adaptation is required with this type of bifocal to develop the selective perception of distance and near vision rays when shifting gaze from distance to near objects. While wearing simultaneous bifocal lenses, the clear image at the point of interest is always surrounded by a slight flare, haze, or blur because of the rays of light coming from objects at other distances. This causes a continuing annoyance to some patients. The

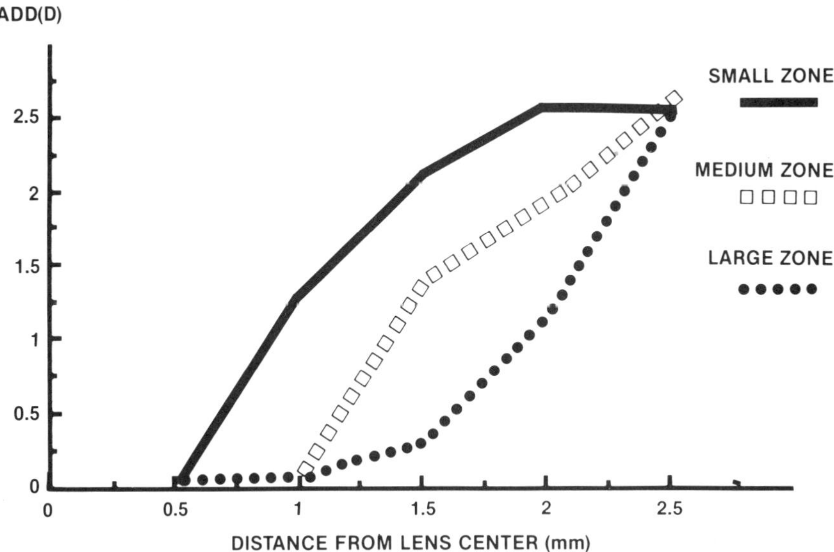

Figure 5-2 Power distribution of concentric bifocals: three lenses with different distance zone sizes.[38] The lens with the small distance zone resulted in good near acuity but substantially reduced distance acuity. The medium-sized zone gave reasonably good distance acuity with a reduction in near acuity of about one line. The large distance zone lens gave excellent distance acuity but very poor near acuity, about the same as obtained with no bifocal add. (Courtesy of G. E. Lowther)

amount of blur surrounding the clear object of regard changes with pupil size, which can lead to problems in conditions of varying illumination levels, such as driving at night or reading outside on a bright summer day. This problem is also exacerbated by the distinctness of the junction between the distance and near portions of the lens, and is less apparent objectively in lenses with well-blended junctions.[35]

Rigid Lenses

SIMULTANEOUS VISION BIFOCAL LENS TYPES

There have been many rigid lens bifocal types of the simultaneous vision form. These have ranged from scleral bifocal lenses to corneal lenses in gas-permeable materials.[3,14,59] It is possible to break down the simultaneous vision rigid bifocal lens design into two principal categories: (1) Those of concentric form with two distinct and constant curvatures on either the front or back surface of the lens, which provide the corrections for distance and near vision; (2) The other form of rigid bifocal design incorporates a central optical zone of distance vision surrounded by an aspheric or quasi-aspheric periphery, which provides increasing plus power with increasing distance from the lens center.

Concentric Bifocal Designs Concentric bifocal lenses first were suggested in 1958 by Collins, and by DeCarle and Moss-Arner.[7,15] These lenses were constructed with a central optic zone of distance vision surrounded by an annulus of reading vision. Both distance and near vision power was ground on the posterior surface of the rigid lens (Fig. 5-3).

The distance vision segment in the Collins lens was 3.5 mm in diameter and that in the DeCarle bifocal averaged 3 mm, although in DeCarle's lens the distance segment size could be varied according to the pupil diameter. Both lenses were made in relatively larger diameters, 9.6 mm for the Collins lens and between 10 mm and 10.5 mm in the original DeCarle version. In

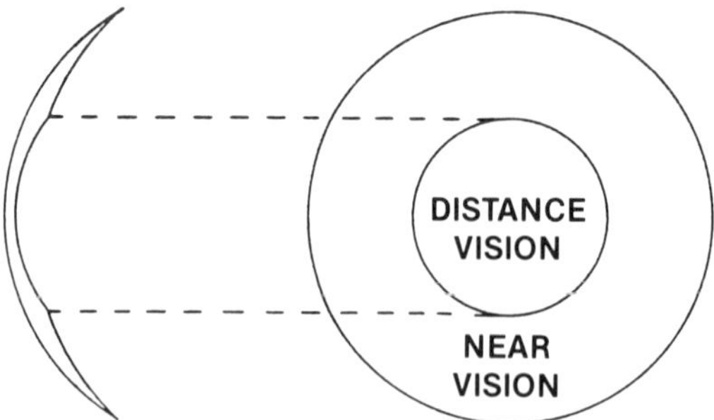

Figure 5-3 The DeCarle concentric simultaneous vision bifocal provides a central zone of distance vision surrounded by an annulus of reading vision. The distance optical zone power is derived from a single radius cut on the posterior surface.

the DeCarle lens the fitting or bearing area of the lens was in the peripheral annulus; in the Moss-Arner lens the central distance vision area provided the fitting area, and the annular curvature was flatter to provide additional power for reading.

All concentric bifocal lens designs require good centration of the lens and the pupil to maintain simultaneous vision. In consequence, all three lenses were fit with alignment fitting relationship to the cornea.

Aspheric Bifocal Lenses In recent years the most commonly fitted versions of simultaneous rigid bifocal contact lenses have been lenses with aspheric or quasi-aspheric peripheral posterior surfaces. The periphery of such a lens provides the additional positive power to correct vision for near. Additive power is provided with eccentricity values of greater than 0.7, and E values of 1.2 to 2.0 give adds of up to 4.5 D.[9] Aspheric lenses have the advantages over concentric, single powered simultaneous vision bifocal lenses of offering intermediate correction from the area of the lens immediately adjacent to the pupil and increasing additive power towards the lens periphery. However, the aspheric lens design has the disadvantage of introducing unwanted cylinder power into the contact lens/eye system.[11]

Versions of aspheric base curve bifocal lenses include the Autofocal, the Fulsite, the Ful-Range, Presbicon, Presbiflex, and the Variable Focus Lens (VFL) (Fig. 5-4).[18,46,56,57] As with the concentric simultaneous bifocal described previously, good lens centration is essential for correct visual perfor-

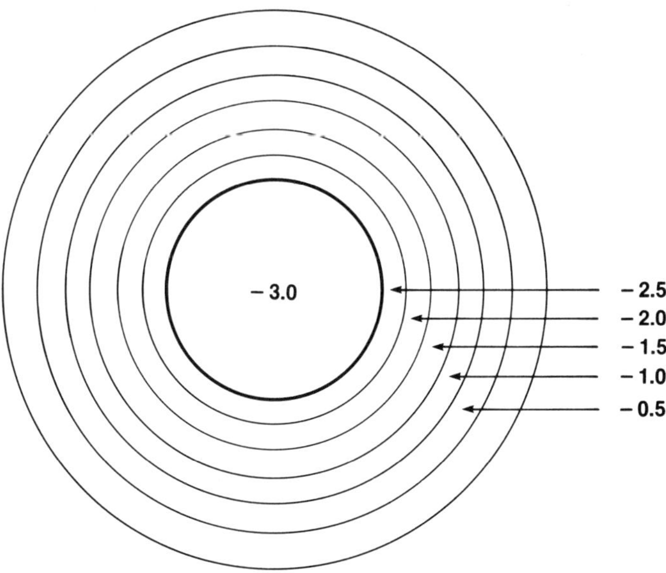

Figure 5-4 Progressive addition concentric bifocal. Diagram shows a lens of −3.00 D distance power, which provides increasing reading additions with increasing distance from the center of the lens.

mance. The usable vision zone of these lenses is approximately 3.5 mm in diameter.[19] In the aspheric back surface lens, there is considerable flattening of the aspheric base curve towards the periphery of the lens.[56] Accordingly, to center these lenses sufficiently to provide good distance and near vision simultaneously, it is necessary to fit them steeper than the flattest corneal curvature by 1.5 D to 3.5 D.[57] In the past this has caused some physiological problems with this type of lens made of PMMA material. However, the introduction of the VFL lens in a gas-permeable hard material has overcome some of these problems.[49] The aspheric bifocal lenses are commonly smaller in diameter than the concentric ones described previously. For example, most are less than 9.0 mm in size, the VFL being most commonly prescribed in 8.7 mm diameters.[54]

FITTING RIGID ANNULAR BIFOCAL LENSES

Simultaneous rigid bifocal contact lenses are fitted most commonly using a trial or diagnostic lens fitting set. For the single powered, peripheral annular lens a fitting set with lenses in overall diameters between 9 mm and 9.6 mm are used. These lenses commonly are fitted on the flattest curvature reading. It is important with simultaneous bifocal lenses of all types to obtain the correct distance vision segment diameter to fit within the pupil area. It may be impossible to fit patients with small pupils with these types of lenses. For larger pupils the lens should be fitted with the distance optic zone inside the pupil diameter so that the distance zone covers about half the pupil area.[23] Accurate measurement of pupil diameter has been advocated by some in fitting these lenses.[31] The average size of the distance optical zone in concentric simultaneous bifocal lens is between 3 mm and 5 mm, and averages 4 mm. With the concentric annular bifocals of the Collins and the DeCarle types, the overall diameter of the lens is large (between 9 mm and 10 mm), which helps the overall centration of the lens.

The fitting of aspheric rigid bifocal contact lenses is similar to the procedure for concentric lenses described previously, in that lenses are required to position over the pupil with as little movement as possible. Because of this need for lens centration, it is necessary to fit aspheric back surface lenses steep by 1.5 D to 3.5 D.[56] On fluorescein examination, apical pooling should be seen under these lenses with the thin intermediate clearance, indicating peripheral tangential touch.

Hydrogel Lenses

SIMULTANEOUS VISION BIFOCAL LENS TYPES

The first of a new generation of hydrogel bifocal contact lenses introduced in the 1980s was the spincast Bausch & Lomb PA1 lens. This spincast version of a former hydrogel single vision lens provides a progressive addition similar to the aspheric rigid bifocal lenses described previously. This variable focus design provides gradually increasing plus power from the lens center to the midperiphery (Fig. 5-5).[33] The effective addition of these lenses is said

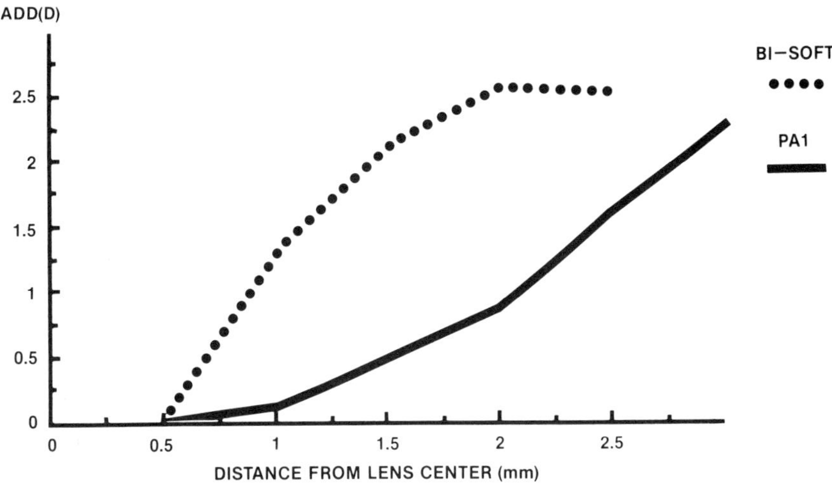

Figure 5-5 Power distribution of the Bausch & Lomb bifocal and Ciba Bi-Soft bifocal as determined by the double aperture technique described by Meier and Lowther.[38] (Courtesy of G. E. Lowther)

to vary between +0.75 D and 1.75 D.[29,38] For this reason it is best suited to early presbyopia.[53]

The requirements for fitting the hydrogel concentric bifocal are similar to those for rigid bifocal lenses. The lens should center well on the eye and be relatively immobile. This is achieved more easily with the larger 13.5-mm diameter lens made from 38% water hydrogel material than is the case with many rigid bifocal lenses. It is also important that the distance optical zone of the lens fit within the pupil area to provide simultaneous distance and near vision. With the Bausch & Lomb bifocal lens it is necessary to have a somewhat larger pupil to give effective near vision than is the case with the other simultaneous hydrogel bifocal, the Ciba Bi-Soft lens.

A second form of simultaneous hydrogel bifocal lens, the Bi-Soft lens was approved by the Food and Drug Administration in June 1982 and introduced shortly thereafter by Ciba Vision Care. Unlike the Bausch & Lomb lens, the Bi-Soft consists of two concentric areas each having a single refractive power (see Fig. 5-5), a central distance optical zone, and a midperipheral annulus for near vision. In this sense, the lens is similar to the concentric rigid bifocal lenses of the Collins and the DeCarle types, but the power of the Bi-Soft lens is located on the anterior surface.

The advantage of the Ciba Bi-Soft lens over the Bausch & Lomb PA1 lens is that it provides a much larger range of near vision, having additions from +1.5 D to 3 D in 0.5-D steps. In addition, the lens also provides a range of base curves of 8.3 mm, 8.6 mm, and 8.9 mm in the 13.8-mm diameter hydrogel form. This allows better control of centration of the lens on the eye. The requirements for fitting this lens are similar to those of all other simultaneous rigid and hydrogel bifocal lenses that require precise centration with minimum movement. It appears that the distance optical zone size in the current Bi-Soft lens gives more distance vision blur but better near vision than is obtainable with the Bausch & Lomb PA1 lens.[34]

Other simultaneous hydrogel bifocal lenses include the Hydrocurve aspheric bifocal lens and the Titmus-Eurocon W38E Hydrophilic bifocal lens.[49] The Hydrocurve II bifocal has its maximum asphericity in the pupil area (diameter 3 mm to 4 mm) to give an effective addition in the region of +1.5 D; distance power range is from +4 D to −6 D. The lens is available in one base curve (9 mm) and a large diameter of 14.8 mm to give good centration. The Titmus-Eurocon lens has two diameters of 13 mm and 13.8 mm as controlling parameters of lens movement, and distance optic zone diameters of 3.2 mm and 3.8 mm for more flexibility in meeting the needs of pupil size variation.

An alternative simultaneous bifocal lens design has been suggested that may provide the basis for simultaneous vision bifocal lenses of the future.[12] This design combines the half wave zone plate and Fresnel lens to produce clear simultaneous distance and near vision images. The design provides these images without the restrictions and requirements of careful lens centration and segment diameter required in other simultaneous bifocal designs. The new design concept allows the distance area of the lens to be approximately one half that of other simultaneous vision lenses. Movements of the lens do not cause visual blur because distance and near vision rays from the center and periphery of the lens contribute to both images. At this time the concept has not been incorporated into an available lens.

FITTING SIMULTANEOUS VISION HYDROGEL BIFOCAL LENSES

The fitting of simultaneous vision hydrogel bifocal lenses is similar to that of annular rigid bifocals. The lenses must center well and have distance optical zone diameters that are smaller than those of the pupil. Good centration is easier to achieve with the larger diameter hydrogel lenses than with rigid versions of these lenses. Modified monovision techniques have also been advocated with simultaneous vision hydrogel bifocal lenses.[33]

ALTERNATING VISION BIFOCAL LENSES

The second method of fitting a bifocal contact lens is that in which distance and near vision portions of the lens are alternately presented in front of the pupil. Such a lens depends on predictable translation or movement across the cornea when the patient changes fixation from a distant to a near object. Ideally, in straight-ahead gaze the patient's pupil falls in the area of the lens corrected for distance vision (Fig. 5-6*A*). On looking down to read the lens moves up, and the pupil occupies the near vision segment (Fig. 5-6*B*).

The advantage of the alternating vision bifocal over the simultaneous vision bifocal is that, providing accurate translation takes place, the alternating vision lens gives distinct vision at distance and near without the attendant problems of blur, haze, or flare surrounding objects of regard. In addi-

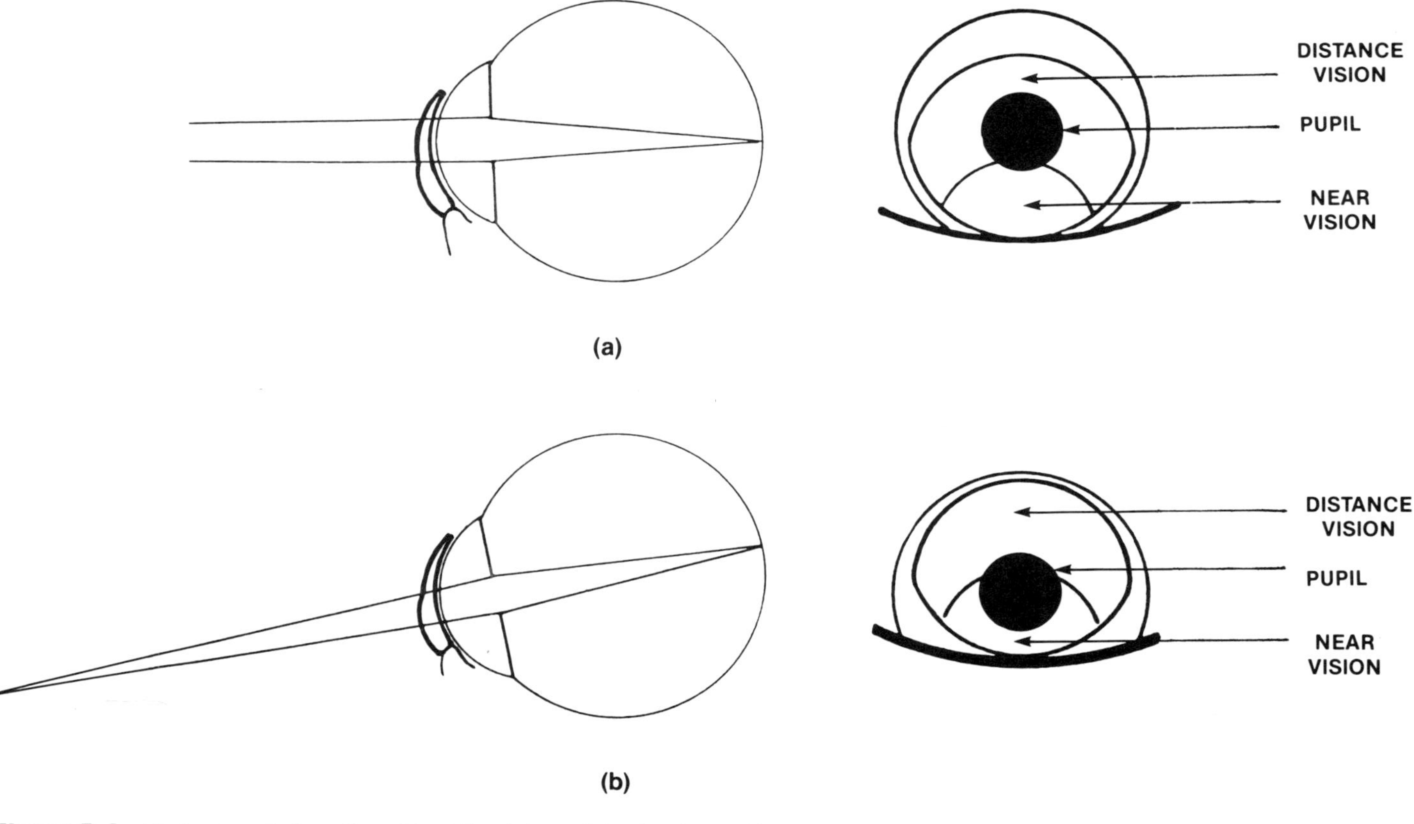

Figure 5-6 Mechanism of alternating vision bifocal. In straight-ahead gaze (*A*), the distance optical zone of the lens covers the pupil. On looking down to read (*B*), the lens translates up to allow the pupil to be covered by the near vision segment of the lens.

tion, the lens design is not as dependent on pupil size for effective performance. Physiologically, this lens can perform better than a simultaneous vision lens because it is not required to fit as tightly to the cornea to center over the pupil. The movement of the lens necessary for the adequate translation of rigid alternating bifocal lenses also facilitates tear interchange behind the lens. This was particularly important in the past when most of these lenses were made from PMMA.

However, there are some disadvantages to the alternating vision bifocal design. This bifocal is highly dependent on the correct lid characteristics for effective performance. For instance, in the presence of a very tight upper lid, or a very loose or low positioned lower lid the lens will not translate or position correctly on the eye. In addition, the necessity of adequate translation with this lens often leads to more subjective discomfort than is found with the simultaneous vision lens. This is particularly the case in rigid and hydrogel versions of the alternating bifocal in which the lens is truncated. In addition, discomfort may result from the head position adopted during near vision. In some patients the correct location of the segment is achieved only when looking directly down with the head kept erect. This can be too restrictive for patients who have the need for a large field of view at near. These are similar to the problems found by some bifocal spectacle lens wearers.

It is possible to categorize alternating vision bifocal contact lenses into two types of lenses depending on the shape of the reading vision zone. These are concentric bifocal lenses and segment bifocal lenses.

Rigid Lenses

CONCENTRIC ALTERNATING VISION BIFOCAL LENS TYPES

The rigid concentric or annular bifocal lenses that have been developed are similar to those described in the discussion of simultaneous vision bifocal lenses. A major difference, however, lies in the size of the distance optical vision segment. In the alternating form this distance portion extends 0.5 mm to 2 mm *beyond* the edge of the pupil in the primary position, because it must cover the entire pupil in straight-ahead gaze under all environmental lighting conditions.[34]

The most commonly adopted form of an alternating concentric bifocal is the Bicon (Fig. 5-7).[23] In this lens the distance optical zone has a diameter from 3 mm to 6 mm and is placed in the center of the lens. The distance zone is ground on the anterior surface of the lens.

Morrison has designed a monocentric alternating bifocal similar in function to the Bicon.[39] It has the distance optical portion ground on the posterior lens surface and is similar to that of the DeCarle bifocal in construction. However, it employs the Bicon type of fit requiring translation to move the pupil from the distance to near vision segments during reading.

Concentric alternating bifocals have been made almost exclusively of

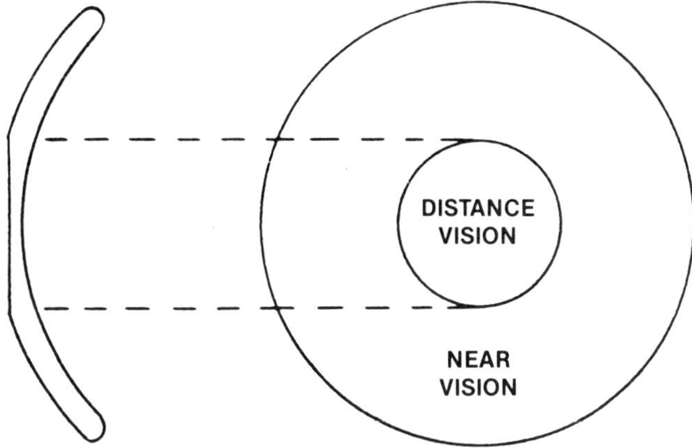

Figure 5-7 The Bicon alternating vision concentric bifocal provides a central zone of distance vision surrounded by an annulus of reading vision. The distance power is ground onto the front surface of the lens.

PMMA, but recently Breger Mueller Welt introduced the lens in a gas-permeable siloxane acrylate (Boston II) material.

An alternating bifocal lens has been described in which the near vision portion of the lens is in the central zone and is surrounded by a distance vision annulus.[10] This Centrad bifocal fits in the inferior portion of the cornea so that distance vision gaze can be obtained through the upper portion of the lens. On looking down, the central near vision zone of the lens is placed in front of the pupil. This type of alternating bifocal is sometimes referred to as a reverse bifocal.

Fitting Rigid Concentric Alternating Vision Bifocal Lenses Fitting the alternating vision concentric bifocal lenses differs from that of simultaneous vision lenses of the same form. These lenses are fitted flatter than simultaneous bifocals to allow for translation. This is achieved by fitting the central optical zone radius 0.5 D to 0.75 D flatter than the corneal curvature.[23] Because the distance optical zone in the center of these lenses is commonly larger than that in simultaneous bifocals, it is sometimes necessary to increase the overall lens diameter to provide sufficient width in the annular zone for near vision. Consequently, these lenses are normally fitted in diameters of 9.5 mm and above. The second of the third curves on the periphery of the lens is fabricated to provide sufficient tear pumping in rigid non-gas-permeable materials.

SEGMENT ALTERNATING VISION BIFOCAL LENS TYPES

The other predominant design of alternating bifocal contact lenses is similar in appearance to the conventional spectacle bifocal lens. In such lenses the reading segment is usually inferior to the distance optical area of the lens.

With this lens there is a need to maintain careful control of the meridional orientation of the lens to ensure that the reading segment is correctly positioned. In addition, these lenses are often made in a bicentric form unlike all other lenses described previously, which are monocentric in construction. However, the bicentric construction can lead to problems in image "jump" being seen on looking down to read. This is an optical effect of a displaced image and diplopia being experienced as the eye shifts from the distance to the near vision portions of the contact lens. The problem can be avoided in segment bifocals, which are made according to the monocentric principle.[36]

To maintain the segment area of the bifocal lens in the correct location on the eye, prism ballast is incorporated with truncation in the construction of the lens. Prism ballast aids lens stabilization by the "watermelon seed effect" created by the differential edge thickness between the upper and lower portions of the lens.[51] Truncation helps stabilize the lens by interaction with the lower lid. In addition, the incorporation of prism and truncation also increases the ability of the lens to translate on the eye.[50]

Segment alternating bifocal lenses can be produced in one of two ways: by cutting two different curves on the anterior or posterior surface of a lens made from a single material; or by fusing into the body of the lens a small segment for reading vision that is made from a material of higher refractive index.

One-Piece Segment Alternating Vision Bifocal Lenses Lenses that have been made from a single material, usually PMMA, have included nontruncated versions in which the distance optical zone is decentered from the center of the round lens, leaving a lower arc of reading area.[23] The benefit of these upswept reading bifocal lenses is that slight rotation of the lens on the eye does not compromise near vision. Lenses of this type have included the concept originated by Black (Fig. 5-8) and the lens marketed as the Ultracon Prism bifocal.[7] An alternative form of a one-piece, lathed bifocal incorporating prism for rotational orientation is the Cinefro Bicentric bifocal.[23] However, in this lens the segment line curves downward rather than upward as in the previous designs. Recently, gas-permeable one-piece crescent segment bifocals have been introduced. Art Optical has made a lens from a

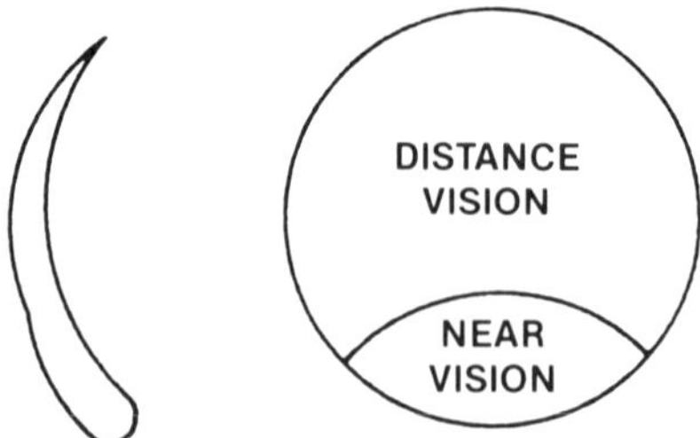

Figure 5-8 The one-piece segment alternating vision bifocal lens is lathe-cut to provide reading addition and prism ballast in the lower portion of the lens.

siloxane–acrylate gas-permeable material (Boston II). The Polycon II bifocal, made from similar material, has been produced in a prism ballasted and truncated form in powers from −0.75 D to −8.75 D with additions of +1 D to 2.5 D. This lens has been investigated for clinical approval by the FDA.

In addition to these commonly used alternating bifocal lens forms, there have been more exotic designs that have incorporated shapes other than those normally associated with contact lenses. For example, the Kontur Three Angle Bifocal lens was triangular with the lower area of the lens forming the reading zone and the upper apex the distance zone. The lower edge of the lens rested along the lower lid.[23] Double truncated rigid bifocal lenses have also been produced, for example, the Ultracon truncated bifocal.[23] The stability of this lens was aided by the incorporation of prism into its construction. Akiyama developed a rectangular lens that was typically 10 mm wide and 4 mm in vertical height.[1] The lens was designed essentially for the emmetropic presbyope who looked above the lens for distance vision and looked down into the lens area to read.

Fused Segment Alternating Vision Bifocal Lenses Alternating bifocal contact lenses may be produced from rigid material by incorporating into the lens area a fused segment for reading vision. This segment consists of a material of a different refractive index from that of the lens body (Fig. 5-9). This bifocal contact lens can be made in a monocentric construction to avoid problems with jump. These lenses are often similar to lathe cut alternating bifocal lenses in that they often incorporate prism and truncation for stabilization of the lens. The fused segment for near vision is usually in the D or upswept crescent shape similar to those adopted in some spectacle lenses. Fused segment bifocal lenses are normally produced in overall lens diameters ranging from 8.5 mm to 9.8 mm. The bifocal segment usually is approximately 6.5 mm wide. The prism ballast incorporated in the lens design usually ranges between 1 D and 2 D. The amount of prism will vary from patient to patient depending on lid configuration and tension. The segment area is often treated with a material that fluoresces under ultraviolet light to allow for determination of the segment position relative to the pupil during fitting.

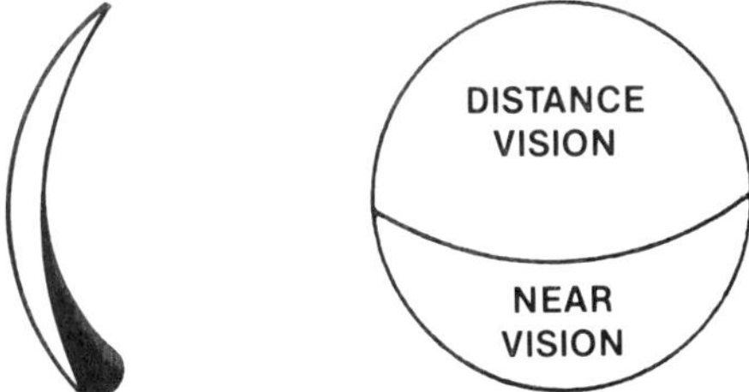

Figure 5-9 In the fused segment alternating vision bifocal a segment of material with a higher refractive index than the body of the lens is fused into the lower portion to give the additive power for reading.

Lenses of this type include the Bi-Site, Contour Comfort, the Jessen Lumicon, the Camp fused bifocal, and the Crescent and Geo Seg designs.[15,17,22,42] All of these bifocal lenses are made with the main body of the lens in PMMA material and the fused segment in a styrene material. The development of gas-permeable hard contact lens materials with different refractive indices is likely to lead to a fused segment rigid bifocal lens being produced in these materials.

FITTING RIGID ALTERNATING VISION SEGMENT BIFOCAL LENSES

In fitting rigid alternating vision segment bifocals it is important to have a diagnostic set of lenses similar in design to that of the eventual prescription lens. For example, if the eventual prescription lens is to be truncated, then so should be the fitting lens, because one of the important determinations to be made in fitting is the position of the segment. This segment height will be dramatically affected by the presence or absence of truncation.

A diagnostic lens that is either on or slightly flatter than the corneal curvature is placed on the eye. This should allow sufficient movement of the lens on the eye to facilitate translation. It is also important in the eventual choice of lens parameters to ensure that the diameter is not so great that translation is hampered by a small palpebral aperture. Some clinicians suggest that the vertical lens diameter be equal to the median vertical palpebral aperture, −0.8 mm.[15] A slightly larger lens is used in some patients to reduce discomfort due to lens impingement on the upper lid margin.

After the lens has been allowed to settle on the eye, the position of the segment top relative to the pupil margin is evaluated. The desired position for the segment top is defined differently by different authors. Most commonly, it is suggested that the lens should have the segment top at the lower margin of the pupil or approximately 1.5 mm below the visual axis.[15,23,42] To some degree the relation between the segment's placement and the pupil depends on pupil diameter. Some clinicians advocated encroachment of the reading zone into the pupil in patients with larger pupils, but avoiding the pupil by placing the segment above the lower pupil margin in patients with smaller pupils.[15] The amount of prism ballast incorporated into the lens depends on the lid tightness and position. Generally speaking, with tight lids it is necessary to incorporate more prism into the lens to obtain rotational stability. More prism is also required in high minus powered lenses.[42] It is suggested that the segment fits 1 mm higher than the pupil margin in plus powered lenses and 1 mm below the pupil in minus lenses.[22]

Hydrogel Lenses

ALTERNATING VISION BIFOCAL LENS TYPES

The most recent development in bifocal contact lens design has been the introduction of alternating vision bifocal lenses made from hydrogel materials. The first of these introduced was the Wesley-Jessen TruFocal lens made from 38% hydrogel HEMA (Fig. 5-10). This lens is 14.5 mm in diameter and is available in three base curves, 8.3 mm, 8.6 mm, and 9 mm.

The lens is available in powers from +4.5 D to −4.5 D and with additions of +1 D to +2.75 D. The lens is an alternating crescent segment bifocal that is lathe cut from the single hydrogel material. The lens in its original form was available with only one segment position. The lens is stabilized with a three quarters prism ballast and a lower truncation to offset meridional mislocation and to aid translation on the eye.[30,48]

Other alternating vision hydrogel bifocal lenses include the Syntex Synsoft and Paris SoftSite bifocals. The Synsoft lens is a concentric annular bifocal (Fig. 5-11) with a prism incorporation in the lenticular flange to aid translation and stabilization of the lens on the eye. This lens is available in two base curves (8.4 mm and 8.7 mm) in each of the two diameters of 13.5 mm and 14 mm. The lens offers distance optical zone diameters of 3.5 mm and 4.2 mm, and is available in distance powers from +4 D to −6 D with additions from +1.5 D to 2.5 D. It is made from a 38% (polymacon) HEMA material. Both the TruFocal and Synsoft bifocals are monocentric to eliminate jump. The prism incorporation in the Synsoft lens is produced by a bal-flange technique.[47] The Softsite bifocal has an alternating vision crescent segment design and incorporates prism ballasting with a modified truncation to provide stabilization and translation. It is made from a 55% HEMA

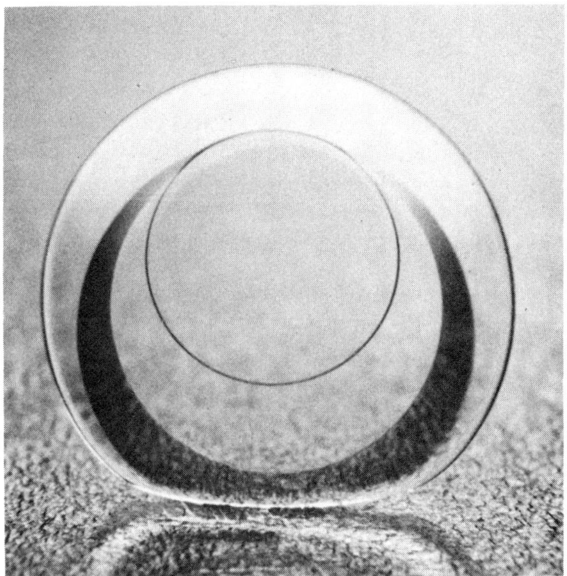

Figure 5-10 Alternating vision crescent segment hydrogel bifocal lens. The distance vision zone is in the center of the lens, and the reading addition is provided by a lower crescent-shaped area. The lens is stabilized with a prism ballast and is truncated for correct location on the eye. (Courtesy of Wesley-Jessen, Division of Schering Corp)

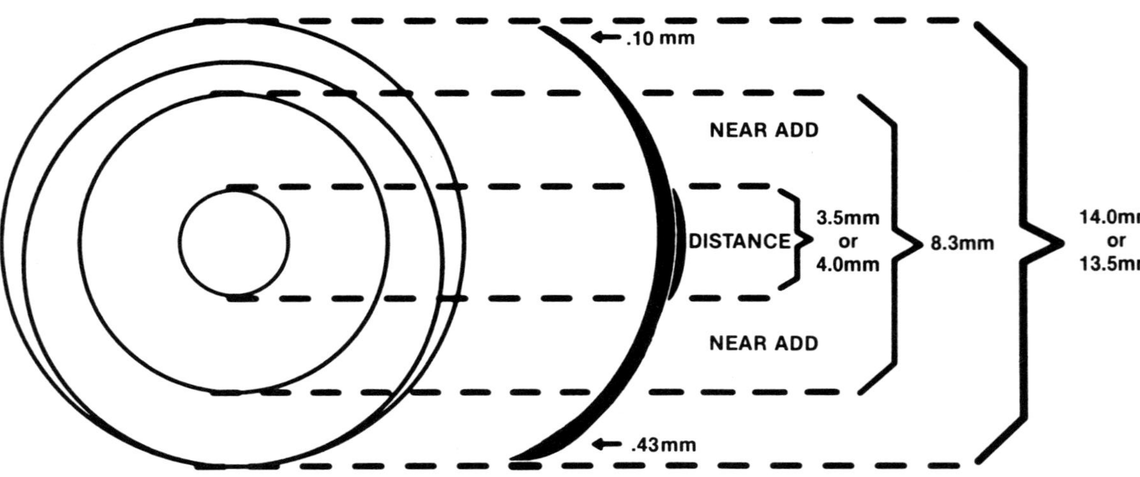

Figure 5-11 Alternating vision concentric hydrogel bifocal. Distance vision is provided by the central zone of the lens, and reading addition by the annulus. This version of the lens is stabilized with a prism ballast. (Courtesy of Syntex Ophthalmics)

material and is available in diameters of 14 mm and 13.5 mm with base curves of 9.5 mm, 9.2 mm, and 8.9 mm. The Softsite lens has a single segment location in each diameter and is available in distance powers of +6 D with additions from +1 D to +2.5 D.

A second generation Wesley-Jessen bifocal, the DuraSoft 2, has been developed. This lens is similar to the original TruFocal but has parameters that incorporate a smaller diameter of 13.5 mm in a single base curve. Recent research has indicated a greater ability to improve translation by changing the diameter rather than the base curve of the hydrogel lens. The newer lens is also made with a thinner lower edge thickness at the truncation for improved comfort. Comparative studies of the original annular simultaneous vision hydrogel bifocal lenses (Ciba Bi-Soft) and alternating truncated bifocal lenses (TruFocal) have indicated significantly better comfort with the simultaneous vision lenses.[2] The DuraSoft 2 bifocal offers two segment height locations to optimize segment location relative to the pupil.

A soft contact lens somewhat similar in shape to the Ultracon Three Angle rigid bifocal lens has been developed under the name of the Vistakon bifocal (Fig. 5-12). Designed by Bayshore, this lens is pear shaped, with the upper edges of the lens at 11 and 2 o'clock removed to aid translation of the lens under the upper lid. The lens is prism ballasted to orientate correctly on the eye.

The advantages of alternating vision bifocal lenses over simultaneous vision hydrogel lenses are similar to those of rigid lenses of the two types.

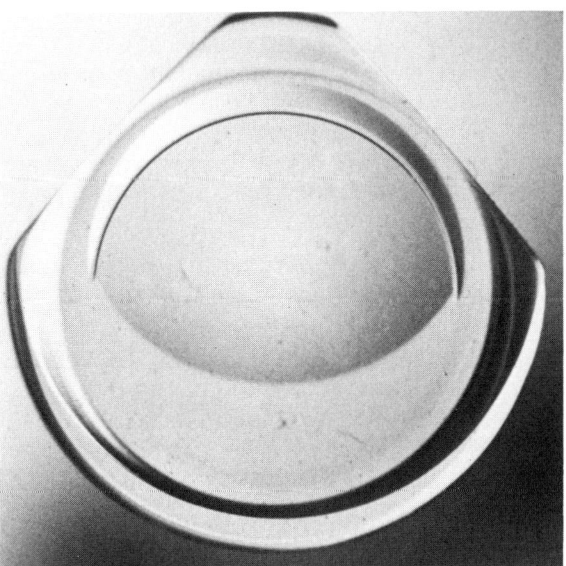

Figure 5-12 This pear-shaped alternating vision hydrogel bifocal was designed by Bayshore. The lens is stabilized with a prism ballast for correct location on the eye and has cutaway sections at the top to facilitate translation of the lens under the upper lid on looking down to read. (Courtesy of Vistakon)

Significantly better quality of vision can be obtained with an alternating vision lens when it translates correctly on the eye. This is particularly the case with the current designs, where distance vision is commonly compromised with the simultaneous vision hydrogel bifocals. Both simultaneous and alternating vision hydrogel bifocals appear to produce good physiological reaction by the cornea.[2] In comparison with rigid alternating vision bifocal lenses, the hydrogels generally provide greater comfort with larger areas for near and distance vision because of their larger sizes.

The disadvantages of alternating vision hydrogel bifocals in comparison with simultaneous vision hydrogel bifocals are reduced comfort and reduction in near vision when inadequate translation takes place.[2] In comparison with the rigid alternating vision bifocal form, the hydrogel alternating lens offers less vertical translation on eye movements because of the greater tendency for the lower edge of the lens to pass under the lower lid, thus reducing lower lid interaction. This reduction in translation ability can be a serious problem in certain patients.

FITTING ALTERNATING VISION HYDROGEL BIFOCAL LENSES

The fitting of an alternating hydrogel bifocal lens will depend on the design of the lens and the available parameters. Before assessing the fit of any hydrogel bifocal lens it is important to allow enough time for the lens to settle on the eye. The necessary equilibration period is required to allow the lens to dehydrate so that it takes up its eventual relationship to the eye before any lens assessments are done.

The intention in fitting the lens is to obtain a segment location such that in the primary position of gaze, the margin between distance and near vision occupies a position at the lower margin of the pupil (Fig. 5-13*A*). Encroachment of the near vision zone into the pupil during straight-ahead gaze can cause doubling of vision (Fig. 5-13*B*). To obtain the correct segment position, a lens with a different segment height may be tried. In lenses with fixed segment locations, a different base curve or diameter may be tried. A larger diameter or steeper base curve is fitted where the reading segment encroaches into the pupil area. If a segment location position is found that is too low on the patient's eye, then the lens probably will not translate up enough to allow near vision on downward gaze. In this case a higher segment is required. If the segment correctly locates on the eye, but the patient reports that near vision is blurred on looking down to read, it is probable that the lens is not translating adequately on the eye. In such a situation, either a flatter base curve or a smaller diameter lens is indicated.

Some fitters have described a method of fitting a crescent-shaped aspheric back surface hydrogel bifocal lens with the near vision segment of the lens encroaching into the pupil area by approximately one third of this area.[26] This bifocal lens is larger in diameter than those employed in the United States and is available with a range of base curves.

In those situations where acceptable vision cannot be obtained at distance or near because of segment position or inability of the hydrogel lens to

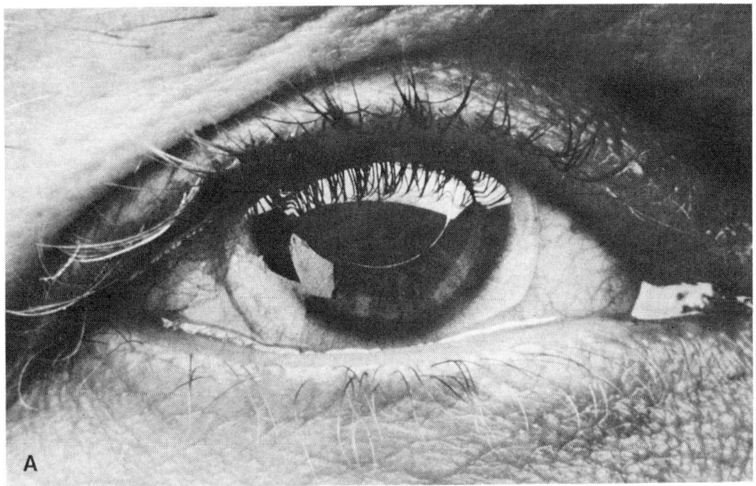

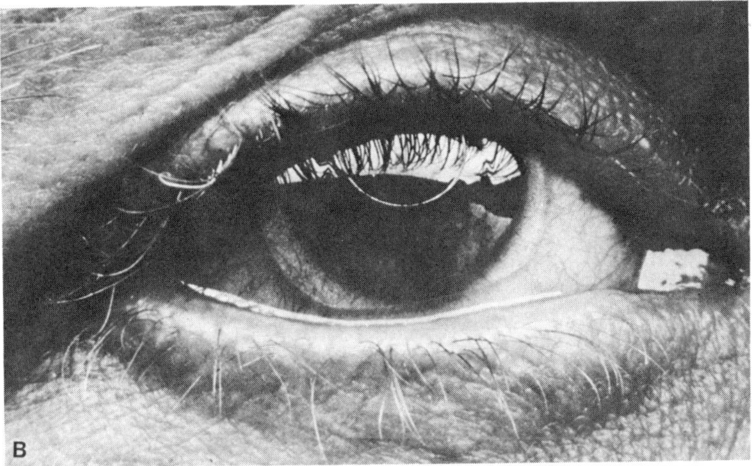

Figure 5-13 Fitting of crescent segment alternating vision hydrogel bifocals. (*A*) This bifocal lens is centered correctly with the distance vision portion completely covering the pupil in straight-ahead gaze. (*B*) This bifocal is positioned too high on the cornea in straight-ahead gaze. The margin between the distance and near vision segments of the lens crosses the pupil. (Courtesy of Wesley-Jessen, Division of Schering Corp)

translate on the eye, the patient should be refitted with an alternative form of presbyopic correction.

PATIENT SELECTION FOR BIFOCAL CONTACT LENSES

The success of fitting any bifocal contact lens depends on the ability of the practitioner to select the appropriate patient. Success rates of over 80% have been claimed with the correct patient selection procedures.[32,34] Generally, however, the success with rigid bifocal contact lenses measured in terms of good physiology, long wearing time with comfort, and satisfactory vision at all distances has been relatively small.[15] Unfortunately, at this stage of development, hydrogel bifocal contact lenses are also difficult to fit and may never be as simple as single vision lenses.[5,24,36] The criteria for selecting a good bifocal soft lens candidate are the following:

1. *High motivation.* It is essential that any patient contemplating the use of bifocal contact lenses in either rigid or hydrogel materials should have sufficient motivation. The necessary adaptation to all bifocal lens forms will tend to reduce patient motivation with time, so it is essential that initial motivation is high.[20,27] It is essential in selecting a patient that the motivation is not simply for "bifocals" but is a distinct preference for bifocal contact lenses.[17] Patients whose only reason for wearing bifocal contact lenses is to get rid of glasses should understand that they may exchange one set of problems with spectacles for a new set of problems with contact lenses.[28]

2. *Previous contact lens wearers.* A patient who has already adjusted to wearing soft or hard contact lenses, and who has reached the age of presbyopia, is already a candidate for bifocal contact lenses.[56,57] The contact lens patient who is particularly appropriate for bifocal lenses is the patient who cannot obtain satisfactory vision with spectacles, for example, the presbyopic keratoconic patient.[57]

3. *Refractive error.* Younger patients with low degrees of presbyopia are somewhat easier to fit than older presbyopes because they are younger and more adaptable to the new lens form. In addition, they may be more aware of the cosmetic appeal of bifocal contact lenses. Patients who have sufficient refractive error to require contact lenses for distance and near are often the best candidates for bifocal contact lenses.[20,28] It is unfortunate that in the present stage of development, no bifocal contact lens is available that will correct for astigmatism.

4. *Occupational requirement.* The ideal bifocal contact lens patient has low demand for near vision, for example, a homemaker.[17,20,33,58] A patient who has a long-term requirement for close near vision, for example, an accountant, a CRT operator, or a secretary, may find the limitations in visual field and stability of near vision in bifocal contact lenses unacceptable.

5. *Cosmesis.* Most patients seeking bifocal contact lenses do so because of the hope of improving their physical appearance. This can be a valuable motivating factor, with the desire to avoid the appearance of aging provided by wearing reading spectacles. In addition, however, some patients are particularly motivated because of occupational needs for a presbyopic correction in contact lens form. These include actors, dancers, and fashion models.[56,57]

6. *Monovision failures.* Patients who have tried monovision correction and have failed to adapt to the monocular visual circumstance may be ideal candidates for bifocal contact lenses.

7. *Realistic expectations.* The correct education of the patient so that the limitations of bifocal contact lenses are fully understood is essential to prepare the patient for the type of vision that will be experienced.[20,53] There is usually some compromise at distance or near vision with bifocal contact lenses.[2,29,30,34,58] The patient with very critical visual requirements is probably not suited to bifocal contact lenses.[20,28,58]

8. *Physiological factors.* These can be divided into several factors that must be considered in fitting certain types of bifocal contact lenses. These are pupil size and lid characteristics.

Pupil size is the most important patient characteristic in fitting simultaneous vision bifocal lenses. Smaller pupils reduce flare or glare effects, but may also cause problems in providing sufficient pupil area to provide simultaneous entry for distance and near vision rays.[20,22] Changes in pupil size may also affect the functioning of simultaneous bifocals during wear. For this reason it is essential that pupil size be measured in normal illumination levels and not under the full glare of the slit lamp.

Lid characteristics, specifically tension and position, are the most important aspects affecting alternating vision bifocal lenses.[20] In a patient with loose lids, the lens may fit beneath the lower lid. In such patients, translation may not be achieved. On the other hand, very tight lids may create too much lift on the lens, resulting in the near vision segment covering the pupil in the primary position of gaze. This will cause diplopia and unacceptable distance vision for the patient.[20,22,23] The position of the lower lid in relation to the limbus is also important with alternating bifocal lens designs. A very low position of the lower lid below the limbal region may not provide sufficient support for the bifocal lens to facilitate translation. The lid aperture size in the vertical direction is also of critical importance in fitting alternating bifocal lenses. A small aperture size may produce insufficient lens movement and inadequate lens translation for near vision.

Taking account of these eight factors, it is possible to match the patient to a particular type of bifocal contact lens with which they are most likely to be successful. Bifocal contact lenses provide a valuable source of practice building, but at the present state of development, no one lens of any type, whether alternating or simultaneous in either the rigid or hydrogel materials, is likely to fit all patients.[13] For these reasons a specialist contact lens practice intending to fit the majority of bifocal patients with the optimum success rate requires the availability of bifocal lenses of all types.

REFERENCES

1. Akiyama K: Study of contact lenses for presbyopia. Contacto 4(5):149, 1960
2. Andrasko GJ: Bifocal soft lenses: A comparison. Contact Lens Forum 9(9):53, 1984
3. Bailey NJ: Contact lens update—2. Contact Lens Forum 7(2):29, 1982
4. Bailey NJ: Contact lens update. Contact Lens Forum 8(2):25, 1983
5. Bailey NJ: Contact lens update. Contact Lens Forum 9(2):31, 1984

6. Bier N, Lowther GE: Contact Lens Correction, 1st ed, a, p318; b, p319. London, Butterworths, 1977

7. Black CJ: Symposium on Contact Lenses, 1st ed, pp 82–87. St. Louis, Mosby, 1973

8. Borish IM, Soni S: Bifocal contact lenses. J Am Optom Assoc 53(3):219, 1982

9. Breger JL: Clinical observation in the use of progressive addition contact lenses for presbyopia. Contacto 25(3):23, 1981

10. Bronstein L: Review of bifocal contact lenses. Optom Weekly 59(25):45, 1968

11. Charman MN: Power variation across concentric multifocal contact lenses. Int Contact Lens Clin 10(5):301, 1983

12. Cohen AL: An improved bifocal lens design. Contact Lens Forum 9(11):21, 1984

13. Davis RL: The bifocal contact lens: A new era. Optom Mgt 18(10):71, 1982

14. Feinbloom W: Patent No. 2129305, U.S. Patent Bureau, Sept. 6, 1938

15. Filderman I, White P: Contact Lens Practice and Patient Management, 1st ed pp 125–135. Philadelphia, Chilton, 1969

16. Fleischman WE: The single vision reading contact lens. Am J Optom Physiol Opt 45(6):408, 1968

17. Girard LJ, Soper JW, Sampson W: Corneal Contact Lenses, 1st ed, pp 294–299. St Louis, CV Mosby, 1964

18. Goldberg JB: Clinical management of the VFL variable focus lens. Contact Lens Forum 2(7):27, 1977

19. Goldberg JB: Aspheric multifocals useable vision zone. Contact Lens Forum 7(10):53, 1982

20. Gwin L: Clinical experience with bifocal soft lenses. Contacto Mini Abstracts 28(1):19, 1984

21. Hales R: Contact Lenses, A Clinical Approach to Fitting, 1st ed, pp 131–134. Baltimore, Williams & Wilkins, 1978

22. Hartstein J: Q & A on Contact Lens Practice, 2nd ed, pp 65–70. St Louis, CV Mosby, 1973

23. Haynes PR: Encyclopedia of Contact Lens Practice: The Fitting of Bifocal Contact Lenses, 1st ed, a, p19; b, p20; c, p24; d, p25; e, p32; f, p35; g, p36; h, p42. South Bend, IN, Encyclopedia of Contact Lens Practice, 1959

24. Health Product Research, Vision Care Survey, 3rd quarter, 1983

25. Hersh J: A novel modality for management of presbyopic contact lens patients. Opt J Rev Optom 106(6):35, 1938

26. Hirst G: Recent developments in hard and hydrophilic aspheric contact lenses, and the use of toric and bifocal hydrophilic lenses. Contacto 24(1):35, 1980

27. Hodur NR: Who should wear soft bifocals. Rev Opt 120(4):47, 1983

28. Jones GH: Fitting the crescent seg bifocal. Contact Lens Forum 9(1):88, 1984

29. Josephson JE, Caffrey B, Pope CA: Bausch and Lomb bifocal hydrogel lens. Contacto 26(6):33, 1982

30. Jurkus J: Bifocals go soft..Rev Optom 120(4):46, 1983

31. Kendall CA: Ultrafocal bifocal contact lens. Contracto 20(1):31, 1976

32. Krajewski RF: Fitting and evaluation of the multifocal aspheric contact lens. Contact Lens J 11(2):22, 1977

33. Kreshon MJ: Fitting the B&L bifocal soft lens. Contact Lens Forum 8(2):49, 1983

34. Lowther GE: Clinical evaluation of a hydrogel bifocal contact lens. Int Contact Lens Clin 9(4):218, 1982

35. Lowther GE: Personal communications, 1984
36. Mandell RB: Contact Lens Practice, 3rd ed, a, p707; b, p708; c, p709; d, p711; e, p715. Springfield, IL, Charles C Thomas, 1981
37. Mazlow B: The pupilens: A preliminary report. Contacto 25(2):128, 1958
38. Meier A, Lowther GE: Measured power distribution across the Bausch and Lomb Soflens PA1 bifocal. J Am Optom Assoc 54(3): 263, 1983
39. Morrison RJ: Morrison Contact Lens Laboratory Fitting Manual. Harrisburg, Pa, 1959
40. Neefe CW: Physiological optics of multifocal aspheric contact lenses. Contact Lens J 10(4):3, 1977
41. Neefe CW: Aspheric multifocals: A major breakthrough. Contact Lens Forum 2(5):44, 1977
42. Neefe CW: Prescribing bifocal lenses. Contact Lens Forum 4(7):19, 1979
43. Neefe CW: Soft bifocal lenses. Contacto 26(2):28, 1982
44. Ong J, Burley WS: Effect of induced anisometropia on depth perception. Am J Optom 49(4):333, 1972
45. Paris Softsite Contact Lens, Inc., Softsite Bifocal Fitting Guide
46. Resler PE: The autofocal lens and esophoria. Contacto 20(1):29, 1976
47. Salvatori AL: Soft lens bifocal design considerations. Contact Lens Forum 7(10):37, 1982
48. Schwartz CA: The saga of the DuraSoft TruFocal. Contact Lens Forum 8(11):61, 1983
49. Titmus Eurocon, Fitting Guide W38E (tefilcon) Hydrophilic Bifocal Contact Lens
50. Tomlinson A, Bibby M: Movement and rotation of soft contact lenses: Effect of fit and lens design. Am J Optom Physiol Opt 57(5):275, 1980
51. Tomlinson A: Succeeding with toric soft lenses. Rev Optom 120(7):71, 1983
52. U.S. Department of Commerce, 1980 Census Report
53. Van Horn PL: Offer guidelines on fitting bifocal lenses. Optom Times 2(3):21, 1984
54. Weinstock FJ: Aspheric multifocal contact lenses. Contact Intraocular Lens Med J 5(1):90, 1979
55. Wesley NK: A new concept in successful bifocal contact lens fitting. Contacto 11(1):71, 1967
56. Williams B: A new hard bifocal lens design. Contacto 20(5):34, 1976
57. Williams B: Fitting aspheric base curve multifocals. Contact Lens Forum 4(7):25, 1979
58. Williams B: Multifocal hard contact lens. Contacto 24(3):15, 1980
59. Williamson-Noble FA: Contact lenses: What of the future? Optician 8:244, 1951

CHAPTER SIX

THERAPEUTIC CONTACT LENSES

JAMES V. AQUAVELLA

The concept of wound binding or applying a bandage to an injured or diseased area of the body probably dates to prehistoric times. The first recorded instance of a bandage specifically for the eye is that of Celsus, who applied a dressing of honey-soaked linen directly to the inferior fornix to prevent the development of symblepharon.[11]

Applying a true "ocular bandage" was revived by Ridley in the second quarter of the 20th century.[21] With meticulous fitting, he was able to use methylmethacrylate "shells" as protective devices in a variety of corneal conditions. Wichterle and Lim reported the use of a cross-linked hydrophilic polymer for contact lenses in 1960.[25] Gassett and Kaufman used this "bandage lens" therapy in a variety of corneal conditions.[17] Since 1970, a number of investigators have contributed to our present concept of therapeutic uses of contact lenses. Such therapy represents a significant addition to the treatment of corneal disease.

The first lenses used by Ridley were compression molded, hard plastic made directly from a cast of the individual eye to be treated. With meticuluous fitting, there was no pooling of fluids and metabolic debris in the interface, fluid exchange being accomplished by blinking as well as by capillarity. Currently, most of the therapeutic lenses employed in ophthalmology are composed of soft materials. However, recent developments of highly oxygen permeable hard materials have created a resurgence of interest in hard shells.

COMPOSITION

The plastic shells used by Ridley were composed of polymethylmethacrylate (PMMA), a synthetic polymer formed by the linear addition of small units (monomer) condensed together to produce a high molecular-weight polymeric chain. Polymerization often is initiated by the addition of a small amount of free radical forming reagent as a catalyst. When more than one monomer is involved (co-polymerization), their appearance in the polymeric chain may be on a completely random basis or may be deliberately structured so that the frequency of component monomer units, as well as their sequence of distribution, is deliberate.[19] A close relationship exists between the inherent chemical composition of the polymer and its physical properties. The ultimate clinical performance of the bandage lens is directly related to one or more specific polymeric properties.

The solubility of the given polymer in a particular solvent may be altered by co-polymerization, and by the extent and nature of the cross-linking.

The property of permeability in hydrophilic polymers depends upon initial solution in the membrane and secondary diffusion. The resistance to diffusion is inversely proportional to the size of the diffusing molecule. This is significant in the use of topical medications in patients who are wearing bandage lenses. The rate of diffusion of the instilled drug molecule through the hydrophilic polymer will proceed according to the general physical rules. It is possible to use bandage lenses as a vehicle for sustained release of medication.

PHYSICAL PROPERTIES

The physical properties, chemical composition, architectural configuration, and specific fitting relationship of the lens to the cornea will determine performance.[4,15] Variations in lens diameter, curvature, thickness, and sagittal depth will produce a variety of fitting situations, which may alter performance. (Fig. 6-1).

In the United States, a number of hydrophilic lenses currently are available for use as bandage lenses. The Bausch & Lomb Soflens and the American Optical Softcon lens were the first to be utilized. They contained 38% and 55% water, respectively. Currently, both thin-membrane lenses and high water content (70% to 85% water) lenses are available and being used as well.

MANUFACTURING TECHNIQUES

The spin-cast process is used by Bausch & Lomb to manufacture its Soflens.[24] In this process, the monomer–polymer cross-linkage agent mixture is poured into its spinning mold while it is polymerized. Only a concave mold is used and the posterior ocular surface of the lens assumes the shape, which varies according to the speed of rotation, the viscosity of the material, and the rate of polymerization. To design the actual contact lens, a combination of mold cord diameter and radius of curvature is selected. Spin speeds and volume of polymer injected are calculated to give the desired values of the finished back vertex power and lens thickness.[14]

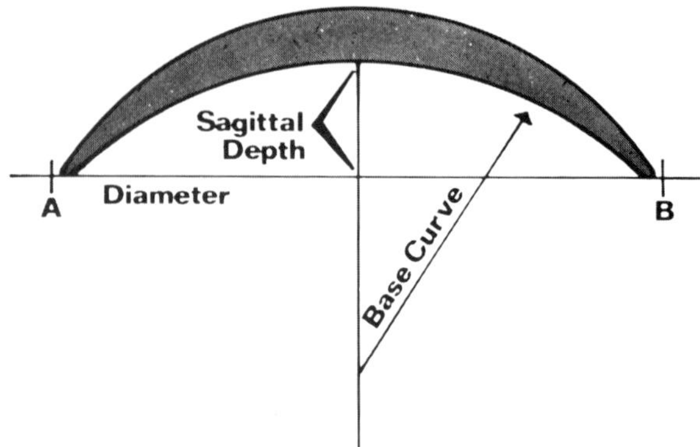

Figure 6-1 The fixed relationship between the diameter and base curve of a contact lens creates a specific sagittal depth. Modifications in the diameter, the base curve, or the sagittal depth will result in altered fitting parameters. However, the sagittal depth may be maintained with modification of both the diameter and the base curve.

The volume of liquid used and the sagittal depth of the mold control the thickness of the soft lens. Slow spin speeds of the mold produce flat lenses with long radii of curvature (oblate), whereas higher spin speeds result in a steeper lens of relatively short radii of curvature (prolate) (Fig. 6-2).

Lathe cutting currently is used by most of the manufacturers of hydrophilic and oxygen-permeable lenses (Fig. 6-3). The hydrophilic material first is polymerized as a rod of plastic.[5] Rods are then cut into buttons, machined, polished, and ultimately allowed to hydrate. Hydration is accompanied by dimensional changes, which proceed according to a fixed formula. The finished product is then stored in buffered 0.9% saline solution. Recently, the lathing process has been automated in an attempt to increase the yield and reduce cost. A cast-molding manufacturing technique currently is being used by some manufacturers.

SPECIFIC LENS CHARACTERISTICS

Despite the ready availability of a large variety of hydrophilic and oxygen-permeable contact lens materials manufactured in a wide range of diameters, curvatures, and thicknesses, lenses specifically approved for therapeutic purposes are limited. The market for therapeutic contact lenses is small and many manufacturers are reluctant to assume the cost of Food and Drug Administration approval. Bausch & Lomb has obtained therapeutic approval for their Plano T, Plano B, Plano U, and Plano O series lenses. All of the lenses are manufactured from Polymacon polymer, which contains 38.6% water. The Plano T lens has a center thickness of 0.17 mm and is manufactured in a base curve of 8.1 mm and a diameter of 14.5 mm. The B series lens is slightly thinner (central thickness, 0.12 mm) and flatter (base curve, 8.8 mm), although it maintains a 14.5-mm diameter. These two lenses have been largely replaced by the U and O series. The U series lenses

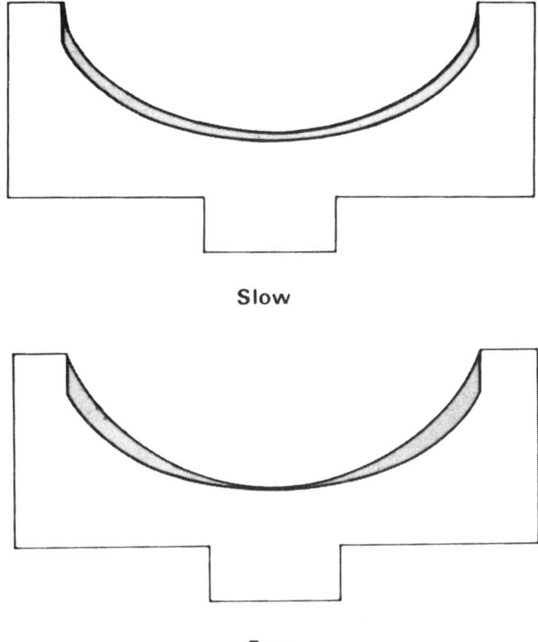

Figure 6-2 Diagram of spin-cast process resulting in either steep or flat lens curvature.

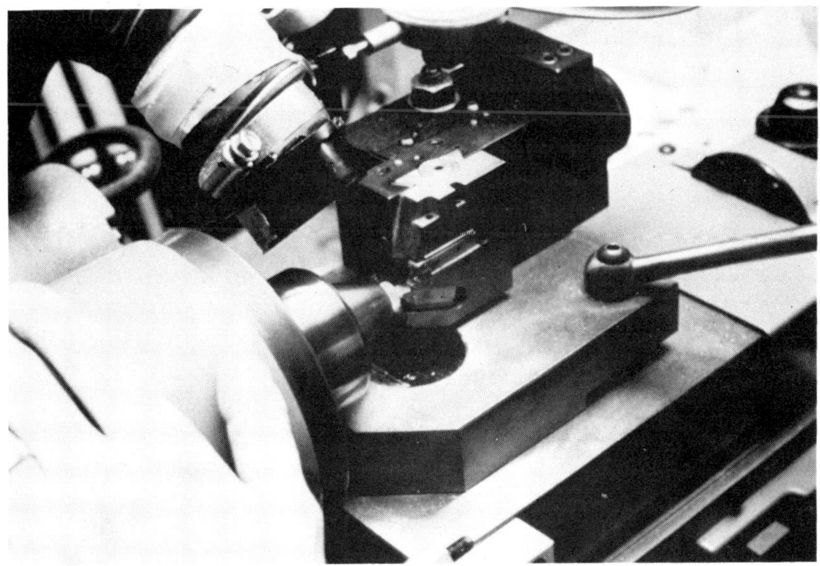

Figure 6-3 Standard lathing process for manufacturing lathe-cut hydrophilic lenses.

are very thin (center thickness, 0.07 mm) and are available in 8.5- and 8.6-mm base curves with diameters of 12.5 or 13.5 mm. The O series has a central thickness of 0.06 mm and is manufactured with a base curve of 8.8 mm and a single diameter of 14.5 mm.

The CSI therapeutic lens manufactured by Syntex is a very thin membrane lens of 38.6% water. It is available in two diameters, 13.8 mm and 14.8 mm, and a variety of base curves from 8.3 mm to 9.3 mm.

The Softcon lens currently manufactured by American Optical has a medium water content of 55%. The original bandage lens was available with a center thickness of 0.35 mm and a variety of base curves from 7.8 mm through 8.7 mm and two diameters (13.5 mm and 14.5 mm). Current models are thinner.

Of the third generation materials, two are approved for therapeutic purposes. Permalens, manufactured by CooperVision, has approximately 71% water and a central thickness of 0.15 mm. It is available in a single base curve (9.0 mm) and a single 15.0 mm diameter. The Softlon/PW lens, manufactured by American Medical Optics, has a 79% water content and a central thickness of 0.18 mm. It is available in a diameter of 14.4 mm with base curves ranging from 8.1 mm through 8.7 mm. More recently, the Revlens, manufactured by Biocontacts, has been submitted for FDA approval. It is composed of a soft acrylic rubber polymer and is less than 1% water by weight, but has a high intrinsic oxygen permeability of 10.4×10^{-9} cm/s. It is available in a 14 mm diameter with a central thickness of 0.15 mm, and is manufactured in base curves ranging from 7.7 mm to 8.9 mm. It is relatively rigid and has been advocated particularly for patients with dry eye problems.

In fitting a therapeutic lens, one should be concerned primarily with the stability, curvature, thickness, and refractive power of the lens selected. Stability is largely a function of diameter. The larger the diameter, the greater the adherence or stability. The stability of the thin-membrane lenses is enhanced by reduced weight.

The curvature of the lens also affects stability. With a smaller radius of curvature (steeper), the lens will exhibit more adherence and stability, whereas with a larger radius (flatter), it will exhibit less adherence and less stability. By varying the geometric relationship between the lens and the underlying cornea, one can achieve great variations in effect.

There are certain basic guidelines for good hydrophilic bandage lens fitting. The lens must center well on the cornea and not tend to decenter with blinking or ocular rotations. Secondly, the lens selected must be comfortable. The presence of a topical anesthetic may mask a basically uncomfortable lens. The edges of the lens should be examined under the slit lamp. Edges that tend to flare may cause increased sensation with blinking, whereas if the edges adhere too tightly, a tight lens syndrome may develop (Figs. 6-4, 6-5).

A large, flat-fitting lens that centers well probably will do the job in most instances. For this reason, many therapeutic lenses are manufactured in one

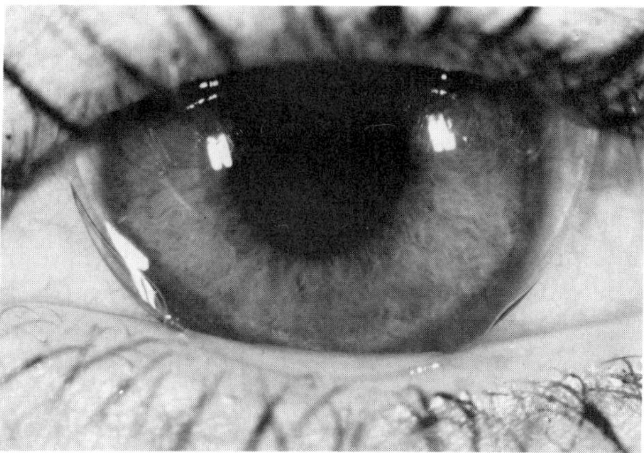

Figure 6-4 A loose-fitting contact lens with the edges flared.

single large diameter. If a painful epithelial defect is present, a slightly steeper fitting lens with a larger interface area may be more comfortable. These large, steep lenses are versatile, but they can produce edema and may have to be changed for a flatter fitting lens as therapy progresses.

ANCILLARY THERAPY

One should not be intimidated by the presence of the lens. The underlying corneal pathology must be treated with the appropriate medications. Antibiotics, steroids, antivirals, and glaucoma medications are employed routinely as indicated in each case.

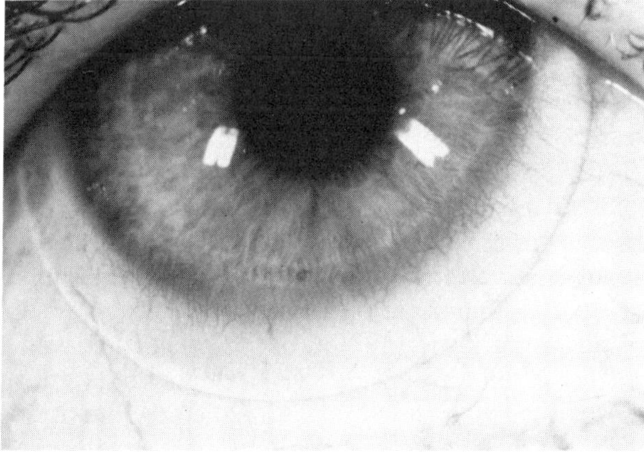

Figure 6-5 A tight-fitting contact lens that does not move with ocular rotations.

Chronic blepharitis, often associated with a variety of chronic corneal problems, may create a hostile environment for the bandage lens. It should be treated vigorously, both prior to and concurrent with bandage lens therapy.

If tear formation is inadequate, a hydrophilic bandage lens will tend to dry out on the corneal surface. Artificial tears or saline solution must be instilled frequently to maintain the hydration of the lens and the underlying cornea. Occasionally, punctum occlusion is of benefit. The use of ultrasonic humidifiers to increase the humidity in the patient's immediate environment also has been of benefit, as have been moist chamber goggles. The selection of a polymer that does not require hydration also has been advocated.

In the presence of lid and conjunctival defects, adequate surgical correction must precede lens fitting if the lens is to be maintained. Thus, symblepharon must be severed or it probably will interfere with wearing the lens. If the palpebral fissure is too wide, a partial tarsorrhaphy may be necessary to support the lens therapy.

Most cases treated with bandage lenses will have some anterior chamber reaction, although it may be difficult to observe through the diseased cornea. Thus, cycloplegics are often used at the onset of therapy and should be continued for the first several days. I advocate the use of standard ophthalmic preparations containing preservatives. The use of medications without preservatives bears an intolerable risk for secondary infection.[8] In many instances, the bandage lens will be worn continuously day and night until the desired therapeutic goal has been achieved. This is particularly true with the higher water content lenses. Although healing can be monitored adequately with a slit lamp without the necessity of removing the lens, it may be desirable to remove the lens during therapy. This usually is accomplished for purposes of cleaning, replacement, refitting, study, or performing various diagnostic tests, such as measuring the intraocular pressure. In some instances, particularly if the lens is causing edema or if there is evidence of neovascularization, it may be desirable to switch to a regimen of insertion and removal.

If the epithelium is fragile, one should take great care to float the lens off by directing a stream of irrigating fluid at the lens margin. The lens may then be lifted off the cornea easily without injury to the underlying tissues. In each instance, the lens should be disinfected before being reapplied. In cases of poor tear formation or in the presence of active infection, it may be advisable to disinfect the lens periodically. In bullous keratopathy, lenses usually are worn for long periods, with routine cleaning and disinfection carried out at 3- to 6-month intervals. In the absence of adequate tear flow, the use of a prophylactic antibiotic is indicated along with disinfection of the lens. Lid scrubs and overall good hygiene are important adjuncts. The bandage lens is not a substitute for routine therapy, but it should be considered the focal point of a comprehensive therapeutic regime.

INDICATIONS FOR BANDAGE LENS THERAPY

There are multiple indications for therapeutic soft contact lenses.[18] They are as follows:

Medical Indications for Hydrophilic Bandage Lenses

Chronic corneal edema

Abrasions, erosions, ulcerations

Filamentary keratitis

Chemical keratitis

Neurotropic keratitis

Neuroparalytic keratitis

Herpes simplex keratitis (stromal disease)

Dry eye syndromes

Ectatic dystrophies

Anterior membrane corneal dystrophies

Entropion, trichiasis, lid defects

Surgical Indications for Hydrophilic Bandage Lenses

Postoperative discomfort

Lacerations

Perforations

Penetrating keratoplasty

Lamellar keratoplasty

Keratectomy

Thermokeratoplasty

A few of the more important conditions will be discussed in this chapter. The three major symptoms indicating bandage lens therapy are pain, reduced visual acuity, and objective corneal pathology. Reduced acuity often relates to anterior regular astigmatism associated with a specific disease entity, or with defects in the tear film, corneal epithelium, or the underlying stroma. Pain relief is afforded in a high percentage of cases where the bandage lens is utilized.[3,6] In those cases where bandage lens therapy could be maintained, approximately 70% show some improvement in the appearance of the corneal lesion as a result of wearing the bandage lens.

Bullous keratopathy is one of the major indications for bandage lens therapy. Nevertheless, one should exhaust traditional means of therapy before inserting the bandage lens. If there is no hope for visual rehabilitation, one has to weigh the long-term effects of bandage lens therapy and give adequate consideration to definitive treatment, such as a conjunctival flap, which does not require support for an indefinite period.

Simple acute corneal abrasions and erosions are best treated by application of a pressure patch. If the epithelial defect persists and pain is a significant problem, a hydrophilic bandage lens may be considered. In syndromes involving deficiencies in the basal epithelium/basement membrane complex, the bandage lens should be worn continuously for 8 to 12 weeks to afford adequate time for complete epithelial healing with a production of new basement membrane.[22] When the bandage lens therapy is discontinued, it is wise to prepare the patient for the possibility of recurrence of the disease. Topical instillation of artificial tear solutions and nighttime use of emollients or hypertonic saline ointment should be maintained for several days following removal of the bandage lens. Lens removal should be planned for a time convenient for both patient and physician, in anticipation of a possible recurrence.

In primary or secondary filamentary keratitis, the application of a hydrophilic bandage lens can afford rapid relief and effect a lasting cure. In herpes simplex keratitis, the use of the lens is usually associated with recurrent stromal disease and persistent epithelial defects.

In the dry eye syndromes, using hydrophilic lenses is not without risk. The incidence of success with these lenses in any of the dry eye syndromes is low in comparison with that evidenced in bullous keratopathy. Nevertheless, when the bandage lens is used as part of a comprehensive therapeutic regimen, it can be an important adjunct. The bandage lens does not eliminate the necessity for frequent application of artificial tear solutions and may require additional topical medication. Moist chamber goggles, punctum occlusion, solid tear substitutes, and environmental humidification are important aspects of a comprehensive therapeutic regimen.

In neuroparalytic keratitis, it is often necessary to reduce the size of the interpalpebral fissure by partial tarsorrhaphy to prevent excessive evaporation and repeated loss of the lens. In addition, patients with dry eyes show a very high incidence of lensopathy.[23]

Hydrophilic bandage lenses should be available in every ophthalmic operating room.[7] They can be inserted immediately following completion of anterior segment ophthalmic surgery performed in infants and young children. The standard protocol for epikeratoplasty calls for a bandage lens. The lenses afford relief from discomfort and facilitate examining the eye postoperatively. Descemetoceles or small corneal perforations without incarceration of uveal tissue may be treated by bandage lens application (Fig. 6-6). A relatively tight-fitting bandage lens often results in rapid reformation of the anterior chamber. On occasion, no further therapy is necessary. The application of the lens is followed by swelling and coaptation of the wound margins. Ultimately, secondary healing ensues. Even when surgical intervention will be necessary, the initial application of a lens enables surgery to be delayed for several hours. Cyanoacrylate adhesive may be applied before inserting the bandage lens (Fig. 6-7). In these instances, the glue must be allowed to polymerize and harden prior to the insertion of the lens.

In penetrating keratoplasty in infants and young children, the application of the bandage lens on the operating table has been a welcome adjunct.

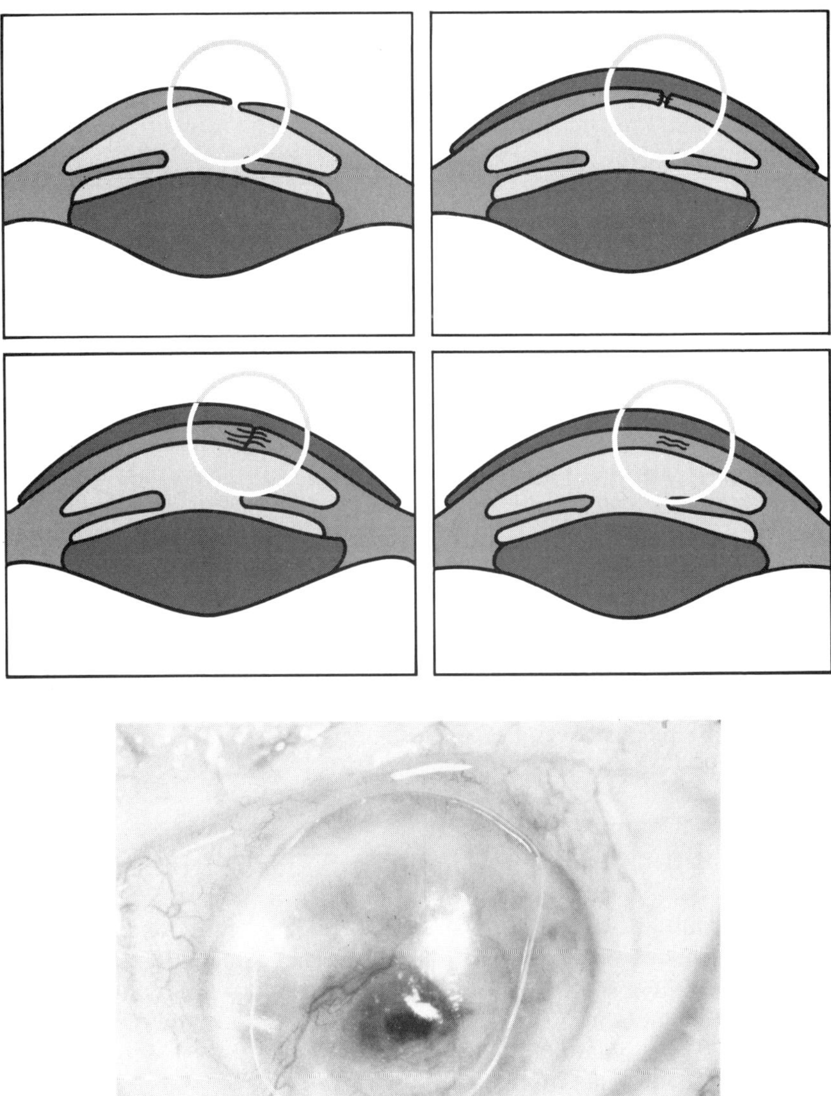

Figure 6-6 (*A*) Diagram showing small corneal perforation (*upper left*). A hydrophilic bandage lens has been applied (*upper right*). This results in coaptation of the wound margins (*lower left*). Ultimately, the corneal tissue heals (*lower right*). (*B*) Clinical example of a corneal perforation treated with a hydrophilic bandage lens. Note the large air bubble in the lens–cornea interface.

Discomfort, blepharospasm, and excess lacrimation all are reduced, and observation and examination are greatly simplified. Another widely held indication for immediate application of a bandage lens in penetrating keratoplasty is chemical keratitis where preservation of donor epithelium is desirable.

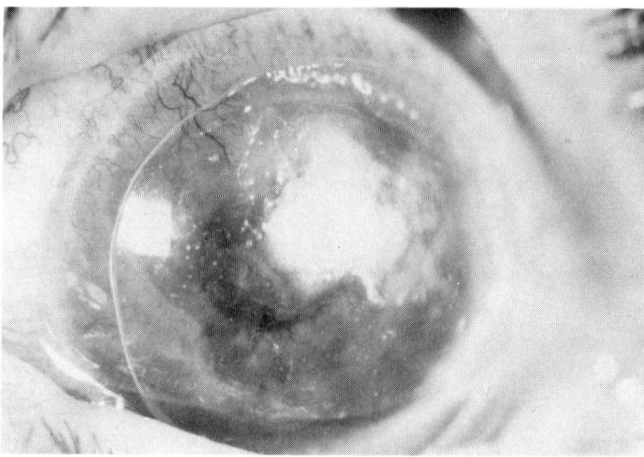

Figure 6-7 A hydrophilic bandage lens applied over cyanoacrylate glue used to treat corneal perforation. Note the large air bubble on the lens–cornea interface.

In lamellar keratoplasty, keratectomy, and epikeratoplasty, application of the bandage lens during the surgical procedure results in a comfortable eye. When using bandage lenses following keratoplasty, one should recall the increased risk for a secondary infection. This is particularly true in the aged, in eyes that have had multiple surgical procedures, and in innervationally deficient eyes. In most instances, the patient should be weaned from the bandage lens as soon as practical.

CONTRAINDICATIONS

The contraindications for hydrophilic bandage lens therapy are the presence of active microbial infection, the lack of adequate follow-up capability, and the inability of the patient to manage lens therapy. Every patient fitted with a hydrophilic bandage lens must have access to ophthalmological care as soon as possible should a problem arise, and must be able to remove the lens or have it removed without serious delay.

INHERENT LENS CHARACTERISTICS

One of the most important characteristics of a good bandage lens relates to its ability to transport fluid and oxygen to the diseased underlying cornea. The fluid permeability of hydrophilic lenses varies from 38% with first generation lenses, through 55% with second generation lenses, to approximately 80% in so-called third generation high-water polymers. It has generally been accepted that a higher fluid content is important in a good bandage lens. This may not hold true for lenses used to treat dry eyes. High fluid content lenses are associated with greater oxygen transmissibility. Some of the harder hydrophobic materials have very high oxygen permeabilities,

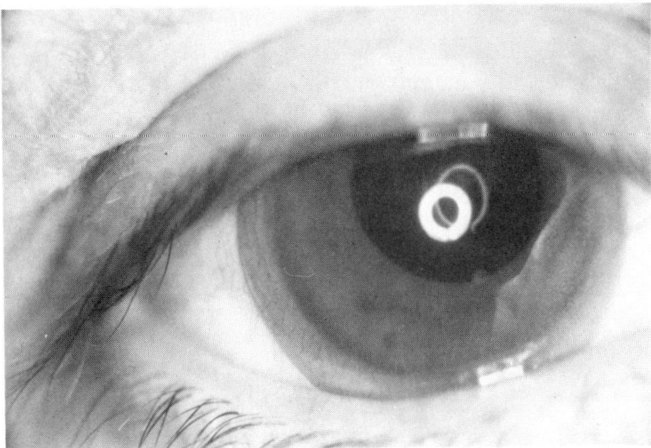

Figure 6-8 Badly discolored hydrophilic lens as a result of treatment with epinephrine.

which may be important in the healing process, whereas most hydrophilic polymers have a relatively low degree of specific gas permeability. Nevertheless, for any given hydrophilic material, the values of fluid and oxygen transmission will be greater as the thickness of the lens decreases.

Primarily because of their larger diameter, properly fitted hydrophilic bandage lenses are not readily lost. Lenses do have a limited life span, which can vary from a few weeks (particularly in the dry eye or neuroparalytic cases) to 1 year or more. Other factors that affect the durability of the lenses relate to damage from handling, instrumentation, or effects of topical medication. Fluorescein and epinephrine products are well known to discolor the lenses (Fig. 6-8). Long-term administration of topical medications ultimately will result in browning and discoloration of the lens. Lensopathies are caused by the deposition of insoluble material on the lens. These materials consist of calcium, mucin, bacteria, or a combination of lipoproteinaceous debris (Fig. 6-9). The deposition is related in part to the surface

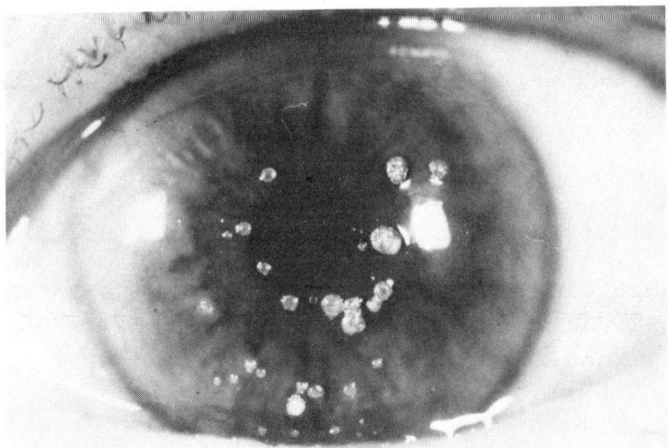

Figure 6-9 Example of lens debris that causes discomfort.

characteristics of the lens–tear film interface, as well as to the tendency for heavier particulate material to plug the pore structure of the hydrophilic polymer.[23] Periodic cleaning with a good surfacting lubricant is indicated. Enzyme cleaning solutions are also available. The use of 3% hydrogen peroxide for disinfection can have a dual beneficial effect in retarding the development of lensopathy. If the debris is relatively minor and is not associated with disturbances in visual acuity or discomfort, the deposits may be allowed to remain. In cases where prophylactic measures do not retard the development of debris and where debris produces side-effects, the simplest mechanism is to replace the lens. This is particularly true with the current low manufacturing cost.

PRINCIPLES OF THERAPEUTIC EFFICACY

A variety of properties of the hydrophilic bandage lenses are thought to be responsible for the therapeutic benefits derived.[2,8,9]

PERMEABILITY

Exchange of drugs and metabolites is not wholly dependent on the permeability of the lens. A pumping action, initiated by the blink reflex, occurs. The pressure of the upper lid tends to collapse the lens–cornea interface with an active expulsion of fluid contents. Secondarily, there occurs a relaxation of the upper lid pressure and active reformation of the interface. In very flat-fitting lenses, exchange also occurs by capillarity.

Topical medication applied over the surface of the lens does not cause concentration of the drug in the lens. For concentration to occur, the lens must be pre-soaked in the drug. In cases of protein debris binding to the lens surface, a concentration of commonly used solution preservatives may occur, resulting in epithelial toxicity and irritation. Although the epitheliopathy may be protracted, the routine instillation of standard ophthalmic preparations containing preservatives has not resulted in irreversible epithelial damage. A far greater danger exists when one dispenses topical medications without preservatives, increasing the risk of secondary infection and permanent corneal damage.

WETTING

The application of the hydrophilic bandage lens tends to trap the interface fluid and assists in assuring the constant wetting of the entire corneal epithelium. Although the contents of the interface are exchanged, a constant and uniform wetting of the entire corneal surface ensues. This is particularly important in cases of instability of the tear film and surface corneal irregularities. The dry eye syndromes are typical of such conditions.

Secondary concomitant blepharitis should be treated vigorously and topical artificial tears instilled as frequently as necessary to maintain hydration of the bandage lens (Fig. 6-10). Although the use of long-term prophylactic antibiotics has been criticized, many agree that prophylactic therapy is indicated in long-term treatment of dry eye syndromes when hydrophilic bandage lenses are used. If the lenses are to be worn 24 hours a day, weekly or biweekly removal of the lens followed by thorough cleaning and disinfection is advisable. Two lenses often are prescribed so that this process may be repeated more frequently while the second lens is on the eye. Superficial sterile infiltrates have been noted to develop under bandage lenses used to treat dry eye syndromes. Such infiltrates are of obscure etiology, but the presence of an active infection must be suspected. Every instance of an infiltrate or ulceration developing under a bandage lens must be examined immediately and treated as an infection until proven otherwise.

VISUAL ACUITY

When a bandage lens is applied, improvement in visual acuity may be related to deturgescence of the edematous corneal epithelium, as well as to replacement of the irregular surface with the smooth, uniform refracting surface provided by the bandage lens.[10] Topical instillation of hypertonic saline solution over the lens may then result in corneal deturgescence. With the control of discomfort, the elimination of glare, and reduction in epiphora and photophobia provided by the lens, visual acuity improves. Acuity can be assisted with either an ordinary plano lens, or a lens with specific power.

In a large series of cases of bullous keratopathy, over 70% of patients were able to achieve some improvement in visual acuity.[6] Eyes afflicted with deep stromal scarring, Descemet's folds with resulting posterior irregular astigma-

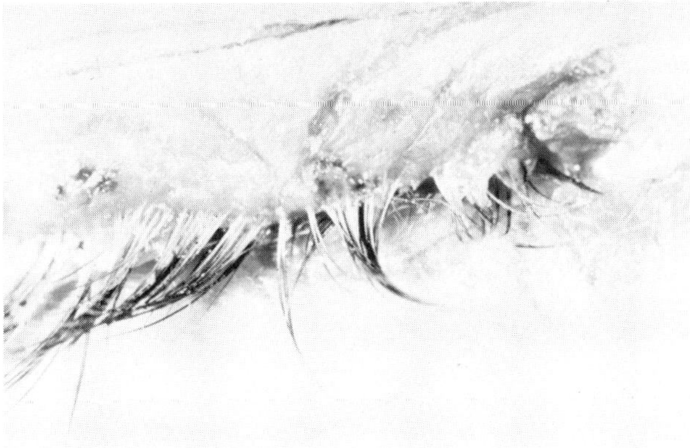

Figure 6-10 Chronic blepharitis, which is often associated with dry eye, may significantly interfere with fitting or wearing a hydrophilic bandage lens.

tism, glaucoma, and posterior segment disorders will not have improved vision.

In monocular aphakia, when fitting with an aphakic lens, the resultant acuity is often significantly better than that obtainable without the contact lens. In practical terms, the improved acuity is due as much to the refractive capacity of the contact lens as to the bandage quality of the lens.

Bandage lenses can be helpful in patients with keratoconus who are unable to wear standard methylmethacrylate contact lenses comfortably. A hydrophilic lens with overspectacle correction often can be maintained for a considerable period of time. Recently in keratoconus, I have used lenses composed of PMMA and silicone (Polycon). A "piggyback" hard lens over a soft cushion lens is possible (Fig. 6-11).[12] A similar system used a cushion lens with a hard lens fitted in a central depression (Flexlens).

Initial optimism was expressed concerning the potential for fitting aphakic hydrophilic bandage lenses following congenital cataract extraction.[16] There are no definitive reports of long-term prevention of amblyopia by using such therapy. One potential drawback is that such eyes are often very highly hyperopic and lenses of very high powers were not available. On occasion, two contact lenses have been fitted (piggyback) to the same eye to provide the necessary power.[6]

The ability to fit an aphakic hydrophilic lens to an eye for extended periods of time has resulted in this technique being offered as a substitute for intraocular lens implantation. It is possible for some patients to maintain extended wear aphakic lenses for periods of several weeks or months without removing them, but success is not uniform and the extended wear of aphakic lenses, particularly in diseased eyes, has not been uniformly successful. Currently, 85% to 90% of all patients undergoing cataract extraction receive an implant.

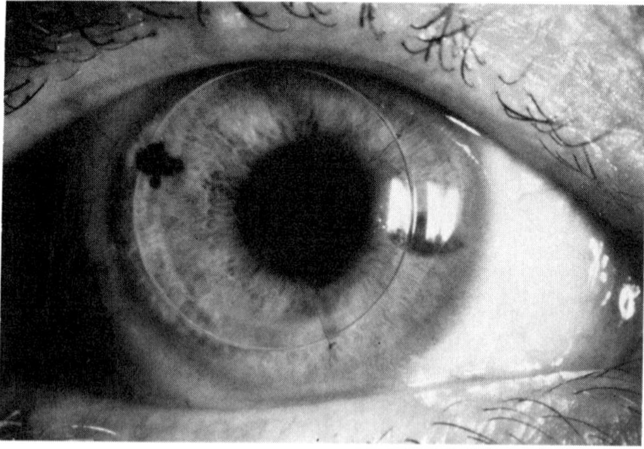

Figure 6-11 Piggyback lens. Note the margin of the large-diameter hydrophilic contact lens (cushion lens). An oxygen-permeable contact lens has been fitted in piggyback fashion.

PROTECTION

The application of a hydrophilic bandage lens protects the underlying cornea not only from desiccation and other effects of the environment, but from any traumatic effects due to the action of the lids and the lashes. Thus, damaged epithelium may heal under the protection afforded by the lens. Even with rapid reepithelialization, a certain amount of time is necessary for a strong bond to form between adjacent epithelial cells and between the basal epithelial cells and newly formed underlying basement membrane. During this period, the cells are particularly vulnerable to minor trauma. Thus, the continued protection by the hydrophilic lens in cases of recurrent erosion is necessary for several weeks.

The use of bandage lenses following alkaline burn or ulceration can prevent damage to corneal epithelium and secondary liberation of destructive collagenase.[13] Large-diameter bandage lenses are of value in protecting the cornea during surgical procedures for the correction of ptosis and lid defects. They may be used in cases of spastic entropion as a temporary measure to obtain comfort immediately prior to surgical repair (Fig. 6-12). In cases of exposure keratitis and filamentary keratitis, the protection of the cornea can result in rapid healing. Protection combined with preservation of tear film is a major reason for applying a hydrophilic bandage lens in postoperative keratoplasty to prevent epithelial drying.

SPLINTING

In instances of full thickness lacerations, perforations, and deep ulcerations, the overlying hydrophilic bandage lens functions as a splint. The body of the lens prevents buckling and distortion in the presence of blinking and blepharospasm. A certain amount of splinting is also afforded in the use of a bandage lens following keratoplasty and to correct a wound leak with shal-

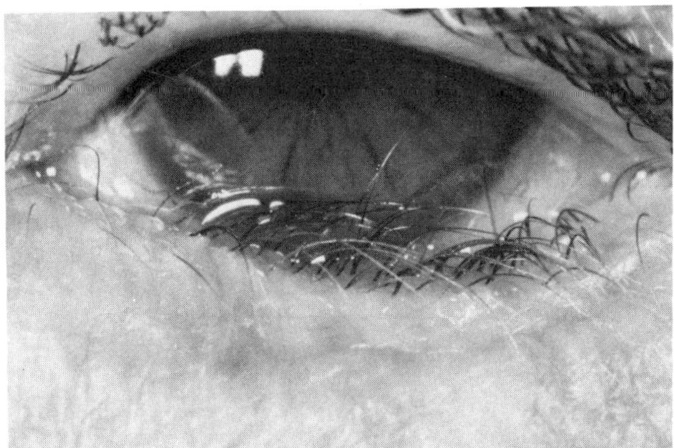

Figure 6-12 Spastic entropion with secondary corneal irritation. Symptomatic relief can be obtained with a hydrophilic bandage lens.

low anterior chamber following cataract extraction. For these purposes, slightly thicker, steep-fitting lenses are utilized. Prophylactic antibiotics, mydriatics, and carbonic anhydrase inhibitors also are indicated as part of the comprehensive therapy. The tight-fitting lens impedes the flow of aqueous through the lesion. Secondary swelling of stromal tissues seals off the leak with subsequent reformation of the anterior chamber. If the anterior chamber has not reformed within a reasonable period of time, adhesives or appositional sutures may be employed.

PAIN RELIEF

Bullous keratopathy, recurrent erosion, and filamentary keratitis are disruptions of the richly innervated epithelium. In these situations, the application of a bandage lens can afford truly dramatic relief. Any of the high water content thin bandages will work well, provided the fit is adequate. Regardless of the manufacturer, it is important to select a lens that centers well over the eye and does not move excessively with ocular rotation and blinking. Such motion can tend to abrade the epithelial surface further and result in secondary anterior uveitis. The combination of little lens movement with a relatively deep lens–cornea interface and prevention of apical touch is particularly suitable for pain relief in the short term. The addition of a cycloplegic during the first few days of therapy will make the situation more manageable by tending to reduce ciliary spasm. For long-term use, the lens that does not move on the surface of the eye can result in a tight lens syndrome.

When initiating bandage lens therapy, it is reasonable to insist that the lens be worn continuously 24 hours a day. Healing can be monitored with the slit lamp without removing the lens. The process of insertion and removal is an open invitation to secondary contamination and the introduction of bacterial elements into the system. Intraocular pressure can be measured reasonably well over the surface of a thin bandage lens, or more properly by rotating the lens off the central cornea for purposes of obtaining an accurate pressure.

Nevertheless, when the painful episode has stabilized, it may be advisable to switch to an intermittent form of contact lens wear. When modifications of the wearing schedule are indicated, they should be instituted. Arbitrary insistence on full-time wear is often not in the best interests of the patient.

DRUG DELIVERY

In the presence of a bandage lens, there is no real impediment to the delivery of medication to the underlying diseased cornea. Evidence indicates that those hydrophilic materials with a high water content may be better vehicles for delivering water-soluble medications. In any event, the rate of entry of the drug into the polymer and subsequent passage into the cornea will depend on the specific physical properties of the drug and the polymer as well as the surface characteristics of the lens–tear film interface, lens thickness, and the state of the lens surface at the time of instillation. Large molecules, such as viruses and bacteria, cannot enter the undamaged surface of the hydrophilic bandage lens. Drugs and topically applied substances, as well as bacteria and debris, may enter the lens–cornea interface by way of the pumping action.

Podos and co-workers have demonstrated that soaking hydrophilic bandages in philocarpine can result in an elevated therapeutic effect that lasts for prolonged periods.[20] Even in the absence of pre-soaking, a hydrophilic lens may actively accumulate the drug, subsequently presenting a uniform surface from which the medication may be pulsed into the cornea. The fundamentals of a versatile drug delivery system are certainly present. However, one would need to know the specific interaction of various drugs and their vehicles with the hydrophilic polymer in question before being able to use this therapy fully. By varying the composition of the polymer, the composition of the drug, the pH of the solution, and the nature of the vehicles and preservatives, an infinite number of dosage and release patterns are theoretically possible. It is also conceivable that the cornea and conjunctival surfaces could act as convenient sites for the administration of a number of drugs whose primary effect is systemic and unrelated to ocular therapy.

Drug delivery relates to the thickness of the lens being utilized. A thinner lens may be expected to allow a greater amount of topically applied drug to pass into the lens–cornea interface. On the other hand, a thicker lens might be expected to store a greater amount of the drug once the equilibrium state had been determined.

DISINFECTION OF HYDROPHILIC BANDAGE LENSES

When the bandage lenses are shipped from the manufacturers, they are in a sterile state, having been autoclaved as mandated by Food and Drug Administration requirements. Until recently, boiling was the only method of approved disinfection. The introduction of dry heat is an attempt to maintain the standards of heat disinfection set up by the Food and Drug Administration and yet eliminate many of the problems involved with boiling. Although both boiling and dry heat are undoubtedly efficacious as disinfection systems, they are certainly cumbersome for both practitioner and patient.

A more important consideration is proper surface cleaning, which may be accomplished by a number of commercially available surfacting cleaners as well as by hydrogen peroxide. The latter technique involves cleaning both surfaces of the lens with a surfacting lubricant, flushing the lens under running tap water, and maintaining the lens in a solution of 3% hydrogen peroxide for 10 minutes, following which the hydrogen peroxide must be eluted from the lens by rinsing with preserved buffered normal saline solution. Usually three or four rinses of a few minutes each in normal saline solution are sufficient to eliminate the hydrogen peroxide and return the lens to an environment of neutral stable *p*H. This will eliminate the sensation of stinging and irritation upon reinsertion. If the saline solution is warm, the process will be accelerated. With the hydrogen peroxide system, lenses may be completely disinfected and reinserted within 30 minutes. An additional benefit of the hydrogen peroxide system is to flex the structure of the polymer and assist in the flushing of the pore structure. Internal cleaning of the lens as well as surface disinfection are thus accomplished. To completely eliminate some spores and fungi, much longer periods of peroxide treatment are necessary. However, if the lens has been surface cleaned and flushed with running water, the potential number of organisms will be greatly reduced and limited exposure to peroxide (in the absence of protein debris) will be sufficient. A number of simplified hydrogen peroxide techniques are available today. Some use a catalytic converter to eliminate residual peroxide.

Cold disinfection systems involve surface cleaning and storage in a solution containing thimerosal, EDTA, chlorohexidine, ascorbate, and other preservatives. The lens is then rinsed with buffered normal saline solution before being inserted into the eye. In chronically inflamed and debilitated eyes, the thimerosal/chlorohexidine systems may be excessively toxic. The toxicity of preservation systems has come under close observation and an effort is being made to reduce the concentration of these drugs. Regardless of the system, it is important to recall that fingers (patient or physician) are the best vehicles for introducing contamination into the system. The hands should be washed well, rinsed, and dried before lens insertion.

COMPLICATIONS

It is important to be aware of the true complications arising from the use of hydrophilic contact lenses. In discussing this aspect, one must differentiate between the use of hydrophilic lenses for correcting refractive error and their use as a therapeutic bandage.

Over the past several years, millions of patients have been fitted with hydrophilic contact lenses for the correction of ametropia. These patients insert their lenses in the morning, wear the lenses essentially all waking hours, and remove them in the evening. Even the relatively new extended-wear lenses have now been worn in large numbers. Misuse of any contact lens, primarily through infrequent disinfection, faulty personal hygiene, or overwear can result in an increased incidence of minor corneal and conjunctival inflammatory episodes. When fitting normal healthy eyes, physicians must insist that products and systems be of low risk. In dealing with the possible complications ensuing through the therapeutic use of hydrophilic bandages, it is important to invoke the concept of risk versus benefit. Thus, in treating severe debilitating corneal disease, the benefits of hydrophilic bandage lens therapy may far outweigh the potential risk factor. It is clear that corneal infection is the major risk of extended wear lenses (Fig.

6-13). Most infected corneal ulcerations that occur in the United States are associated with contact lens wear.

Severe cases of neurotropic keratitis and Stevens–Johnson syndrome are characterized by the frequency of secondary infection due to the inadequacy of the defense mechanisms of the eye. When such a patient is fitted with a hydrophilic bandage lens and an infection occurs, it may be a direct complication. However, a certain percentage of these infections would have occurred in the absence of bandage lens therapy.

The main complications of bandage lens therapy are discomfort, intolerance, secondary infection, neovascularization, and lensopathy.

Lenses may be lost, torn, or discolored. They may also become coated with insoluble debris. Such cases of lensopathy may entail replacing the lens at frequent intervals, which tends to increase the cost of maintaining the patient on this form of therapy.

In my experience, no irreversible corneal damage has occurred from the routine use of topical medications containing preservatives in conjunction with bandage lens therapy. To the contrary, there is a far greater risk from contamination when these preservatives are withheld. Thus, in treating corneal pathology with hydrophilic bandage lenses, standard ophthalmic medications are preferred in almost all cases.

The patient who is wearing a hydrophilic bandage lens successfully may develop discomfort as a result of a deposition of insoluble material on the lens. If these depositions are on the posterior surface or the lens periphery, they may be particularly annoying.

Some patients cannot be made comfortable with a hydrophilic bandage lens regardless of the pathology involved. As the depth of experience of the fitter increases, the number of cases that cannot be fitted comfortably decreases. On rare occasions, the application of a hydrophilic bandage lens has produced a true intolerance evidenced by sterile hypopyon and increase of ocular inflammation. Such cases are of extremely rapid onset, and should

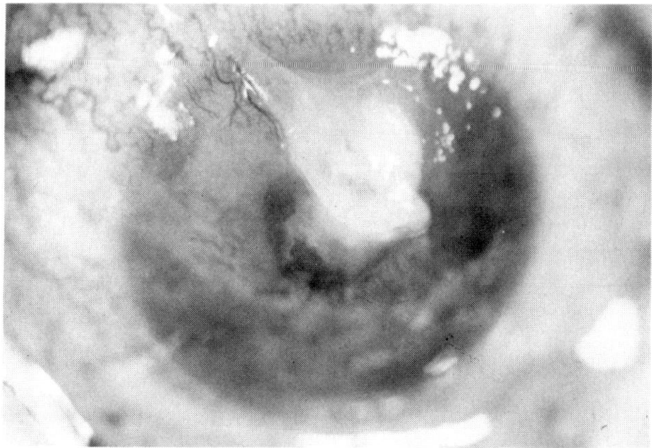

Figure 6-13 *Severe corneal infection is a dreaded complication of bandage lens therapy.*

not be confused with secondary infection. In recent years, the role of the ocular immunological system in complications related to contact lens wear has been highlighted.[1]

Neovascularization evidenced with bandage lens use may be superficial or deep. Most physicians believe that it is related to decreased oxygen tension in the presence of a constantly worn hydrophilic lens, whereas others implicate the direct traumatic effects of wearing the lens. In normal eyes that have been fitted with daily-wear hydrophilic lenses for corrective purposes, neovascularization is frequent. In cases of painful pathology when the pain has subsided, it may be advisable to switch to intermittent wear and have the patient remove the lenses at bedtime. In the final analysis, each case must be judged on its own merit. Typically, thinner, high water content lenses will cause fewer instances of neovascularization than thicker and relatively low water content lenses.

AVOIDANCE OF COMPLICATIONS

To avoid complications from wearing bandage lenses, I recommend the following routine.

PRELIMINARY STEPS

1. Attempt to determine the visual potential of the eye prior to fitting the bandage lens. An accurate refraction, fundus examination, and estimation of the degree of corneal irregularity, opacity, and scarring should be made.

2. *Intraocular pressure:* Elevations in intraocular pressure should be ruled out, and if present, should be treated with appropriate systemic and topical medications. If ephinephrine is being used to control the intraocular pressure (as is often the case in aphakic bullous keratopathy), an alternative means of glaucoma control should be employed in the course of bandage lens therapy.

3. Chronic iritis is often a component of chronic corneal disease. In many cases, the degree of corneal opacity precludes an accurate diagnosis. These cases should be treated with cycloplegics and topical steroids when necessary.

4. An estimation of corneal sensation is important. Neurotropic keratitis carries an increased risk.

5. Treat pre-existing blepharitis.

LENS INSERTION

An attempt should be made to select an initial lens that has great potential for being the definitive lens used in therapy.

1. No anesthetic should be used in the eye prior to fitting the lens. The presence of a topical anesthetic precludes an accurate assessment of the comfort afforded by the bandage lens. If a patient is discharged before the effects of the anesthetic have worn off, secondary discomfort may develop.

2. The fitting of the lens should be evaluated after a period of at least 20 minutes to allow for the lens to settle down. Lacrimation may cause a lens to have excessive initial movement.

3. A relatively thin, high water content lens should be used for initial therapy even if an aphakic lens may be indicated later. The patient should be stabilized initially with a thin, high water content lens.

4. Before actually inserting the lens, the physician should wash, rinse, and dry his hands.

5. Insertion technique is important. If the patient is prone and the lens inadvertently falls from the fingers, it will tend to land in the eye rather than on the floor.

6. A steep-fitting lens generally should be avoided unless specifically indicated. Such a lens will demonstrate very little or no movement on the eye although it may initially appear to be very comfortable for the patient. If the lens is too loose fitting, it will demonstrate excessive movement (several millimeters) and will not tend to center with the blink or with ocular rotations. This type of lens will be uncomfortable in the long run.

PATIENT INSTRUCTION

A number of complications can be avoided by accurately explaining to the patient what is expected of him in caring for his lens and what he should anticipate in wearing the lens.

1. Written instruction should be provided, in booklet form if possible, stating how to remove the lens. Specific instruction in insertion and removal should be given to the patient or to a member of his family even if the lens is to be worn on a full-time basis.

2. The patient must have the telephone number of an ophthalmologist or another individual who may be contacted should he get into difficulty during the first several days of bandage lens therapy.

3. The comprehensive medical regimen should be fully explained to the patient and written down if possible. One should address blepharitis, iritis, and glaucoma, as well as the specific therapy indicated for the disease.

4. The patient must be aware of the date and time for the return visit to the physician.

5. In the event of pain, increased redness, reduced vision, corneal opacity, or infiltrates, the patient must be seen as soon as possible.

EVALUATING AND REFITTING THE LENS

In cases where improvement in visual acuity is possible with bandage lens therapy, and following stabilization of the situation, an attempt to refit the contact lens should be made.

1. Generally speaking, a flatter fitting contact lens will afford the best possibility for improvement in visual acuity.

2. Overrefraction is often facilitated when the keratometer reading is taken over the anterior surface of the lens.

3. If the corneal edema and irregularity have stabilized, consider switching to a high water content aphakic contact lens in cases of monocular aphakia associated with bullous keratopathy.

4. The patient should insert and remove the thicker aphakic bandage lenses on a daily basis. Extended wear may be possible, but corneas that are marginally compensated require adequate oxygen.

5. The patient should be re-instructed on long-term good hygiene, and evaluated for compliance with lens care practices.

ULTIMATE REEVALUATION OF THERAPY

If relief of pain is inadequate, lens therapy may be discontinued and alternatives considered (conjunctival falp or penetrating keratoplasty). If the vision is inadequate for the patient's needs, keratoplasty may be specifically indicated.

In the final analysis, the use of bandage lenses, although not a panacea, continues to have an important place in therapy.

REFERENCES

1. Allansmith MR, Baird RS, Greiner JV: Number and type of inflammatory cells in conjunctiva of asymptomatic contact lens wearers. Am J Ophthalmol 87:171, 1979

2. Aquavella JV: Bionite hydrophilic bandage lenses in the treatment of corneal disease. In Gasset AR, Kaufman HE (eds): Soft Contact Lenses: Symposium and Workshop of the University of Florida, Gainesville, pp 190–198. St Louis, CV Mosby, 1972

3. Aquavella JV: Chronic corneal edema. Am J Ophthalmol 73:201, 1973

4. Aquavella JV, Jackson GK, Guy LF: Therapeutic effects of Bionite lenses: Mechanism of action. Ann Ophthalmol 3:1341, 1971

5. Aquavella JV: Lathe cut versus spin cast lenses. Ophthalmol Times 2(5): May 1977

6. Aquavella JV: New aspects of contact lenses in ophthalmology. Adv Ophthalmol 32:2, 1976

7. Aquavella JV, Shaw EL: Hydrophilic bandages in penetrating keratoplasty. Ann Ophthalmol 8:1207, 1976

8. Aquavella JV: The soft contact lens. I. Therapeutic experience with the Softcon lens. Int Ophthalmol Clin 13:167, 1973

9. Aquavella JV: Therapeutic uses of hydrophilic lenses. Invest Ophthalmol 13:484, 1974

10. Aquavella JV: Treatment of Chronic Corneal Edema. New York, Medcom, 1973

11. Arrington GE: A History of Ophthalmology. New York, MD Pub, 1959

12. Baldone JA: The fitting of hard contact lenses onto soft contact lenses in certain diseased conditions. Contact Lens Med Bull 6:15, 1973

13. Brown SI, Bloomfield SE, Pearce DB: A follow-up report on transplantation of the alkali-burned cornea. Am J Ophthalmol 77:538, 1974

14. Clements D: Soft Contact Lenses: Clinical and Applied Technology, pp 435–442. New York, Wiley, 1978

15. Dorman-Brailsford MI: The importance of sag heights when fitting Bionite lenses. Ophthalmol Opt 12:1047, 1972

16. Enoch JM: The fitting of hydrophilic (soft) contact lenses to infants and young children. II. Fitting techniques and initial results on aphakic children. Contact Lens Med Bull 5:41, 1972

17. Gasset AR, Kaufman HE: Therapeutic uses of hydrophilic contact lenses. Am J Ophthalmol 69:252, 1970

18. Mobilia EF, Dohlman CH, Holly FJ: A comparison of various soft contact lenses for therapeutic purposes. Cont IOL Med J 3:9, 1977

19. O'Driscoll KF: Polymeric aspects of soft contact lenses. In Gasset AR, Kaufman HE (eds): Soft Contact Lenses: Symposium and Workshop of the University of Florida, Gainesville, pp 3–15. St Louis, CV Mosby, 1972

20. Podos SM et al: Pilocarpine therapy with soft contact lenses. Am J Ophthalmol 73:336, 1972

21. Ridley F: Therapeutic uses of scleral contact lenses, Int Ophthalmol Clin 2:687, 1969

22. Stark WJ, Fogle JA, Kenyon KR: Damage to epithelial basement membrane by thermokeratoplasty. Am J Ophthalmol 83:392, 1977

23. Tripathi RC, Tripathi BJ, Ruben M: The pathology of soft contact lens spoilage. Ophthalmology 87:365, 1980

24. Uotila MH, Gasset AR: Fitting manual for Bausch & Lomb and Griffin lenses. In Gasset AR, Kaufman HE (eds): Soft Contact Lenses: Symposium and Workshop of the University of Florida, Gainesville, pp 285–313. St Louis, CV Mosby, 1972

25. Wichterle O, Lim D: Hydrophilic gels for biological usage. Nature (London) 185:227, 1960

CHAPTER SEVEN

SPECIAL REFRACTIVE PROBLEMS

KENNETH A. POLSE and EMILY KENYON

Ametropias that are not normally corrected with spectacle lenses and those refractive conditions that require special contact lens fitting techniques are discussed in this chapter. Rather than approach it by lens type (*e.g.,* torics, gas-permeable lenses), we chose to discuss this topic by refractive condition. Included are residual astigmatism, high corneal astigmatism, keratoconus, irregular astigmatism, aphakia, and presbyopia. For each refractive condition, the optimum fitting method is discussed, although other techniques not mentioned might certainly be important alternatives. Also, some conditions might fall into several categories. For example, post-penetrating keratoplasty could be included in high corneal astigmatism or irregular astigmatism, and either of the fitting techniques might apply to the penetrating keratoplasty (PKP) patient. We have attempted to use a systematic fitting approach, although we recognize that no "cookbook" formulary will work with these complicated conditions and that practitioner experience will ultimately be the best guide to achieving a successful fitting.

RESIDUAL ASTIGMATISM

Residual astigmatism is the astigmatism that remains uncorrected when a spherical contact lens is worn. The amount of residual astigmatism depends upon the interplay of a number of factors, including the type of spherical lens worn (hard or flexible), the degree of lens flexure following the blink, the degree of tilting or decentration of the contact lens with respect to the visual axis, the amount of corneal toricity, the amount of lenticular toricity, the presence of lenticular lens tilting, and the presence of an eccentric position of the fovea in relation to the visual axis. Although an accurate differential diagnosis of the source of the astigmatism is often difficult to make, it is possible to determine whether residual astigmatism is present. Most clinicians maintain that amounts of residual astigmatism greater than 0.75 D often result in reduced visual acuity and patient discomfort, especially in those patients who have previously worn glasses with good vision.

ESTIMATING RESIDUAL ASTIGMATISM

As a general rule the clinician should expect residual astigmatism (1) if the corneal cylinder and refractive astigmatism do not match; (2) if there is contact lens displacement so that the optic center of the lens does not coincide with the center of the patient's pupil; (3) if there is significant corneal cylinder and thin (<0.14 mm) gas-permeable lenses are used; (4) if there is refractive astigmatism and gel lenses are used; or (5) if there is an unusual corneal shape (*e.g.,* following PKP or cataract surgery).

For many patients, it is possible to estimate the amount of residual astigmatism by comparing corneal toricity to the total refractive astigmatism. For example, if a patient's total spectacle astigmatism is 1.5 D and there is no measured corneal toricity, a residual astigmatism of approximately 1.5 D would be expected. This amount could be modified by the lens position or any lenticular astigmatism, but in general the prediction is fairly accurate. The best way to determine residual astigmatism, however, is to place a spherical lens on the eye and perform an overrefraction.

Once the amount of residual astigmatism is known, the clinician can select the lens type that might best reduce or eliminate the astigmatism. For example, if there were no measured astigmatic refractive error, but the keratometry readings showed 1.5 D of corneal toricity, it would be expected that the "tear lens" under a hard lens would create about 1.5 D of residual astigmatism. A soft lens, however, would not be expected to cause any residual astigmatism because the lens would conform to the cornea without creating a tear lens.

METHODS TO CORRECT RESIDUAL ASTIGMATISM

Before residual astigmatism can be corrected, the total refractive astigmatism must be measured, keratometer readings taken, and a spherocylindrical refraction performed over a spherical lens of the type being considered (rigid or soft). These measurements will help the clinician determine the appropriate lens correction. Listed below are methods used to correct the residual astigmatism, depending on the type of lens being fitted.

Soft Lenses

If a soft lens is used to correct residual astigmatism, lens rotation on the eye must be prevented. Several methods are used to stabilize the lens. These include truncation, prism ballast, and thin circular peripheries. No single method is the best, and frequently the practitioner may have to try several nonrotating types of lenses to find the one that fits best for a particular patient. Even with the best stabilization, the lens usually will not locate exactly in a perpendicular position; therefore, before prescribing the axis and power of the front cylinder, it is necessary to determine the degree of rotation. This is best done by using spherical trial lenses with the type of lens stabilization desired. The lens is placed on the eye and the orientation (degree of rotation) and stability of the lens can be assessed by noting the position of small markings placed on the lens surface. If the lens does not rotate, the position will remain fixed even after several blinks. It is important to assess the degree of rotation after the lens has been on the eye for sufficient time (10 to 15 minutes) for the patient to be comfortable and blinking normally. Following insertion, there is usually reflex tearing, which causes the lens to position differently from when there is normal tearing. Most often, the lens positions so that the lens markers have rotated in a clockwise or counterclockwise direction towards the horizontal position (180°) corneal meridian. Rotation presents no problem as long as the position remains stable and does not change with each blink. If the lens is stable, then a spherocylindrical overrefraction will determine the best corrected visual acuity. When the final lens is ordered, the amount of lens rotation must be either added to (if rotation appears clockwise to the fitter) or subtracted from (counterclockwise) the patient's cylinder axis (in minus cylinder form). In the majority of cases the bottom of the lens rotates toward the patient's nose, so the axis for the right eye must be reduced and the axis for the left eye increased.

Most manufacturers provide axes in five-degree steps and cylinder powers in half-diopter steps to about 2 D to 2.5 D. More parameters are being introduced, and some laboratories are planning to make "custom" designed lenses that will provide cylinders in many axes and powers. The front toric lenses being produced today are considerably improved over those of several years ago, and many patients who could not be fitted previously can now achieve good acuity and comfort with the current toric lens designs.

Hard Lenses

There are several possible methods to correct residual astigmatism using hard lenses depending upon the degree of residual astigmatism and the amount of flexure in the lens. The most common method is to use a nonrotational lens with the desired cylinder ground onto the front surface. Lens stability is controlled by grinding 1 D to 1.5 D prism into the lens (Fig. 7-1). Such lenses are referred to as prism-ballast lenses. Although somewhat heavier than spherical lenses due to increased thickness, they are usually comfortable. Some practitioners also truncate the lens, although this technique may make the lens uncomfortable and is not usually necessary to achieve lens stability. Prism-ballast PMMA lenses often caused poor physiological response because of the reduction in tear pumping that occurs with

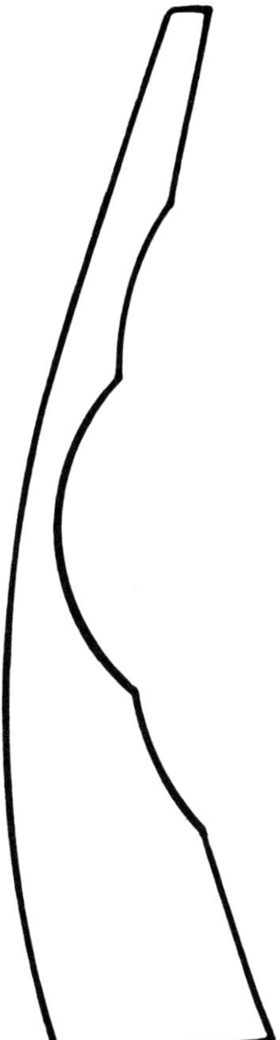

Figure 7-1 Cross-sectional view of prism-ballast lens showing base-down prism to stabilize the lens on the cornea.

the prism-ballast lenses; however, the gas-permeable materials provide sufficient oxygen transmission so that corneal physiology is usually unaffected.

Both the amount of prism and the cylinder power and axis must be determined before prescribing these lenses. A spherical, prism-ballast lens should be tried first. If the practitioner does not have trial prism-ballast lenses, most laboratories will supply trial lenses on loan. Select the base curve based on a spherical (nonprism) trial fit. Most prism-ballast lenses need to be at least 9 mm in diameter because they tend to ride slightly low and the patient may experience blur if the diameter is too small. The base of the trial prism lens will be marked so that the degree of lens rotation can be noted. As with the soft lens, it is important that the lens not rotate with every blink. If the lens does rotate, more prism is needed (increase prism by about ½ prism diopter [PD]). The prism usually does not orient exactly vertical; therefore, the degree of rotation must be added or subtracted from the final prescription when ordering the cylinder axis for the front surface. Patients often take slightly longer to adapt to prism-ballast lenses than to the thinner spherical design. The initial lens awareness usually subsides with increased wearing time over a 2 to 4 week period.

Sometimes careful attention to the base curve–corneal fitting relationship will allow the practitioner to overcome residual astigmatism by using a thin spherical lens. Herman has shown that the steepness or flatness of the fit significantly affects the amount of lens flexure on a with-the-rule cornea.[5] Lenses fitted flatter than flat K will flex less, or even in an against-the-rule direction. Lenses fitted steeper than flat K will begin to flex significantly in a with-the-rule direction. Therefore, if residual astigmatism occurs with a cornea whose toricity closely resembles the refractive astigmatism, it is possible that the cause is lens flexure, and the clinician may be able to reduce the residual astigmatism by fitting the lens slightly flatter than flat K by about 0.37 D. Conversely, if the cornea has more with-the-rule toricity than refractive astigmatism, a fitting relationship that is slightly steep should allow lens flexure, reducing the tear lens cylindrical power and reducing the expected induced astigmatism. The same study has not been reported on against-the-rule corneas, but here the range of acceptable fitting relationships from a lens centration standpoint is far narrower, and correction of residual astigmatism by varying the fitting relationship may not be possible.

Summary

Residual astigmatism is a common refractive problem and occurs in normal corneas as well as those eyes that have had disease or surgery. These small amounts of uncorrected refractive error can be a constant source of patient complaint. If the patient must wear contact lenses (*e.g.,* keratoconus, post-PKP, aphakia) and there is residual astigmatism that cannot be corrected easily in the contact lens, it is possible to include the correction in a pair of spectacles to be worn over the contact lenses.

HIGH CORNEAL ASTIGMATISM

Corneas with high toricity are sometimes difficult to fit satisfactorily because of excessive lens movement, lens decentration, and patient discomfort. One fitting solution for some patients is to prescribe a lens with a toric back surface. Conditions that most often require toric back-surface lenses are listed here.

With-the-rule corneal toricity over 3 D

Against-the-rule corneal toricity over 2 D

Post-penetrating keratoplasty with high toricity

Aphakia with high toricity

Advanced keratoconus

Radial keratotomy with high toricity

Corneal scarring from injury or disease

Frequent lens displacement on toric cornea

Lens decentration (nasal or temporal riding position) on toric cornea

The best way to assess the need for a toric back-surface lens is to observe the fit and listen to patient symptoms. The patient will usually complain of frequent lens displacement or loss, or of lens awareness, which is caused by the excessive movement and contact of the lens edge with the lower lid. The slit lamp examination will show a toric fluorescein pattern and considerable lens movement. Also, there is often marked edge standoff due to the rocking effect of the lens. Finally, visual acuity is frequently reduced because of lens movement and tilting that occurs with spherical power lenses placed on a highly toric cornea.

CORRECTING HIGH ASTIGMATISM

It is possible to construct a back-surface toric lens that more closely conforms to the corneal topography. These lens designs usually require a front toric surface (bitoric lenses) to obtain satisfactory vision. These bitoric designs are available with rigid lenses but not with the flexible lens materials (*e.g.*, HEMA materials). Because these lenses often are thicker than comparable spherical lens designs, it is important to select the material with the highest oxygen transmissibility (Dk/L) available. Most of the currently available silicon–acrylate lenses have Dk/L values in the range of 12 to 15 $\times$ 10^{-9} (cm/sec) (ml O_2/ml $\times$ mmHg) and provide adequate oxygen if a proper tear pump (peripheral and secondary curve system) is designed and the lens thickness is kept at a minimum (0.25 mm or less). If these design features are not included, corneal edema may result.

Although usually heavier than spherical lenses, toric back-surface lenses can be made to position and center properly. Also, the toric base curve usually results in less lens movement and better comfort compared with a spherical lens on the same cornea. It is possible to incorporate other lens design features into the lens, such as lenticulation (see discussion of Aphakia) or prism (see discussion of Residual Astigmatism), thus making this design applicable to a wide range of refractive errors. It is important to understand that a toric back surface is prescribed to solve a physical fitting problem and not to improve visual acuity. In fact, one of the problems with back-surface toric lenses is in obtaining satisfactory visual acuity.

The fitting of this lens requires a diagnostic fitting with toric lenses. It is not possible to predict the fitting relationship accurately based on observations from spherical lenses. As a general rule, the first trial lens should have base curves that are about 0.5 D (0.10 mm) flatter than the flattest meridian and from 0.5 D to 1.5 D (0.1 mm to 0.3 mm) flatter than the steepest meridian, depending upon the amount of corneal toricity. The greater the corneal toricity, the flatter the base curve from the steepest meridian. From a manufacturing standpoint, it is often difficult to lathe lenses with toricities greater than 6 DK. Once the diagnostic lens is placed on the eye and sufficient time is given for the patient to become comfortable, the fit can be evaluated. If the lens is fitting properly, there should be good centration, 1 mm to 2 mm of slow movement following the blink (during the intrablink period), and a fairly even distribution of fluorescein under the lens.

The criteria used for fitting spherical lenses should also be applied with regard to changing base curves, diameter, and peripheral and secondary curves. For example, if the lens appears too steep, both curves should be flattened, or if the lens rides low (as may happen with plus lenses or a very loose upper lid) a minus-carrier lenticular, toric base curve should be prescribed. Color Figure 7-1 shows two examples of corneas with high with-the-rule toricity fitted with spherical lenses (Color Figs. 7-1 *A* and *C*). Note the highly astigmatic pattern, which is characterized by a vertical band of fluorescein. When these corneas were refitted with toric base curve lenses (Color Figs. 7-1 *B* and *D*), the fluorescein patterns show an even distribution of dye under the lens. Lens movement and rocking are also greatly reduced with the back-surface toric design.

After the diameter and curves are selected, the front curves must be chosen to correct visual acuity. This is one of the most confusing aspects of fitting a back-surface toric lens. In most cases, the keratometry readings of a highly toric cornea will closely approximate the spectacle astigmatism. Therefore, the theoretically desired lens would be a spherical lens, with the astigmatic correction coming from the tear lens. When a toric base, spherical front surface lens is fitted, the cylindrical power of the tear lens is reduced. The resultant cylinder usually does not correct the astigmatic refractive error and in some cases can increase the astigmatic error. Thus, it is usually necessary to design a bitoric lens with a spherical power effect to correct the induced astigmatism.

Sarver has shown that this calculation is straightforward if the spectacle astigmatism matches the corneal astigmatism.[11] Figure 7-2 is constructed to show how the calculation is made. A cross should first be drawn indicating the actual corneal curvatures and the spectacle powers in each meridian (Fig. 7-2*A*). Next, a cross representing the lens is drawn, incorporating the toric base curve chosen (Fig. 7-2*B*). Each meridian is then treated like a simple spherical lens problem. To determine the back vertex power of the lens in each meridian, the power contributed by the tear lens must first be calculated. In the example, the 90° meridian of the lens (40.5 D) is fitted 0.5 D flatter than K (41 D), so the tear lens in that meridian contributes −0.5 D of power. Therefore, the lens power in that meridian should be increased by +0.5 D over the spectacle power in the 90° meridian (+0.5 + plano = +0.5). Similarly, the lens in the example is fitted 2 D flatter than steep K (at 180°), so the contact lens power in that meridian must be +2 D greater than the spectacle power (+2 − 7 = −5). These calculated powers are now added to the crosses (Fig. 7-2*C*). To assure that the calculation has been done correctly (to provide a spherical power effect), the lens cross should be

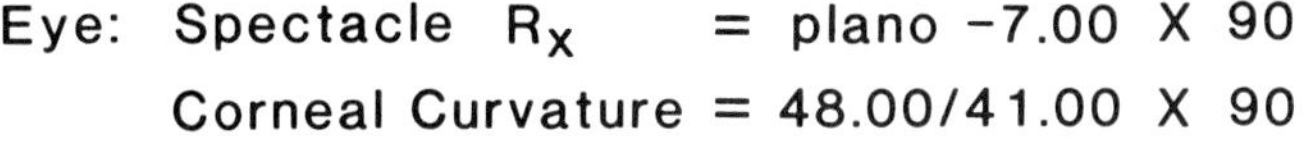

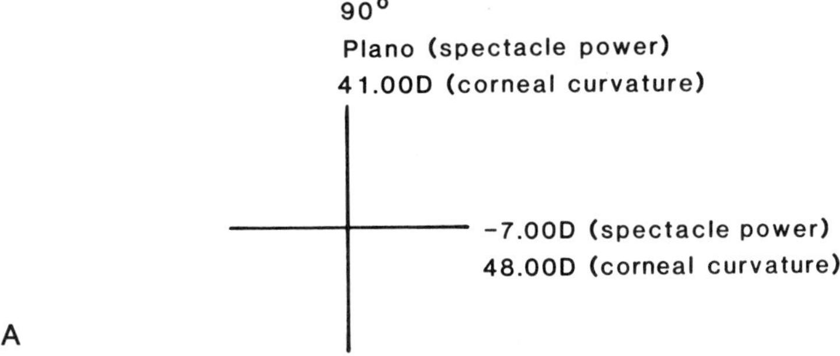

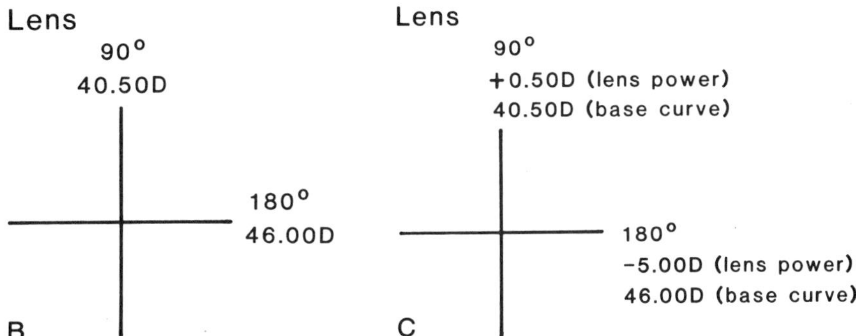

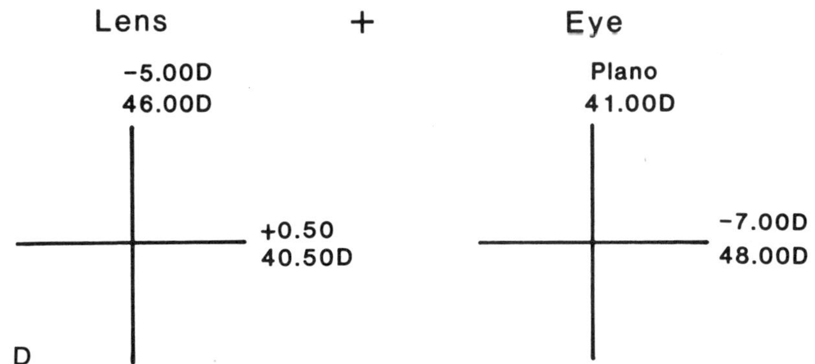

Figure 7-2 (A) A cross is drawn to represent the prescription of the eye in the flattest (90°) and steepest (180°) meridians, and the corresponding corneal curvature readings. (B) A cross is then drawn to represent the lens curvatures (in diopters) that are chosen for fitting purposes. (C) After the power of the tear lens is taken into account, the power needed in each meridian is added to the lens cross. (D) To check the calculation of the prescribed lens power, the lens cross is rotated and added to the eye cross. In this orientation, the contact lens plus the tear lens still should accurately correct the eye's refractive error.

turned 90° and added to the eye cross (Fig. 7-2*D*). In the example, the lens turned 90° is now 5 D steeper than the corneal curve at 90°. The tear lens thus provides +5 D of power and the lens provides −5 D; the total power is 0 D, which is the power required to correct the eye in that meridian. Similarly, the lens is now 7.5 D flatter than the cornea in the 180° meridian and provides −7.5 D of tear lens power, which added to the +0.5 D of lens power gives −7 D, the power needed by the eye in the 180° meridian. Note that the prescription of the contact lens, written in spherocylindrical form (+0.5 − 5.5 × 90) has an astigmatic correction equal to the difference in base curves of the lens (46 − 40.5 = 5.5).

This type of design is satisfactory as long as the corneal toricity is close in power and axis to the total amount of refractive astigmatism. For example, if the refractive astigmatism is −3 D at 180° and the corneal toricity is 2.5 D steeper in the 90° meridian, most of the astigmatism is due to corneal toricity and the spherical power effect lens design will usually work satisfactorily. If a toric base curve is necessary for fitting purposes and a "spherical" lens does not adequately correct the astigmatism, additional cylinder may be added to the front surface. In this case, a spherical effect, toric base trial lens should be placed on the eye and checked for rotational stability. If the lens does not rotate and rests with its flattest meridian aligned with the flattest corneal meridian, the additional cylindrical power (in minus cylinder form) may simply be added to the steeper meridian. Such a perfect result is rare, however, and it is generally simplest to use a spherical effect lens and supplementary spectacles.

KERATOCONUS

One important therapeutic indication for contact lenses is the correction of keratoconus. The neutralization of the irregular corneal surface by the tear lens usually corrects vision to normal levels. Even when normal acuity (20/20) is not achieved, there is a marked improvement in contrast detection, which greatly improves the patient's vision.

FITTING

There are many important considerations in fitting the keratoconic patient, including curvature, size of cone, corneal thinning, corneal scarring, corneal irregularity, and refractive error. Each of these ocular characteristics may influence the lens fit. There are some general fitting guidelines that increase the chances for success. First, if possible, use a gas-permeable material. The increased oxygen availability often improves the physiological result and may prevent or slow some of the scarring that often accompanies advancing keratoconus. Second, with the gas-permeable lenses, it is possible to use lenses of overall diameters between 8.8 mm and 9.3 mm, which is considerably larger than the 7.8 mm to 8.4 mm size used with PMMA lenses. The larger diameter usually improves comfort and often provides better vision than the smaller diameter PMMA lenses. Third, the lenses should be fitted with as little apical touch or pressure as possible. Recent studies have suggested that the marked apical pressure that often occurs with the small PMMA lens fit seems to cause or aggravate corneal scarring. This progressive scarring may be prevented or slowed by using slightly steep gas-permeable lenses.[6,7] Finally, gas-permeable materials allow the secondary and peripheral curves to be fitted slightly steeper than those of PMMA lenses. This is because the oxygen reaching the cornea is not entirely dependent on the tear pump. Reducing peripheral curve radius and width reduces edge standoff, thereby usually improving comfort compared with the flatter and wider curves that are sometimes necessary with PMMA lenses.

Although many methods of fitting have been proposed, there is really no one correct fitting philosophy. Every keratoconic cornea is unique, and the lens fit can only be determined from a diagnostic fitting, which should include a careful overrefraction to obtain the appropriate spherical lens power. The method listed below is a guideline, and the practitioner's own experience and observations should be the final determinant in lens selection.

Begin by attempting to measure the corneal curvature. Often the curvature is beyond the range of the standard keratometer. The scale can be extended by placing a +1.25-D lens over the target mires, which extends the range approximately 9 D. For example, if a 46-D reading is made with the added minus lens, the actual reading is 55 D. Accuracy of this method can be improved by measuring the four standard steel spheres that come with the keratometer both with and without the minus lens. From these measurements a calibration curve can be constructed, which compares the normal and expanded ranges.

After the curvature is determined, the diagnostic lens can be selected. Start with a lens that is close to the flattest corneal meridian and add about 0.25 D to the base curve for each diopter of corneal toricity. For example, if the measured curvature is 45/50, select a base curve of 46.5 D. For curvatures under 48 DK, use a diameter between 9 mm and 9.2 mm. As the curvature increases, the diameter must be reduced (*i.e.,* for curvatures of 48 DK to 54 DK, use an 8.8 mm to 9 mm diameter; and beyond 54 DK, use a diameter of 8.8 mm or less). If possible, use diagnostic lenses that are gas permeable. The flexing characteristics of these lenses are considerably different from those of the PMMA lens, and therefore the overrefraction and subsequent visual acuity is most accurately assessed using the same material that will be prescribed.

After the lens has been in place long enough for normal tearing to resume, fluorescein pattern observations are made. It is important to record all the parameters of the trial lens (*e.g.,* thickness, peripheral and secondary curves), because the selection of subsequent diagnostic lenses and the final prescription will be based not only on base curve, diameter, and power considerations, but also on the peripheral curves, optic zone diameter, and thickness. Characteristics of an optimum fit are shown in Color Figure 7-2, and are listed as follows.

Good centration following blink

1 mm to 2 mm slow lens excursion during intrablink period

Minimum apical touch

No air bubbles under lens

Adequate peripheral curves (0.3 mm to 0.5 mm wide)

Minimal edge standoff

Because the use of two or more peripheral curves is needed to achieve an optimum fit, the optic zone diameter is usually small. Therefore, the lens must center well over the pupil if vision is to be corrected properly. One problem with keratoconic fits is that the lens sometimes moves excessively following the blink. It is important that the lens move (for tear replenishment under the lens) but not excessively, which causes discomfort and reduces vision. With the patient in primary gaze, try to obtain aobut 1 mm to 2 mm of slow vertical movement following the blink. Use a base curve that does not bear heavily on the corneal apex. This can best be assessed by observing with a thin optic section. Points of hard bearing will appear dark, without any fluorescein. Make certain there is an adequate peripheral and secondary curve system by looking for the characteristic outer green band, which should be about 0.3 mm to 0.5 mm wide. There must be some observable curve present or the lens will fit too tightly and may actually cause compression lines on the cornea. On the other hand, if the peripheral curves are too flat, there will be a large green band, which will usually have air bubbles trapped in the tear reservoir. This curve may result in too much edge standoff and also cause the air bubbles to get trapped under the center of the lens. If the pattern has this appearance, the peripheral curve radius, width, or both should be reduced.

Several diagnostic lenses may have to be tried before a reasonable pattern can be obtained. Once the best fitting lens is selected, an overrefraction is performed. If the spherical power of the lens is close or corrects the refractive error, the final power of the lens can be accurately calculated. However, if the overrefraction indicates that an additional 4 D or more is needed, it is possible that the final lens may give a different visual acuity than that measured with the trial lens and the overrefraction. In addition to vertex distance effects, part of the reason for this difference between measured and actual power needed is attributable to the flexing characteristics of the gas-permeable polymers. Lens flexing is influenced by the lens center thickness, which is somewhat dependent on the lens power. Also, as the lens becomes higher in minus, the edge becomes thicker, which may cause the lens to position differently and thereby result in a different refractive power effect. For these reasons, it is best to use diagnostic lenses close to the required power. If such lenses are not available, the prescribed lens will at best be an estimate and a second lens may have to be ordered.

The above methods are meant only as a guideline. The final lens selection will be determined by many factors, including patient comfort, vision, and follow-up examination of corneal tolerance. In some cases the keratoconus is too advanced for a hard lens fitting. This is usually the case when the lens will not stay on the eye or when comfort is so poor that the patient must discontinue wear in spite of the visual handicap. Only two choices remain. The first is to consider a corneal transplant, and the second is to try a piggyback lens fit (soft–hard lens combination; see discussion of Irregular Astigmatism). Sometimes the piggyback lens works well, especially as an interim measure while keratoplasty is being considered or if a transplant is contraindicated.

IRREGULAR ASTIGMATISM

Irregularities of the anterior corneal surface usually result in substantial visual loss that is not correctable with spectacles or flexible contact lenses. Causes of these irregularities include keratoconus, corneal scarring, irregular astigmatism, penetrating keratoplasty, epithelial disease, and trauma. These irregularities can usually be neutralized by the tear lens that is formed when a hard (nonflexible) contact lens is placed upon the eye.

In practice, the clinician first should try a hard contact lens on patients with anterior surface irregularities to determine if the vision is correctable. However, in many cases, the hard lens cannot be tolerated due to mechanial irritation, or lens instability. In these patients the use of a hydrogel lens would appear to be an ideal solution, because it would tend to drape over the corneal surface and be much less irritating than the hard lens. Unfortunately, hydrogel lenses do not correct the surface irregularity, and therefore vision is usually unacceptable.

A solution to avoiding the instability and mechanical irritation of the hard lens while still maintaining good vision is to fit a hydrogel lens over the cornea and then place a hard gas-permeable lens over the gel lens. This technique is referred to as *combination lens fitting* or *piggyback fitting,* and was first reported by Westerhout in 1973 and more recently by others.[1,2,12] Different methods have been suggested, including steep and tight hard lenses, loose fitting hard lenses, and gel lenses with a concavity in the front surface to act as a carrier for the hard lens. Whatever the method used, the limiting factor seems to be the physiological tolerance of the cornea to the reduced oxygen. Most currently prescribed gel lenses (*e.g.,* thin, low-water or thick, high-water lenses) provide about 55 mmHg to 65 mmHg (7% to 9%) oxygen tension to the cornea when the eye is open. Although these lenses provide sufficient oxygen to meet the metabolic needs of the epithelium when the eyes are open, a hard lens placed over the gel lens further reduces the available oxygen at the anterior corneal surface.[3,10]

Several steps can be followed to optimize the oxygen delivery to the cornea. First, select a gel lens that will provide the highest possible oxygen transmission (Dk/L). High-water lenses usually do not work well for combination systems, and therefore a thin (30 μ or less) low- or medium-water lens (38% to 45% H_2O) should be used. Second, if there is a substantial myopic refractive error, prescribe as much minus as possible in the gel lens, because this will decrease lens center thickness (thereby incresing the *Dk/L*). Incorporating most of the minus power in the gel lens will also make the hard lens somewhat more comfortable because of reduction in edge thickness. Third, select a hard gas-permeable lens of the highest available *Dk/L*. Currently, several manufacturers have experimental silicon–acrylate lenses with *Dk/L* values two to four times higher than presently available materials. Use these lenses, if available, because they will greatly increase oxygen delivery to the cornea. Finally, use an optimum fitting hard lens with a good peripheral system to provide the maximum tear pump. Following these steps should provide sufficient oxygen to meet physiological requirements.

There is no single correct method to fit combination lenses. The following suggested procedures can be used as a guide.

Select appropriate gel lens (good centration, little movement)

Measure curvature over gel lens

Select initial hard lens based on "over K" reading

Place hard lens over gel lens

Observe fluorescein pattern using Fluorexon

Overrefract

First select a gel lens that covers the cornea and limbal areas and does not have excessive movement. This lens should have as little edge standoff as possible. After the gel lens has been selected, take keratometer readings over the lens. Although there will probably still be some distortion, the mire appearance should be improved compared to the reading made directly on the cornea. If the mire images are not clearer, another gel lens (steeper or flatter base curve) should be tried. Using the "over K" as a guide, select a hard lens. Fit the lens to the flattest K allowing an increase in base curve of 0.25 DK (0.05 mm) for each diopter of toricity measured with the gel lens in place. Observe the fit of the hard lens over the soft using Fluorexon dye. (This dye is a fluorescein dimer that is large enough to prevent penetration of dye into low and medium water hydrogel lenses.) Use the criteria that are usually evaluated for hard lens fits, including: (1) good centration after the blink; (2) 1 mm to 2 mm of slow downward lens movement during the intrablink period; (3) minimum apical clearance; (4) an even distribution of dye under the lens; and (5) a bright green peripheral pattern, which indicates that there is a optimum tear reservoir for good tear pumping. Once the optimum fit has been determined, measure the refractive error over the combination. If there is a substantial need for increased (or decreased) minus power, try to make the adjustment in the gel lens. Ideally, the hard lens should have a power of −2 D to −3 D with the remainder of lens power prescribed in the gel lens.

Using these fitting procedures should provide the best chance for a good fit. The hard lens is handled (inserted and removed) in the standard fashion. Many patients ask whether the gel lens can be prescribed as an extended-wear lens. This decision depends on the corneal condition and rests with the physician. Generally, however, it is best if both lenses can be removed because extended-wear lenses fitted even to normal corneas can result in complications.

It is important to have the patient build up wearing time gradually and return regularly for follow-up care. Changes in lens parameters will be based on observations similar to those made when hard lenses are normally fitted. If the patient is carefully monitored and care is taken to achieve an optimum hard lens fit, it is possible to obtain an excellent visual and corneal result.

APHAKIA

Contact lens correction of aphakia is an important rehabilitative procedure for those patients who are not fitted with intraocular lens implants or who are currently wearing spectacles and could benefit from contact lens wear. Several types of contact lenses can be used to correct aphakia. Rigid lenses may be designed from gas-permeable materials to prevent physiological disturbance, using either a single-cut or a minus-carrier design. Hydrogel lenses also may be used, with the choice of either extended-wear or daily-wear regimens. In the near future, extended wear of hard gas-permeable materials may also be an option.

Hydrogel correction is often less complicated than fitting rigid lenses, but for many patients it may not provide as optimal a result. For example, hydrogel lenses are more fragile, require more frequent replacement, do not correct corneal astigmatism, and require more cumbersome handling procedures than do rigid lenses. Thus far, aphakic hydrogel lenses have not been available in toric designs, and therefore aphakic patients with significant residual astigmatism must either be fitted with rigid lenses or be given supplementary spectacles that incorporate the astigmatic correction. If gel lenses can be fitted, most patients prefer the excellent comfort they provide. Also, if indicated, extended wear of gel lenses is excellent and convenient.

Hydrogel fitting procedures are discussed in Chapter 3; the following discussion is limited to the design and fitting of rigid lenses. Rigid aphakic contact lenses can be divided into two designs: single-cut and lenticular minus-carrier lenses (Fig. 7-3). Both lens types are useful, each having its advantages and disadvantages depending on the particular patient.[4,9,13] The following list compares criteria for selecting lenticular or single-cut lenses.

Lenticular Preferred	*Single-cut Preferred*
Cornea flatter than 45 D	Cornea steeper than 45
1.5 D or more against-the-rule toricity	With-the-rule toricity
Wide palpebral aperture	Narrow palpebral aperture
Loose upper lid	Tight upper lid
Lower lid below inferior limbus	Irregular or large pupil
Ectropion	

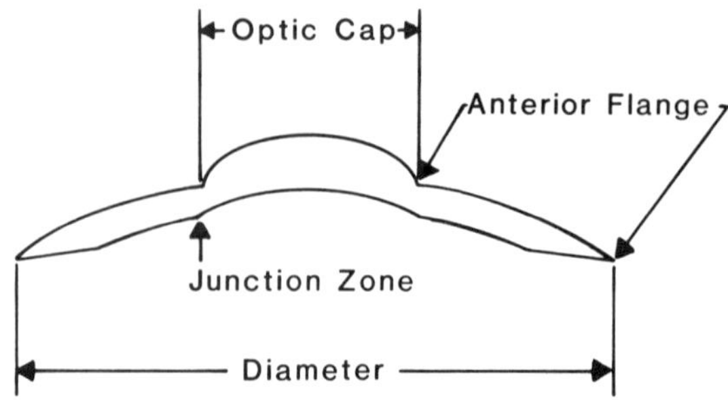

Figure 7-3 Diagram of lenticular lens showing optic cap, anterior flange, junction zone, and diameter.

If the corneal curvature is flatter than 45 D or if there is 1.5 D or more against-the-rule corneal toricity (vertical meridian flatter than horizontal), minus-carrier lenses are usually indicated because they provide better centration and movement. For corneas steeper than 45 D or with-the-rule toricity (vertical meridian steeper than horizontal), a single-cut lens should be considered. A single-cut lens can usually be made smaller than a minus-lenticular lens, and therefore may provide a better physiological result on steep corneas. The added weight because of increased center thickness of a single-cut lens also helps prevent excessive upward decentration of the lens that may be caused by with-the-rule toricity or excessively tight eyelids.

The width of the palpebral aperture also affects the choice of minus-carrier versus single-cut lenses. A wide aperture or lower lid margin that touches below the corneal limbus is an indication for a minus-carrier lens. The ability to make a smaller lens in a single-cut design makes them more appropriate for very narrow palpebral apertures. The thicker edge of the minus-carrier lens causes it to be held by the upper lid, and therefore it is not as dependent on the lower lid for positioning. A loose upper lid can usually grasp a minus-carrier lens and give good positioning where a single-cut lens would tend to drop excessively; conversely, a tight upper lid may cause excessive upward decentration of a minus-carrier lens, and a single-cut lens should be tried.

Lenticular lenses can be fitted to round, well-centered pupils, but large keyhole, wedge-shaped, or irregular pupils usually do better with single-cut lenses because the junction zone of the minus-carrier lens may cross the pupil, causing visual disturbance.

FITTING

The period after surgery before a patient can be successfully fitted with a rigid lens depends on the type of surgery. Patients who have undergone phacoemulsification are usually ready for contact lens fitting in 4 to 6 weeks, whereas patients who have had intracapsular cataract extraction require about 12 weeks. The decision is usually based on several factors: stability of keratometric measurements and lack of mire distortion; stability of the manifest refraction; and slit lamp examination of the cornea. It is usually sufficient to measure corneal curvature and refraction every 2 weeks until two successive readings show no change.

Fitting a Single-Cut Aphakic Lens

A single-cut aphakic lens is fitted in the same manner as any spherical single-cut lens. However, it is important to use an aphakic trial set, because the added weight from the increased center thickness makes these lenses ride much lower, on average, than myopic lenses. If a single-cut lens can be made to center well, it is preferable to use this lens design because of the ease of manufacture.

Fitting a Minus-Lenticular Aphakic Lens

The following are some guidelines for selecting various lens parameters.

Diameter Overall diameter usually ranges from 8.2 mm to 9.4 mm, depending on corneal curvature, corneal diameter, lid characteristics, and optic cap size (see below). Flat or large corneas generally require lenses near the large end of the range; steep, small corneas or small palpebral apertures require smaller lenses. Loose lids or low-hanging lower lids are also indications for large lenses, whereas tight upper lids may indicate small lenses. The overall lens diameter should be 1.5 mm to 2 mm larger than the optic cap size so that there will be an adequate lenticular flange for the lids to grasp.

Base Curve The same criteria are applied to selecting base curve for an aphakic spherical lens as are used for phakic spherical lenses (*i.e.,* begin the trial fitting with a base curve close to the flatter corneal reading). In many aphakic patients, however, it may be necessary to select a lens 0.5 D to 0.75 D steeper than the flat corneal reading because corneal surgery often seems to leave the cornea with a steeper periphery than normal. For each diopter of corneal toricity, the base curve can be increased approximately 0.25 D. High corneal toricity may require a toric base curve (see discussion of High Corneal Astigmatism). It is important to use an aphakic trial set and do a trial fitting because of the contour changes often seen after surgery, and because aphakic lenses are much heavier than standard myopic trial lenses and will tend to ride much lower than myopic lenses.

Optic Zone Diameter The optic zone should be larger than the pupil size by about 2 mm to 3 mm, if the lens centers well and the pupil is round. A lens that decenters significantly or a pupil with a significant sector defect within the palpebral aperture will require a larger optic zone. In general, a minimum optic zone diameter of about 6.5 mm is required.

Optic Cap Size The size of the front optic cap is usually selected very close to the optic zone diameter. The cap size limits the effective optic zone; therefore, the optic zone is usually not made larger than the optic cap, except to tighten the fit. The larger the optic cap, the thicker the lens; therefore, the smallest optic cap size consistent with good vision should be selected.

Anterior Peripheral Curve Radius The anterior curve of the lenticular flange should be 1 mm to 3 mm flatter than the base curve radius to provide an adequate edge thickness for lid control. The positioning of the lens can be controlled by varying the flange width and radius (Fig. 7-4).[8] The longer the radius or the wider the flange, the higher the lens will tend to ride. Conversely, the shorter the flange radius or the narrower the flange, the lower the lens will ride. A lenticular aphakic lens fitting will allow the practitioner to check a first approximation of the fit and vary the final lens specifications as needed.

Thickness The thicknesses of two points in the profile of a lenticular aphakic lens are important for a good physiological response and optimum fitting. To optimize physiological response, most aphakic rigid lenses should be prescribed in gas-permeable materials with as thin a center as possible, because the oxygen transmissibility (Dk/L) is inversely related to lens thickness. In addition, a thinner lens will help reduce lens dropping and discomfort. However, reduction of center thickness is limited by the fragility of the lens at the junction zone. A junction thickness of less than 0.13 mm may lead to lens breakage; therefore, it is best to specify a junction thickness of 0.13 mm and the center thickness will be determined automatically by the optic cap size and junction thickness. It should be remembered that any extra thickness at the junction zone will automatically add center thickness, making the lens heavier and less transmissible to oxygen.

Peripheral and Secondary Curves The use of trial lenses and fluorescein is the best method of determining the width and radii of the secondary and peripheral curves. These curves must be flat enough to provide an adequate interchange of tears under the lens, but the use of gas-permeable materials allows the practitioner latitude to select a tight enough fit to achieve good stability.

Power The highly hyperopic refractive error of aphakia makes an overrefraction over an *aphakic* trial lens important. If a calculation based on a spectacle refraction is used to determine the lens power, small errors in vertex distance measurement can cause significant errors in power. If the

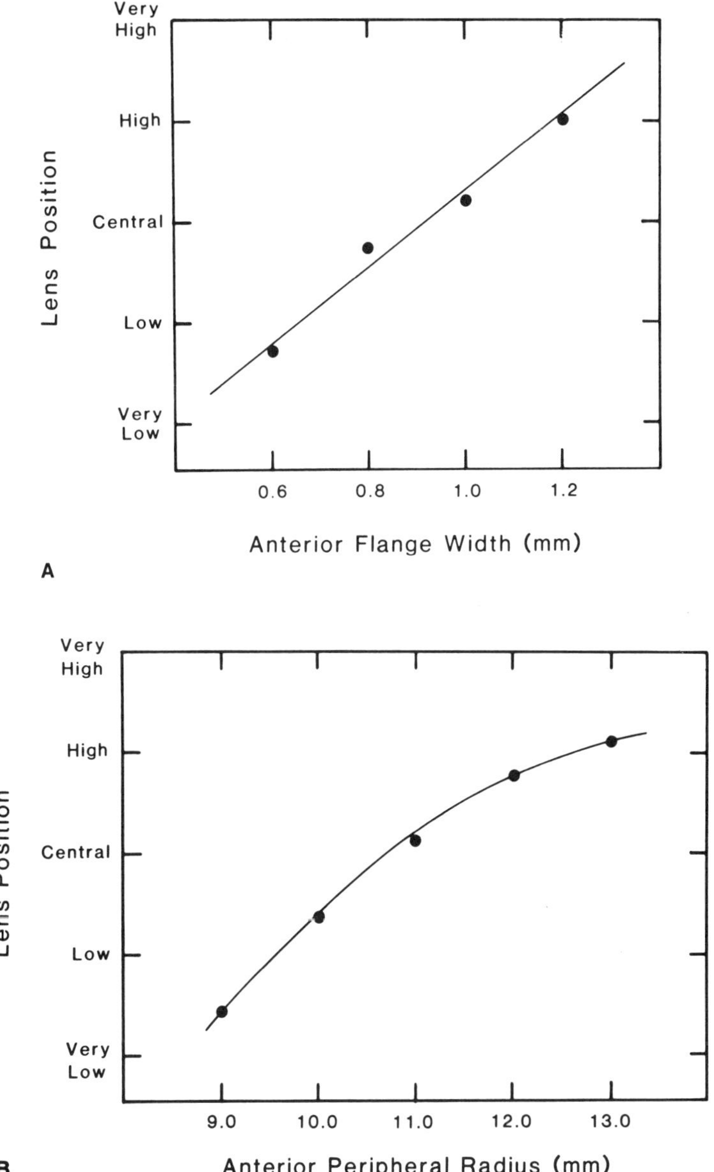

Figure 7-4 (A) Relationship between anterior flange width and lens riding position. (B) Relationship between anterior peripheral curve radius and lens riding position. (Redrawn from Nelson G, Mandell RB: The relationship between minus carrier design and performance. Int Contact Lens Clinic 2(2):75, 1975)

trial lens selected gives an overrefraction of more than ±4 D, another trial lens should be selected and the overrefraction repeated. An overrefraction of less than ±4 D can be added to the power of the trial lens, and vertex distance can be ignored. If a trial lens of the correct base curve is not available for the overrefraction, but one of approximately the correct power and a fairly close base curve is available, it may be used as long as the lens is stable enough for a good overrefraction. In this case, the induced tear lens must simply be calculated and its effective power incorporated into the correction. For example, if the base curve desired is 42 D and an aphakic lens of 42 D and +11 D power gives an overrefraction of +4.75 D, it is safer to repeat the overrefraction with another trial lens of 43.25 D base curve and +15 D power. In this case the tear lens contributes 43.25 − 42.00 = +1.25 D of power. If this second lens gives an overrefraction of −0.25, the correct power to order is +15.00 − 0.25 + 1.25 = +16.00. Note that the power ordered is 0.25 stronger than would have been ordered if the trial fitting had stopped after the first lens.

It is also important to perform a spherocylindrical refraction over the trial lens. In general, the easiest way to incorporate the residual astigmatic refractive correction is in a pair of supplementary spectacles, because the patient will require a near correction in any case. Unless the patient will be unable to function without his supplementary spectacles, it is safest to wait until the patient has begun adapting to his lenses before prescribing the spectacle correction.

PRESBYOPIA

Perhaps no type of lens design has created more consumer and practitioner interest than the bifocal contact lenses. There is a large potential market for well-fitting soft and hard bifocal lenses, and therefore lens manufacturers are spending considerable time and effort on research and development of bifocal contact lenses. Although several bifocal lenses have been introduced, there is no single lens material or type that provides both good distance and near vision to satisfy the needs of most patients.

Bifocal lens designs can be divided into two general categories: simultaneous and translating vision lenses. The simultaneous vision bifocal is constructed with a concentric (annular) lens design (Fig. 7-5) or an aspherical form. The annular design consists of a small central optic center usually about 2.25 mm in diameter and a large peripheral portion. The central portion usually corrects the distance vision, while the peripheral portion is constructed to correct the near vision. As the name "simultaneous" implies, there are two foci on the retina at the same time. This type of lens is currently available in soft materials in a considerable range of plus and minus distance powers with near adds up to +2.5 D. The lens can also be made in a rigid gas-permeable material, but no laboratories are producing such lenses at present.

The aspheric simultaneous vision lens depends on a constant change in power (more plus and less minus) from optic center to the periphery. The

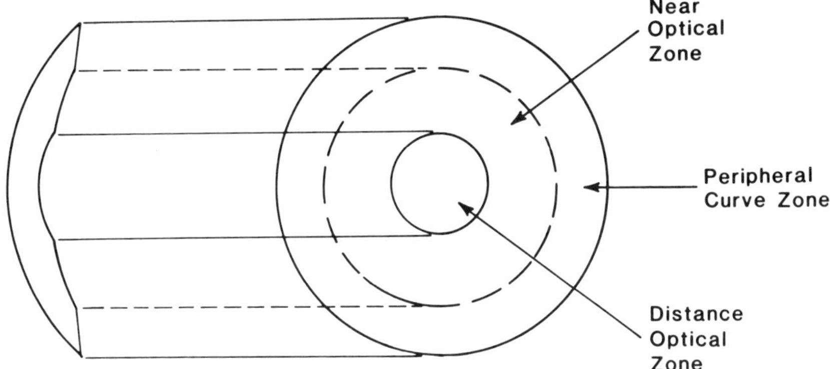

Figure 7-5 Cross section and front view of annular simultaneous vision bifocal contact lens. Distance objects are viewed through the small central optic and near objects through the mid-peripheral area. Patient has both near and distance vision focused simultaneously on the retina.

central area of the lens provides the distance vision while the changing aspheric periphery provides the near visual acuity. Because of the limitation on aspheric design, the effective add is limited to about +1.5 D. This lens is made in hydrogel material; however, aspheric bifocals are not currently available in any rigid material.

Both types of simultaneous bifocal lenses have clinical limitations. For example, it is not possible to have two simultaneous foci that can provide good vision at both distance and near. The annular lens gives somewhat better near vision, whereas the aspheric design seems to provide better distance vision. Some practitioners have recommended that an annular lens be fitted to one eye and an aspheric lens to the other eye. This is really a variation of the monovision approach. Such an approach can be effective if the clinician is careful to determine whether near or distance vision is more critical for the patient and prescribe accordingly. For example, if the patient primarily wants to use the lenses for reading, then the annular lens should be fitted to the dominant eye; if the lens is to be used mainly as a distance lens, then the aspheric design should be fitted to the dominant eye.

The translating type of bifocal depends upon the lens moving on the eye so that, as the patient looks into downgaze, the near portion of the lens is viewed through the pupil (Fig. 7-6). These lenses theoretically work the best because they take advantage of normal eye movements (*i.e.,* when the eye moves into downgaze for reading, the bifocal is pushed into the pupillary axis by the lower lid). The translation type of bifocal has a crescent-shaped segment that comes into position when the patient directs his gaze downward. The lens must not rotate and must be prevented from sliding under the lower lid so that the bifocal segment is shifted into place when the patient looks down. To meet these requirements the lens is usually made with prism and is truncated. These two lens features add considerable mass

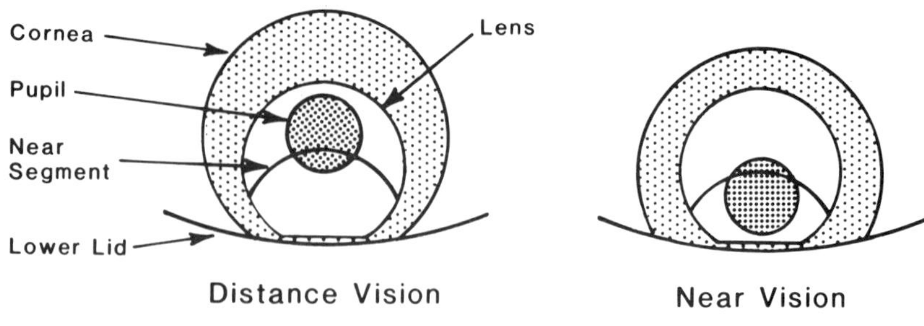

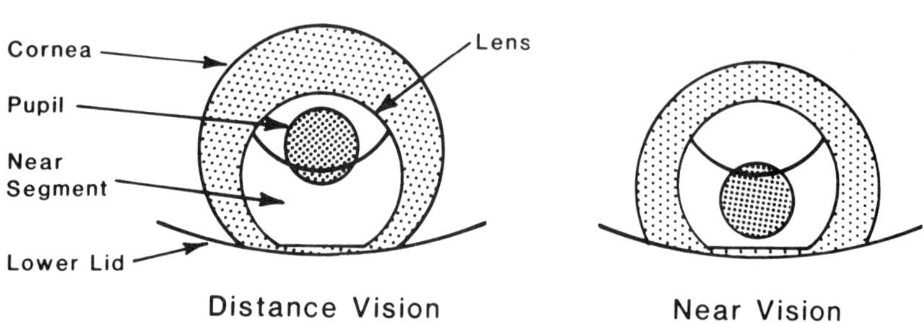

Figure 7-6 Diagram of translating bifocal contact lenses. In primary gaze the distance portion of the lens is positioned in front of the pupil. As the patient looks downward, the lid pushes the lens up, bringing the near segment in line with the pupil.

to the lens, often making it uncomfortable compared to the simultaneous vision lenses. Also, because of the increased lens thickness, the oxygen transmission is reduced, causing some patients to develop adverse physiological responses when wearing the lenses for long periods of time.

Rigid bifocal lenses thus far are all of the translation type. When PMMA lenses are used, a material of a higher index of refraction can be used for the bifocal crescent, thus achieving the needed power without substantially increasing lens mass. The silicon–acrylate lenses are available in only one refractive index, and therefore the bifocal power must be ground into the lens. This adds to the lens mass, but the silicon–acrylate materials can be designed more easily to provide sufficient oxygen to meet physiological requirements for daytime wear.

FITTING BIFOCALS

Bifocal lens designs are limited at present, and many patients cannot be fitted successfully. There are at least two important considerations in the successful fitting of bifocal contact lenses: patient selection and proper choice of lens type (*i.e.,* flexible versus rigid, translating versus simultaneous). Indications and contraindications to prescribing bifocal contact lenses for a particular patient are listed below.

Indications	*Contraindications*
High motivation	History of contact lens failure
Definite need for vision correction	Emmetropia
Successful hard lens wearer	Bifocal spectacle failure
Successful soft lens wearer	Large pupils
Moderate to high myopia	Loose lower lid
Successful spectacle bifocal wearer	Lower lid below inferior limbus
	Anterior segment disease

If these indications and contraindications are carefully adhered to, the chances for selecting a successful bifocal wearer will increase substantially.

Most fitters agree that the single most important factor in bifocal success is the patient's motivation and willingness to accept something slightly less than "perfect" vision. The patient should have a dependence on a visual correction. If the patient needs correction only for reading, there will be less motivation to wear contact lenses. Also, if the patient requires absolutely clear vision (comparable to spectacles or single vision contact lenses), currently available hard and soft bifocal lenses may not be acceptable because distance or near visual acuity is slightly reduced with these lenses. An additional indication is current success with contact lenses. If the patient has not previously worn contact lenses, then moderate to high myopes may do better than hyperopes because lens thickness can be reduced, thus improving the chances for physiological tolerance.

Among those patients who may be poor bifocal candidates are those with previous history of contact lens failure. These lenses are not usually quite as comfortable as single vision lenses; and also, because of their increased mass, physiological acceptance may be marginal. Patients with pupils larger than 3 mm do not do well because larger pupils tend to result in increased flare and reduced vision. For a translating type of bifocal, the lower lid must be relatively tight and tangent to the lower limbus. If either of these factors is not satisfied, the lens may not position correctly when the patient looks down to read. Finally, the presence of certain anterior segment problems such as dry eye, endothelial disease, or chronic lid inflammatory disease may limit the physiological tolerance of these lenses.

Once the decision has been made to try bifocal contact lenses, the clinician must determine what type of bifocal lens should be selected. If the patient is a successful hard or soft lens wearer, it is best to keep the same lens type; only if that lens type cannot be fitted should the alternate material be tried.

If the patient has no previous contact lens experience and no strong preference for one lens type, the chances for an optical success are probably slightly higher using the gas-permeable hard lenses. The clinician can try a diagnostic lens and evaluate the patient's response to the hard lens. If it is unacceptable, then a soft lens can be tried. With regard to the soft lenses, the best lens design seems to depend on the particular patient. The clinician will most likely have to try several lens types in the office before determining what type of flexible lens, if any, will work best.

Because the determination of the appropriate lens type must be done on a trial and error basis, a large inventory of lenses is usually necessary. For rigid lenses, the segment height can be varied and small changes can be critical in achieving success. With hard lenses, diameter, base curve, power, and so forth can also be varied, and therefore the number of trial lenses is more than most practitioners could maintain in an inventory. Most laboratories will loan trial bifocals or allow the practioner to order the lenses on a per case basis, giving the clinician a chance to see if the patient can adapt to the bifocal. For soft lenses, only trial and error will determine the best fit. On some patients, it is sometimes possible to fit one type of soft bifocal on one eye and another type of lens on the other, giving maximum vision for both distances. This modified "monovision" approach is sometimes acceptable to highly motivated patients. It is also possible to fit a spherical lens to one eye and a bifocal to the other, which works quite well for some patients.

In summary, a successful bifocal fitting requires high patient and practitioner motivation. Several lens changes may be required and the patient must be willing to tolerate something less than what he obtained with his single vision glasses or contact lenses. Considerably more research and development is needed before the optimum bifocal lens is available to provide the quality of vision that most patients expect.

REFERENCES

1. Baldone JA: The fitting of hard lenses onto soft contact lenses in certain diseased conditions. Contact Lens Med Bul 6(2–3):15, 1973
2. Dutescu M: Results of pick-a-back contact lens fitting. Contact Lens J 5(5):10, 1976
3. Fatt I, St. Helen R: Oxygen tension under an oxygen-permeable contact lens. Am J Optom Arch Am Acad Optom 48(7):545, 1971
4. Fraser JP, Gordon SP: The "apex" lens for binocular aphakia. Ophthal Optician 7(23):1190, 1967
5. Herman JP: Flexure of rigid contact lenses on toric corneas as a function of base curve fitting relationship. J Am Optom Assoc 54(3):209, 1983
6. Korb DR, Finnemore VM, Herman JP: Apical changes and scarring in keratoconus as related to contact lens fitting techniques. J Am Optom Assoc 53(3):199, 1982
7. Korb DR: Recent developments in fitting contact lenses for keratoconus. J Am Optom Assoc 55(3):172, 1984

8. Nelson G, Mandell RB: The relationship between minus carrier design and performance. Int Contact Lens Clinic 2(2):75, 1975
9. Polse KA: Contact lens fitting in aphakia. Am J Optom 46(3):213, 1969
10. Polse KA, Decker MR, Sarver MD: Soft and hard contact lenses worn in combination. Am J Optom Physiol Opt 54(10):660, 1977
11. Sarver MD: A bitoric gas permeable hard contact lens with spherical power effect. J Am Opt Assoc 56(3):184, 1985
12. Steele E: A preliminary report on the fitting of cases of high astigmatism with hydrophilic lenses. Contacto 20:36, 1976
13. Welsh MD, Welsh J: The Second Report on Cataract Surgery, pp 23–37; 48–57. Miami, Ed. Press, 1971
14. Westerhout D: The combination lens. Contact Lens 4(5):3, 1973

CHAPTER EIGHT

EXTENDED-WEAR CONTACT LENSES

GULLAPALLI N. RAO

The concept of extended-wear contact lenses was introduced based on the premise that the normal physiologic requirements of the cornea can be maintained in the presence of a contact lens in the eye for longer than 24 hours at a time. Significant advances have been made in contact lens technology since then, and extended-wear contact lenses have become a reality, not just a concept. The idea was originated with the introduction of therapeutic lenses and was later extended for the correction of aphakia and myopia. Investigations are currently under way on the use of extended-wear lenses to correct astigmatism and presbyopia. The original materials used for extended wear were, by and large, hydrophilic, but new hard, gas-permeable materials appear to have great potential. At the present time, only hydrophilic lenses and lenses made of silicone elastomers are being used for extended wear.

PHYSIOLOGY OF EXTENDED WEAR

The normal physiology of the cornea and the alterations that occur with extended-wear contact lenses have been discussed in detail in Chapter 1. However, it is important to review a few basic principles.

Although our knowledge of corneal physiology is far from complete, some basic factors related to extended wear have been identified. One of the most important is the oxygen availability to the cornea, because this is crucial for maintaining normal corneal metabolism, and hence transparency. Oxygen is normally supplied to the cornea by three routes: atmosphere, limbal capillaries, and aqueous. In the closed eye state, these routes may be supplemented by the lid vasculature. For atmospheric oxygen to reach the cornea, the lens should have adequate oxygen transmissibility along with mobility to allow the lens pump mechanism to work.

Lack of optimal oxygen supply can lead to hypoxia with all its attendant adverse effects on the cornea. Although adequate oxygen transport does not guarantee the success of extended wear, it is a basic requirement.

BASIC APPROACH TO EXTENDED WEAR

A number of lens-related and patient-related factors have to be considered to achieve success with extended-wear contact lenses. These, along with a basic understanding of corneal anatomy and physiology, will enhance the chances of optimizing the conditions for extended wear.

LENS-RELATED FACTORS

Lens-related factors include the specific lens material, its method of manufacture, the architectural configuration of the finished lens, and the fit of the lens to the corneal surface. The basic lens variables have been identified to include the polymer, durometer factor, lens diameter, thickness, water content, and edge design. To these factors, one can add the important consideration of surface characteristics. Inherent polymeric composition bears a direct relationship to the manufacturing technique, as well as to the specific design of the finished contact lens. Each polymer is associated with identifiable physical properties. One of the most important requisites for extended-wear contact lenses is gas transmission. In addition, patient comfort is important. The comfort can often be increased by increasing the water content of the lens. High water content lenses are also associated with higher degrees of oxygen transmission. The disadvantages of such lenses appear to be a greater degree of fragility and susceptibility to surface contamination.

In selecting a material and designing a lens to be used for extended wear, the contact lens manufacturers have utilized six basic approaches.[1]

Surface Characteristics

A highly wettable, hard surface will facilitate the circulation of tears around the lens and consequently assist in oxygen delivery to the underlying epithelium. There is evidence to indicate that such surfaces impede the deposition of mucoproteinaceous and mineral debris. The refractive characteristics of such a surface are good, and generally provide stable acuity and good correction of astigmatism. Cellulose acetate butyrate (CAB) has been shown to be oxygen permeable, yet to a significant extent, its success as a lens for extended wear relates to a highly wettable surface, contributing to rapid exchange of metabolites at the tear film–corneal interface and little interference with the tear film. The CAB lens also has a higher degree of heat conductivity with a consequent lower requirement of oxygen.

High Oxygen Transmission

Because of its high inherent oxygen transmission, silicone material offers a great potential for extended wear and has been found to be an excellent material for this purpose. Despite its great potential for extended wear, the necessity for creating a stable hydrophilic surface has been a significant impediment to the use of silicone for extended-wear lenses.

Thin Membrane Lenses

When dealing with hydrophilic lenses, there exists the well-known inverse relationship between oxygen transmission and lens thickness. Both Bausch & Lomb and Corneal Sciences Industries (CSI) have been instrumental in developing thin membrane lenses with hydrophilic polymers of relatively low water content. The main difficulty has been the handling characteristics of these very thin lenses, and the inherent problems of lens design involved in producing a thin lens with high plus aphakic power. The advantages to this approach, however, are the good vision afforded by a polymer with relatively low water content.

Medium Water Content Hydrophilic Lenses

Both Hydrocurve II and Softcon lenses are manufactured with polymers having approximately 55% water content, approved by the Food and Drug Administration for extended wear. These medium water content lenses have been used clinically for several years and generally produce stable optics and have relatively good fitting characteristics. They are available in a wide range of parameters. The combination of the medium water content, relatively low inherent oxygen permeability of the polymers, and necessity for relatively thick lenses, all tend to produce a situation that, when considered by the parameter of corneal oxygen requirements alone, can be considered marginal. Consequently, the percentage of potential extended-wear patients successfully fitted without adverse corneal effects is somewhat limited.

High Water Content Hydrophilic Lenses

Both Permalens and Sauflon have been the main advocates of high water content lenses in the United States. They use materials of high water content (70% to 85%), which consequently have greater oxygen transmission than conventional hydrophilics. Higher water content is also associated with a more comfortable lens.

Combination Lenses

The combination of silicone and polymers, such as silicone/PMMA, and mechanical combinations consisting of high water content or thin membrane skirts with central harder materials have been advocated by a number of investigators. Saturn II utilizes an oxygen-permeable hard center and a medium water content soft skirt. It has recently been approved for sale.

None of the commonly available hydrogel lenses meets the ideal level of oxygen transmissibility. The silicone elastomers and other high Dk/L gas-permeable materials offer great potential in this direction and appear to be very promising for extended wear. This aspect has been discussed in detail in Chapter 1.

Available Lenses for Extended Wear

All the currently available contact lenses for different conditions are listed in appropriate chapters. These include lenses for aphakia, myopia, hyperopia, and toric lenses.

PATIENT SELECTION

Successful wear of extended-wear contact lenses relies significantly on a number of patient-related factors in addition to an understanding of physiologic principles and lens-related factors. These include patient selection, patient instruction, and follow up.

Factors Influencing Patient Selection

A number of factors have to be considered in selecting patients for extended wear of contact lenses.

Age The age of the patient has to be considered in making a judgment about fitting extended-wear lenses, because alterations in the structure and function of the eye as a function of age may affect the decision about extended wear. Alteration in the normal defensive mechanisms in the aging eye, such as tear film dysfunction and a decrease in the corneal functional reserve, are examples. In addition, factors such as the decrease in corneal sensitivity may delay the development of subjective symptoms in the older age group, leading to greater degree of ocular morbidity following contact lens wear. This is borne out by the evidence that aphakic patients have a higher incidence of complications compared with the younger population.

Lifestyle In fitting extended-wear contact lenses, it is particularly important that one is conscious of the general lifestyle of the patient. Patients who are constantly exposed to working conditions that are likely to adversely affect the performance of extended-wear lenses should not be considered for extended wear. Also significant is the patient's general lifestyle where compliance with instructions is likely to be poor.

General Health The general health of the patient has to be considered before fitting with extended-wear contact lenses. Patients who have debilitating conditions such as chronic alcoholism or poorly controlled diabetes mellitus with evidence of complications, and others on immunosuppressive therapy constitute a high-risk category for problems such as infection. Such cases are characterized by low resistance and inability to appreciate early symptoms and to seek prompt professional care. In addition, corneal surface defenses may be impaired, with changes in the epithelial structure and precorneal tear film, and marked decrease in corneal sensitivity. Patients who have evidence of any general infectious processes or foci of infections in other parts of the body should particularly avoid extended-wear contact lenses.

Insertion and Removal Although the lack of need for insertion and removal of contact lenses is considered the main advantage of extended-wear contact lenses, either the patient or someone in the patient's environment should be able at least to remove the lens in an emergency. This will minimize the risk of severe complications.

Hygiene Persons with poor personal hygienic habits should be scrupulously avoided for extended-wear contact lenses. Any complacency in hygiene can lead to devastating complications with a high degree of ocular morbidity.

Ocular Environment One of the important factors in the development of infections in the eye is the presence of microbial flora on the lid margins. These opportunistic organisms, which are the normal inhabitants of the lids, can become more virulent and produce fulminant infections where conditions are optimal for the proliferation of these organisms. This risk is particularly more pronounced in the aphakic age group. Because of the host's impaired defense mechanism, special attention should be given to the following aspects.

Lids: Detailed examination is mandatory and any evidence of lid infections should be evaluated carefully.

Blink response: It is not uncommon to see patients with incomplete blinking. Because tear exchange is one of the primary requirements for the maintenance of extended-wear contact lenses, normal blinking is essential.

Interpalpebral area: In patients in whom the blink response is incomplete, the exposed interpalpebral area should not be too wide because of the risks of excessive drying of the lens as well as the potential for loss.

Corneal sensitivity: Corneal sensitivity is diminished following contact lens wear of all types. Because corneal sensitivity is essential for the recognition of early symptoms, corneal integrity should be assessed prior to the contact lens fitting. Patients with a marked decrease in corneal sensitivity are not good candidates for extended-wear contact lenses. In addition, the epithelium of hypoesthetic corneas may be abnormal and may increase the risk of some of the epithelial problems in these patients.

Evaluation of the Corneal Surface Prior to Fitting With Extended-Wear Contact Lenses

Evaluation of the corneal surface includes an assessment using stains such as rose bengal and fluorescein. Attention should be directed to the thickness of the cornea. Any suspicion about increased thickness should be confirmed by pachymetry. Corneal endothelial status should be evaluated by slit lamp biomicroscopy. Whenever any doubt exists about the status of endothelial cell morphology, it has to be verified using the techniques of specular microscopy.

Proper fit: During the patient selection process, once the decision has been made to go ahead with the fitting of the extended-wear lens, appropriate evaluation of the fit is extremely important.

Follow up: It is absolutely mandatory for all patients who are fitted with extended-wear contact lenses to adhere to a strict follow-up schedule. If the patient is unlikely to comply, this constitutes a contraindication for extended-wear contact lenses.

Follow-up Schedule

In all patients with extended-wear contact lenses, our recommended routine follow-up schedule is evaluation of the eye and the fit 1 hour, 1 day, 1 week, and 1 month following the fitting of the lenses. Once this has been established, the patient is reevaluated again after 3 months. Subsequent exams are scheduled every 3 months during the first year and every 6 months thereafter. The patient is instructed about the symptoms of blurring, redness, and irritation, which warrant an immediate call to the ophthalmologist. Instruction is important to eliminate the risk of serious complications. During the follow-up period for patients with extended-wear contact lenses, one has to look for tight lens, dirty lens, ocular intolerance, or reduced visual acuity.

Ocular intolerance is characterized by pain, redness, and irritation and objective signs of lid edema, decreased lens mobility along with steepening of the lens, epithelial problems such as erosions and edema, and endothelial changes in the form of bedewing.

If any of the symptoms appear, it is imperative for the ophthalmologist to advise discontinuing lens wear. Once the symptoms resolve, the fit may have to be modified, or in some cases, the type of lens that is given to a particular patient may need to be changed. During the initial period after the refitting, the patients have to be monitored very closely to study the adaptation of the new lens and to elicit any signs of recurrence of the problems. In all these patients, particular attention has to be paid to the problem of insertion and removal.

In the routine follow up of all extended-wear contact lens patients, the following factors have to be specifically assessed, particularly in those for whom extended wear is considered a risky proposition. Visual acuity should be recorded at each follow-up visit, and assessment of corneal status with a slit lamp evaluation is of paramount importance. The conjunctiva should be examined, particularly at the upper tarsal conjunctiva, for any evidence of problems such as giant papillary conjunctivitis. In addition, the fit of the contact lens has to be assessed periodically along with the measurement of corneal thickness using pachymetry whenever altered corneal function is suspected.

COMPLICATIONS OF EXTENDED WEAR

A number of complications associated with the use of contact lenses are also seen with extended-wear contact lenses. However, the incidence of complications with extended wear is higher than with daily-wear contact lenses. These include the entire constellation of complications such as lens deposits, problems of anoxia, lens failure, infection, giant papillary conjunctivitis, and lens intolerance. Because of the risk of sight-threatening sequelae associated with some of these complications, it is important for the clinician to be aware of all the basics related to extended wear, and to pay special attention to all the factors of lens selection, patient follow up, and instruction that have been outlined in this chapter.

CONCLUSION

In the ultimate analysis, improvements in our understanding of corneal physiology as well as lens technology will continue to contribute towards minimizing complications. The idea of an ideal extended-wear lens that is thin, antimicrobial, laminated, highly oxygen permeable, and with a deposit-resistant surface is still being pursued. This in concert with the concept of a "disposable" lens may have a significant beneficial impact on the complication rate.

REFERENCES

1. Aquavella JV, Rao GN: Which lens: contact lenses currently available for extended wear in aphakia. Ophthalmology 87:151, 1980
2. Lembach RG, Wilson LA: Extended wear contact lenses. In Dabezies OH (ed): Contact Lenses: The CLAO Guide to Basic Science and Clinical Practice, pp 61.1–61.19. New York, Grune & Stratton, 1984

CHAPTER NINE

COMPLICATIONS
OF CONTACT LENSES

GULLAPALLI N. RAO and JAGJIT S. SAINI

Contact lenses play a very significant role in the management of refractive as well as therapeutic problems. The diversity of contact lenses available makes this modality very popular. Contact lens technology is in a constant state of mutation, gradually approaching the development of the most "optimal" lens; however, the occurrence of complications is a continuing cause for great concern. All types of lenses were shown to have the potential to produce deleterious effects of varying degree on the ocular structure. The complications secondary to contact lens wear can be either alterations in the refractive status of the eye or pathologic alterations of varying severity resulting in different degrees of morbidity. Although a better understanding of the corneal anatomy and physiology and the alterations induced by contact lenses have helped to elucidate the pathogenesis of some of the complications, we are still unclear about some forms of contact lens induced external eye disease. The increasing awareness of these complications, both among ophthalmologists and patients, has helped to minimize their incidence to some degree.

Complications are reported with all forms of contact lenses and with both daily-wear and extended-wear regimens. In general, it is accepted that extended wear of contact lenses tends to increase the incidence of complications.

Complications induced by the presence of contact lenses are influenced by both lens-related and patient-related factors. Although all types of contact lenses have the potential to produce adverse effects on the eye, more complications are reported with hydrophilic soft lenses, a phenomenon exaggerated with extended-wear lenses. Most problems related to hard contact lenses are secondary to anoxia, but the gamut of corneal and other external eye problems occurs in soft contact lens wearers. The underlying factors appear to be either anoxia, allergy, or infections. With gas-permeable lenses, the problem of hypoxia has been obviated. These differences are due to the type of lens material, its surface, structural characteristics, and the cleaning solutions employed. Each of these complications can be triggered by a single factor or can be the cumulative effect of several factors.

Soft contact lenses are the most popular type of contact lenses in the market today. Lenses of different parameters and with varying degrees of oxygen transmissibility are available. The increasing popularity of these lenses is paralleled by the concern about the complication rate associated with them.

In this chapter, we will address some of the most common complications encountered in contact lens wearers and discuss their early recognition, prophylaxis, and management.

LENS-RELATED COMPLICATIONS

The lens-related problems include lens splitting, lens spoilage with formation of deposits on the lens surface, and fitting problems characterized by the clinical entity of tight lens syndrome. Another notorious and often vexing problem is the loss of lenses. The spectrum of ocular complications may range from subtle alterations in the normal physiology to gross structural damage resulting in sight-threatening sequelae as exemplified by some corneal ulcerative processes. Conjunctival and corneal changes of allergic, anoxic, infective, and toxic etiology have been described.

LENS SPLITTING OR DAMAGE

Soft contact lenses are inherently fragile; therefore, splitting is not uncommon. The degree of fragility varies for different lenses and depends to a great degree on factors such as water content. The Permalens with a water content of around 71%, for example, has greater fragility, which may result in the development of cracks in the edges of the lenses. Although the damage seems to be seen more frequently in the periphery along the edges of the lenses, other parts of the lenses are equally vulnerable.[74] Lens damage is usually due to improper handling, lens fatigue, or a combination of these factors.

Although asymptomatic patients do not warrant treatment or change in the lens, patients who develop symptoms should be given proper attention in the form of a new replacement lens. This problem is reported to occur in about 20% of all daily-wear patients.[12]

LENS SPOILAGE

Of the lens-related complications, spoilage is the most frequent and has the greatest potential for initiating adverse ocular responses. The incidence of lens deposits has been shown to vary widely, and this is due to each physi-

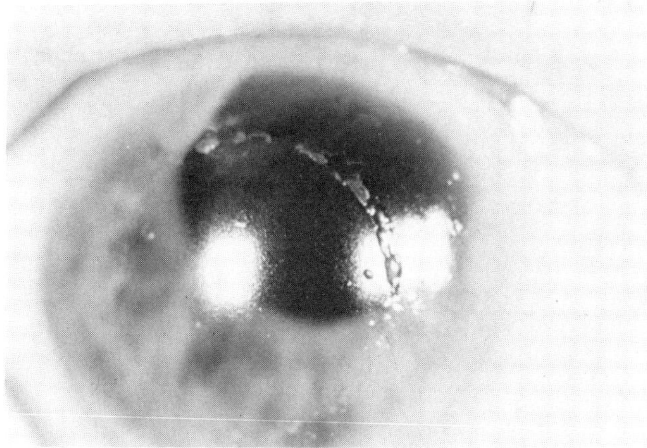

Figure 9-1 Mucoid lens deposits at the junction of the optical zone and the carrier portion of the contact lens in a 78-year-old aphakic patient.

cian's criteria for the diagnosis of lens spoilage. There have been several anecdotal reports claiming the superiority of one lens over another in minimizing the problem, but no scientific data are available to support this contention. The problem is encountered more commonly with extended-wear contact lenses.

Clinically, lens spoilage may manifest either as a diffuse coating of fine proteinaceous debris on the surface of the lens, or as a collection of mucoid material (Fig. 9-1), or in the form of large deposits that are resistant to all forms of cleaning (Fig. 9-2). This constitutes the most difficult problem encountered in patients using extended-wear contact lenses.[20]

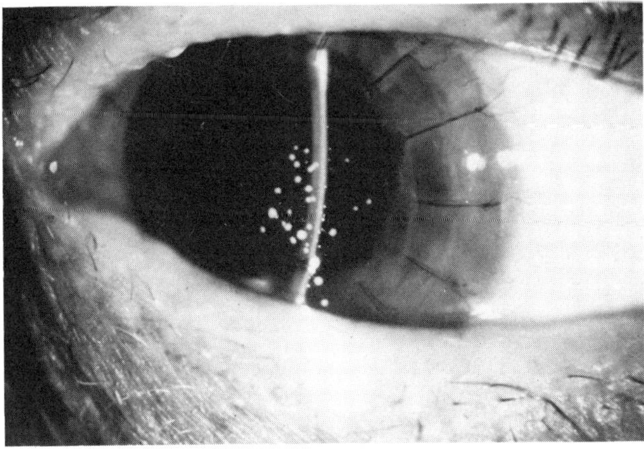

Figure 9-2 Accumulation of calcareous deposits in the central part of the lens.

Predisposing Factors

For successful wear of soft contact lenses, the integrity of the lens surface is a significant factor. The normal smooth surface is important to maintain the optical characteristics of the contact lens, as well as for the comfort of the patient. A number of factors may predispose to contact lens spoilage, but the exact etiology and the pathogenic mechanisms responsible are not clearly defined. Although clinicians are aware of the common occurrence of this problem, no definite solution is available for its management.

The various factors that contribute to deposit formation can be either lens related or related to the environment within the patient's eye. Lens handling, lens cleaning, the use of cosmetics by the patient, the general environment in which the patient lives and works, and the history of topical or systemic drug use can all significantly influence the occurrence of the deposits.

Composition

For a proper understanding of the pathogenesis of lens spoilage, one of the important prerequisites is knowledge about the composition of the deposits. Tripathi and co-workers have demonstrated that lens deposits are composed of a variety of substances and can be inorganic, organic, or mixed in composition.[75] Microbial contaminants and other factors such as manufacturing and physiologic defects, purity of the polymer, and aging and decaying changes in the lenses contribute to this phenomenon.[66,75] A detailed analysis undertaken by the above investigators have given us some insight into the possible composition of the different categories of deposits. Clinical correlation of these observations has indicated that a number of patient-related factors may be responsible for this phenomenon. These include the following:

1. The status of the patient's eyelids, with particular reference to the presence of meibomitis or blepharitis

2. Lagophthalmos, which may produce excessive drying of the lens surface, making it vulnerable to deposit formation

3. Tear film dysfunction

4. Any conjunctival inflammatory process

5. Relative dry eye leading to concentration of tear proteins, which coat the surface of the lens. In the absence of adequate tear circulation around the lens, this may lead to excessive deposit formation. Calcification of contact lenses has been reported in patients with dry eye and increased tear concentration.[34]

The hydrophilic lens material has been shown to have an attraction for tear proteins, especially lysozyme, as well as other amino acids and glycoproteins.

The ocular factors alone do not lead to the formation of lens deposits. Lens-related factors that favor the buildup of deposits include the quality of polymer material; the presence of manufacturing defects; aging changes in the lens; and type of cleaning regimen.

Diagnosis of Lens Spoilage

Although the advanced forms of lens spoilage can be diagnosed easily because of the presence of obvious changes on the lens surface, early detection of lensopathy or lens spoilage is often difficult. A number of clinical and laboratory investigations can be performed to facilitate early diagnosis. The information available in the literature from different types of microscopic techniques can perhaps be used to develop an understanding of the clinical phenomena associated with these changes. The clinical evaluation can be performed by detailed biomicroscopy of the contact lens surface. Specular microscopy can be an important additional tool. The different types of deposits and the characteristics of different types of spoilage have been elucidated by Lohman and co-workers using the technique of specular microscopy.[42]

Clinical Manifestations

EFFECTS OF LENS SPOILAGE ON THE CONTACT LENS

Spoilage can induce many changes in the contact lens. These include characteristics such as alterations in lens fit, thickness, or texture; changes in the contact with the cornea; altered fitting characteristics of the lens; irregularity of the surface of the lens, resulting in changes in optical characteristics of the lens; development of wrinkles and shrinkage of the lens; defects of the edges of the contact lens; cystic formations on the lens; and refractive changes secondary to these problems.

Optical Manifestations

The following optical alterations may manifest secondary to lens spoilage: change in visual acuity; loss of quality of the image; restriction of the size of the visual field; development of ghosting and distortion; osmotic effect of some lenses; subjective complaints of seeing halos around lights; development of polyopia; visual aberrations; photophobia; and astigmatic errors.

Ocular Manifestations

The manifestations in the eye could vary from mild tear film abnormalities and discharge to the most prominent forms of corneal ulcerative processes. The following are some of the ocular manifestations of lens spoilage: tear film abnormalities; increasing incidence of discharge from the eyes; epiphora; ocular irritation; change in the blink rate; constant foreign body sensation in the eye with increasing intolerance to the lenses; conjunctival changes, including mild hyperemia, allergic conjunctivitis, giant papillary conjunctivitis, follicular conjunctivitis, and infective conjunctivitis; and corneal changes, including various forms of superficial keratitis, aseptic ulceration, and infective corneal ulcers.

All these manifestations can occur secondary to anoxia, hypoxia, or allergic processes that can be initiated by deposits and protein, which act as antigens, on the surface of the lens.

Management

The management of lens spoilage is one of the most frustrating problems for the ophthalmologist and the patient. Very often, the only effective way of eliminating the problem is by replacing the lenses; however, this can cause significant financial hardship to the patient. This problem is ameliorated to a certain extent by new policies initiated by contact lens manufacturers.

Prophylaxis The best way of delaying lens spoilage is by proper patient selection, patient instruction in lens care, and follow up. In patient selection, one has to be particularly conscious of not fitting people with obvious tear film and lid abnormalities with extended-wear lenses.

Cleaning Frequent and thorough cleaning of the contact lens surface will minimize spoilage. However, these measures may not have any effect in controlling the problem. Once the lens deposits occur, it is very difficult to remove them.

Enzymatic Cleaners Frequent use of enzymatic cleaners is recommended for persons with whom lens deposits occur rapidly.[12] However, there is no documented evidence of the value of this technique.

Lens Replacement Replacement is perhaps the only effective way of managing lens spoilage. The decision to replace a lens depends on the symptoms it causes. Any blurring or irritation with objective signs of ocular response constitute indications for lens replacement. In any patient with whom frequency of lens replacement due to deposits becomes excessive, the use of extended-wear lenses should be reevaluated.[15]

TIGHT LENS SYNDROME

Tight lens syndrome is a condition often reported in aphakic patients using extended-wear contact lenses.

Clinical Manifestations

The typical patient with tight lens syndrome has been fitted with contact lenses within the past 48 to 72 hours. The patient has a sudden onset of pain, redness in the eye, and blurred vision. The ocular signs may vary from an immobile lens on the eye, to acute inflammatory reaction of the anterior segment of the eye. This is characterized by lid edema, ciliary injection, corneal edema, epithelial erosion with entrapment of epithelial cells under the contact lens, and inflammatory reaction in the anterior chamber (Color Fig. 9-1). Very minimal or no movement of the lens is seen. Often, this might lead to the development of an imprint at the limbus. A considerable amount of mucoid material along with epithelial debris from the desquamated epithelial cells may have accumulated under the lens.

Pathogenesis

Although the exact pathogenesis is not clear, a number of factors may be incriminated in the development of tight lens syndrome. A number of alterations in the ocular environment can steepen the lens. Alteration in tear pH is a factor that often affects the lens structure and thereby the lens fit.[44,49] Dehydration of the lens can also lead to similar problems. Hypoxia induced by a steep lens can produce epithelial problems such as epithelial denudation, as well as lead to corneal edema due to imbibation of excessive fluid into the corneal stroma through metabolic changes initiated by hypoxia.

Treatment

In the initial stages where the symptoms are limited to discomfort in the eye, the only treatment needed is the discontinuation of the lens until the eye returns to normal. If there is any evidence of inflammation, it should be treated according to severity. In those cases where there is severe iridocyclitis, the eye should be treated with cycloplegics and sometimes may even require the use of topical glucocorticoids. Once the eye has become quiet, refitting of the contact lens has to be decided depending on the motivation of the patient and the overall situation of the eye. If a decision has been made to refit an eye with a lens, this has to be accomplished using a flatter lens either with higher water content or with increased oxygen permeability. In those cases where the extended wear of contact lenses is not mandatory, the patient may be encouraged to switch to daily-wear contact lenses.

Recurrences of this syndrome have been reported. In such cases, use of eye drops with alkaline pH may be of help. Unisol, which is a preservative-free saline, can be used. In cases where recurrences are common, a change to a different type of lens may be indicated.

LENS LOSS

Loss of lenses is one of the most serious problems causing considerable economic burden to patients. Patients, particularly aphakic patients, who are fitted with extended-wear contact lenses require frequent replacement, which may be a financial burden. The exact causes of lens loss are not clear. The anatomical configuration of the eyelids and the eye, the contact lens fit, lens spoilage, and keratoconjunctivitis sicca all may contribute to easy lens loss.

There is no simple remedy for this problem. One measure is patching the eye at night. Frequent application of lubricants such as artificial tear substitutes may help to minimize the incidence of lens loss by keeping the lens moist and thereby *in situ.*

OCULAR COMPLICATIONS

Ocular responses to contact lens wear vary from milder forms of conjunctivitis to serious complications leading to loss of vision.

The most common clinical manifestation is the development of red eye, where the basic causes are essentially the same as in non-contact lens wearers. However, the presence of a contact lens renders the eye more vulnerable to exogenous insults. Conjunctivitis can be of different types in these patients, ranging from allergic reaction to protein on the contact lens surface, to toxic reaction to contact lens solutions, to infective process from contaminated contact lens solution, or to factors related to patient hygiene.[3,21,57,64,79]

CONJUNCTIVAL REACTIONS

Conjunctival reactions may vary from minimal conjunctival hyperemia to the most acute forms of conjunctivitis. Reactions can be allergic, toxic, or infective in origin.

Allergic Conjunctivitis

The clinical presentation of allergic conjunctivitis takes diverse forms, and includes simple forms of conjunctival hyperemia to giant papillary conjunctivitis.[3] Allergic conjunctivitis rarely leads to any visual deficit.

SYMPTOMS AND SIGNS

In the simple forms of allergic conjunctivitis, the symptoms include itching, excessive tearing, and excessive mucus secretion. Objective evaluation reveals limbal hyperemia with conjunctival chemosis (Fig. 9-3), collection of mucoid material in the conjunctival cul-de-sac, and papillary and follicular changes in the tarsal conjunctiva. In addition, some cases have been reported with Tranta's dots at the limbal area.[47] In the more advanced stages, the upper tarsal plate is covered with giant papillae.

PATHOGENESIS

The basic mechanism is believed to be an allergic reaction to protein on the contact lens surface, which acts as an antigen.[3,64] Allergic reaction may also occur secondary to exposure to contact lens solutions.[51,52]

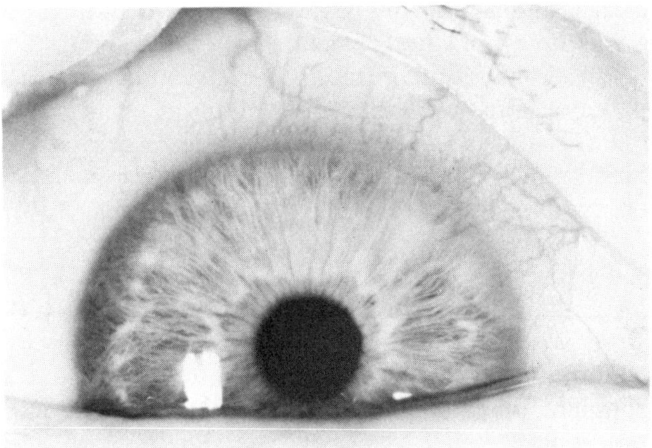

Figure 9-3   Limbal hyperemia with chemosis in a patient who developed allergic conjunctivitis.

MANAGEMENT

Allergic conjunctivitis of any origin is not amenable to any particular treatment regimen. No specific drug is available to control this problem effectively. The best method of management is to cease wearing contact lenses. The patient's comfort can be increased by frequent instillation of lubricants (artificial tear substitutes). In patients who have excessive mucoid secretion, mucolytic agents such as acetylcysteine in 10% dilution may give relief. Recently, cromolyn sodium in 4% concentration has been reported to be beneficial in these cases.[46] Combined with replacement of the contact lens, this appears to be particularly beneficial. There is some tendency to use topical glucocorticoids for treating this problem. In general, however, these drugs arc not of any significant help in these cases.

Once the condition has improved, the question of resuming contact lens wear should be addressed. The contact lens can be refitted according to some basic principles. The lens has to be replaced with a new lens, and the cleaning regimen has to be modified.[30] In addition, a lcns of a different edge type may be of help. Lubricating agents used regularly may minimize surface deposition. In those patients who use lenses on an extended-wear basis, switching to a daily-wear regimen may be of significant help.

Giant Papillary Conjunctivitis

The development of giant papillae on the upper tarsal conjunctiva in contact lens wearers can be a significant problem. This complication was reported originally by Spring and has been elucidated further by the work of Allansmith and colleagues.[3,71]

This syndrome is much more prevalent in soft contact lens wearers compared with hard contact lens wearers, but it can occur at any age without any sex predilection.[3] The exact incidence is not known, but it is speculated that it occurs in 1% to 5% of hard contact lens wearers and in 10% to 15% of soft contact lens wearers.[26] In a prospective study conducted on 200 hard contact lens wearers from a selected population, an incidence of 10.5% was noted.[36] The time of onset may range from a few weeks to several years.

The predominant symptoms are increasing awareness of the lens, increasing irritation, itching, blurred vision, and a marked degree of lens movement. Classically, these signs include the development of giant papillae on the upper tarsal conjunctiva, mucus strands in the conjunctival cul-de-sac, and a contact lens coated with proteinaceous debris. Soft and hard contact lens wearers have similar symptoms. Variations in severity are common. In a typical sequence, mild discomfort and itching are accompanied by a gradual increase in eye secretion, ultimately leading to complete intolerance of the contact lens in the eye. The clinical picture has been recognized to pass through several stages of evolution. Allansmith has described the different stages of giant papillary conjunctivitis.[3]

Stage 1 is characterized by the presence of a minimal degree of mucus, usually confined to the nasal corner of the eye and noted upon arising in the morning, along with a mild sensation of itching. These symptoms often can be elicited only by direct questioning and the patient may not volunteer any information. This stage is typically characterized by the absence of any signs.

Stage 2 demonstrates increasing intensity of the symptoms in terms of increased visual blurring with a gradually increasing intolerance to the lens. In addition, there is a considerably greater degree of mucus formation along with itching. It usually occurs after several hours of contact lens wear, and most often towards the end of the normal wearing time. Objective evaluation would reveal an increase in the diameter and elevation of papillae on the upper tarsal conjunctiva, which can be detected by biomicroscopic examination. The conjunctiva is usually thickened, edematous, and hyperemic, and tends to obscure the fine vascular distribution. Towards the end of stage 2, enlarged giant papillae become visible with biomicroscopy (Fig. 9-4). These giant papillae are not the result of enlargement of normal papillae, but rather a substructure derived from the deep tarsal conjunctiva.

Stage 3 is characterized by an increase in the severity of mucus secretion, itching, and excessive lens movement on blinking. Additionally, one can see a marked degree of coating of the contact lens surface, with both mucus and debris. The duration of lens tolerance is often diminished. An evaluation of the eye would reveal a marked increase in both the number and the size of the papillae on the upper tarsal conjunctiva, and the apices of the papillae may take fluorescein staining. Mucus strands usually can be seen in the conjunctival cul-de-sac.

Stage 4 is marked by an increased degree of severity of the symptoms, with complete intolerance to the contact lens. The lenses become coated almost instantaneously upon insertion into the eye. Extreme intolerance will not allow the lens to remain in the eye for any length of time. The

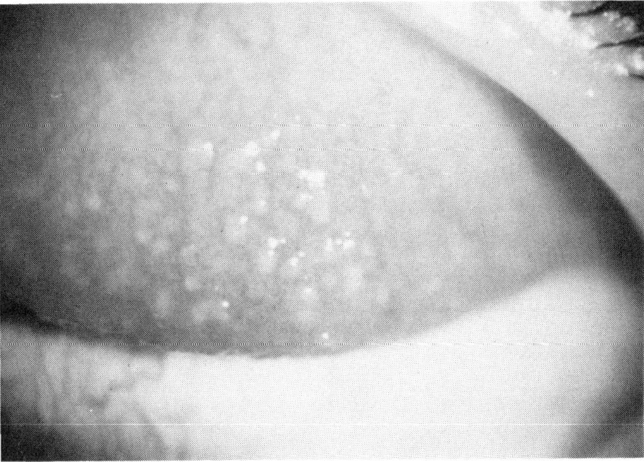

Figure 9-4   Stage 2 of giant papillary conjunctivitis demonstrating the gradual emergence of papillae in the upper tarsal conjunctiva with hyperemia of this area.

mucus secretion becomes excessive, and the patient may complain of gluing of the lashes in the morning. Objective evaluation demonstrates flattening of the apices of the papillae (Fig. 9-5) with positive fluorescein staining. The contact lens becomes heavily coated with deposits and the lens is often seen to be decentered.

When giant papillary conjunctivitis is analyzed further, some degree of difference in its characteristics can be found between hard and soft contact lens wearers. The number of papillae is usually fewer in hard contact lens wearers. Also, the apices of the papillae present a greater elevation in con-

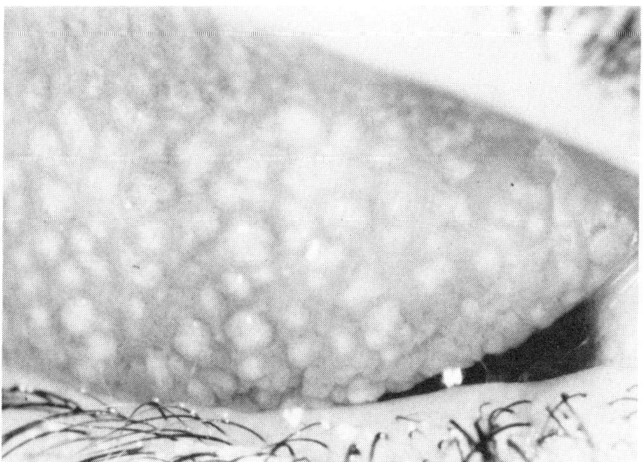

Figure 9-5   Stage 4 of giant papillary conjunctivitis in a 62-year-old aphakic patient who had been using extended-wear contact lenses for 3 years. The entire upper tarsal conjunctiva is coated with evidence of papillary reaction.

trast to the round, flatter morphology of the papillae in soft lens wearers. According to Korb and co-workers, there is a difference in the zonal distribution of papillae between the two different types of lenses.[35,37] Whereas the hard contact lens wearers usually develop the papillae initially in the zones of tarsal conjunctiva closer to the eyelid margin, the soft lens wearers typically develop them closer to the tarsal fold. This phenomenon seems to correspond to the area of tarsal conjunctiva that comes in contact with the periphery of the lens. Unilateral development of these changes is seen very rarely.

In advanced stages, one can see the development of papillae occupying all the zones of tarsal conjunctiva in both hard and soft lens wearers. In such patients, the clinical picture very closely resembles that of vernal conjunctivitis.

Giant papillary conjunctivitis can recur with similar signs and symptoms. These develop much more rapidly than the initial onset even after apparent cessation of contact lens wear for several years.

PATHOLOGY

Greiner and associates employed scanning electron microscopic techniques to demonstrate alterations in surface morphology of the upper tarsal conjunctiva in contact lens wearers.[25] According to Greiner and associates, giant papillary conjunctivitis appears to be only an extension of changes that are normally seen in all contact lens wearers. Contact lens wear with its mechanical action on the tarsal conjunctiva seems to be responsible for alterations in the morphology of this region. In most lens wearers, this response rarely leads to any clinical manifestations. Indeed, the conjunctival surface may remain stable for long periods of time. On the contrary, in giant papillary conjunctivitis, the underlying papillae seem to increase the epithelial surface area twofold. The exact pathogenesis of this is not clear. It leads to marked distortions in cell shape accompanied by changes in conjunctival morphology.

Giant papillary conjunctivitis in contact lens wearers is characterized by a distinct cell profile, which has been summarized as follows by Allansmith and co-workers.[4]

1. Mast cells in the epithelium
2. Eosinophils in the epithelium and substantia propria
3. Basophils in the epithelium and substantia propria

Although the total number of lymphocytes and plasma cells increases, this reflects only an increase in total mass of conjunctiva. The presence of the above cell types represents that giant papillary conjunctivitis is an immunologic reaction, and the presence of basophils points to a type of delayed hypersensitivity called *cutaneous basophil hypersensitivity.*

PATHOGENESIS

Although the exact pathogenesis of giant papillary conjunctivitis is not known, it is commonly believed to be an immune reaction. In addition, the mechanical factor of the contact lens edge rubbing against the tarsal conjunctiva is considered to play a significant role in the development of this clinical picture.[27] However, this does not satisfactorily explain the sudden onset of this syndrome after several years of successful contact lens wear. Greiner and co-workers suggest that the mechanical trauma from the contact lens edge rubbing against the tarsal conjunctiva produces some alterations in the normal surface epithelium of the conjunctiva, resulting in degranulation of mast cells.[27] Such trauma also disrupts the epithelial surface, which normally acts as a barrier to the tear film and external environment. The coated contact lens then serves as a vehicle for the presentation of environmental debris (antigens) to this compromised epithelium. Such a combination of factors may result in the release of mediators of inflammation in the lymphoid conjunctival stroma and may initiate the changes observed in the inflammatory cells. It is likely that the newly acquired lymphatic cells are deposited in the stroma, where there already is a preexisting aggregation of lymphoid cells, which in turn results in follicular-like formations. Increased accumulation of lymphocytes in these areas would lead further to expansion of the stroma and overlying epithelium, and any further growth of the papillae would result in the formation of surface papillae.

TREATMENT

There is no effective means of treating giant papillary conjunctivitis. Several approaches can be tried, either singly or in combination, which may alleviate the patient's symptoms.

Cessation of Lens Wear Because contact lenses are the cause, the results of discontinuing wear are obviously encouraging. In the early stages, where the symptoms and signs are minimal, one could continue lens wear and still obtain some degree of resolution, either complete or partial, by measures such as more frequent cleaning of the lenses along with using enzymatic cleaners such as papain.[38] Removing the lens from the eye more frequently also helps the situation. If the lenses show evidence of gross degree of lens spoilage, the lenses need replacement. When replacement is considered, thought should be given to using a lens of different edge design to correct the mechanical factor. These measures may allow the continuation of lens wear. However, if the clinical picture becomes worse use of the lenses should be discontinued. This measure often leads to resolution of the symptoms with a gradual decrease in severity over a few weeks. Improvement in symptoms, change in the inflammatory reaction of the conjunctiva, and fluorescein staining of the papillae are helpful signs to assess the improvement in the condition. However, papillae will remain for weeks, months, or years.

Medical Therapy No drug is effective in controlling giant papillary conjunctivitis. Use of lubricants or vasoconstrictors may add to the comfort of the patient.

The use of cromolyn sodium 4% eyedrops has been shown to have some beneficial effect.[46] Although this does not alter the natural course of the disease, this might give symptomatic relief to the patient. In addition, using this drug concurrent with a new lens may allow early return to contact lens wear.

Use of topical corticosteroids is limited to the control of severe degrees of inflammation, and should be discouraged in view of the potential for adverse effects of this drug.

Infective Conjunctivitis

Different types of conjunctivitis of infectious origin (bacterial, fungal, or viral) can occur following contact lens wear. Their occurrence appears to be more frequent in soft lens wearers. Any red eye seen in contact lens wearers needs prompt attention and should be considered to be of infective origin unless otherwise proven. Although the exact cause of infection is often not found, lenses have the potential to transmit the organisms into the eye, and therefore can be incriminated as causative factors. There are reports in the literature showing that hydrophilic lenses can harbor microbial organisms, particularly in spoiled lenses.[2,6,22,26] However, there is no direct evidence thus far to link the presence of these organisms on the lens surface to the manifestation of a clinical problem. The problem may very well be limited to the development of inflammatory reaction without any overt infection. Reports in the literature do not corroborate the common belief that eyes with extended-wear contact lenses may indeed favor the existence of more microorganisms. Smolin and co-workers have observed that there were more microbial flora in the eyes of preoperative cataract patients compared with the eyes of aphakic patients using extended-wear contact lenses.[70] There was a report suggesting that aphakic contact lenses tend to harbor more fungi than other organisms because these lenses are thick.[6]

CLINICAL SYMPTOMS AND SIGNS

The patient may often complain of irritation, redness, and excessive tearing along with a history of crusting upon awakening in the morning. There may not be any pain associated with these symptoms in the form of lid edema, blepharitis, or the presence of diffuse conjunctival injection. If the infection is severe, conjunctival chemosis may be seen.

MANAGEMENT

The management is institution of appropriate measures, including microbiological studies to isolate the causative microorganisms, followed by initiation of antibacterial therapy. The contact lens use has to be discontinued. The selection of an appropriate antibiotic depends on the causative organism, but initial therapy with broad spectrum antibiotics such as erythromycin ointment or gentamicin may be effective. If microbiologic evaluation reveals that the organism is not susceptible to these antibiotics and no improvement in visual status is apparent, specific antibiotics should be started.

Toxic Conjunctivitis

In recent years, one of the most commonly encountered forms of conjunctivitis following contact lens wear is toxic conjunctivitis. It is very often secondary to the preservatives in contact lens solutions.[10,51,52]

The exact pathogenesis of this condition is not clear, but it is commonly believed that the preservative adsorbed onto the contact lenses may be a determining factor. In the lower water content lenses, it has been shown that the adsorption capacity for the preservatives is equal to the water content of the lens.[16] The lenses that have a tendency to adsorb greater degrees of these preservatives may have a greater potential for toxic effect compared with those with a smaller adsorption capacity. A number of commonly used lens solutions contain toxic substances that may produce epithelial problems. Chief among these is benzalkonium (BAK), used in approximately 50% of all ophthalmic solutions.[53]

CLINICAL PICTURE

The clinical picture of toxic conjunctivitis resembles other forms of conjunctivitis. The patient complains of irritation and redness, usually of sudden onset but occasionally seen after a change in the contact lens solution, or after changing from hard contact lens wear to soft contact lens wear in the immediate past. On examination, there is usually marked hyperemia of the conjunctiva with some degree of chemosis. The tarsal conjunctiva is usually free of any papillary or follicular reaction. The corneal changes include infiltration, pannus formation, and epithelial keratopathy. An appearance similar to viral keratoconjunctivitis has been described in patients who developed keratitis secondary to toxicity to solutions. The thimerosal sensitivity presents a classic clinical picture that can be diagnosed easily. A characteristic clinical syndrome is typified by the superior limbic keratoconjunctivitis seen in contact lens wearers.

Superior Limbic Keratoconjunctivitis

A new syndrome seen in contact lens wearers has been described where there is involvement of the superior limbal area along with the superior part of the cornea. Because of its similarity in clinical appearance and location to superior limbic syndrome described by Theodore, it is often called *contact lens-associated superior limbic keratoconjunctivitis*. The phenomenon is due to exposure to thimerosal in the contact lens solutions. It was first described by Miller and colleagues, and corroborated by other reports in the literature.[48,68,80,81]

CLINICAL PICTURE

The typical clinical picture is characterized by symptoms of irritation, tearing, and redness of sudden onset in a patient who has worn contact lenses successfully for several months or years. Some patients may complain of difficulty in keeping the lenses in the eye as well as keeping them clean. The other typical history is that of a change in the contact lens cleaning regimen or a switch from several years of successful hard contact lens wear to soft contact lenses. There are usually no visual complaints, unless the problem extends to the central part of the cornea. The patient may complain of considerable light sensitivity and inability to keep the eyes open.

OBJECTIVE SIGNS

Clinical evaluation reveals the presence of signs of inflammation more or less confined to the superior limbal area of the conjunctiva with hyperemia and some degree of elevation of the conjunctiva due to edema. In addition, there may be papillary reaction of the upper tarsal conjunctiva with inflammation of this area in some cases. The superior aspect of the cornea demonstrates hazy epithelium in the shape of a wedge with a clearly defined margin that separates it from the adjacent normal epithelium (Color Fig. 9-2). Intense superficial vascularization of the adjacent cornea is seen. There is positive fluorescein staining both of the conjunctiva in the superior limbal area and the corneal area that is involved in the disease process. Very rarely, this condition extends into the visual axis. Opacities at the level of the Bowman's membrane may be seen occasionally.

Superior limbic keratoconjunctivitis is usually bilateral but rarely can be unilateral with one eye showing minimal changes.

MANAGEMENT

Cessation of contact lens use may result in remission. However, it may require several weeks for the tissues to return to their normal appearance. The patient should be warned of such a possibility.

Once resolution has been achieved, patients may have to be refitted and the cleaning regimen has to be changed. As a rule, thimerosal-free solutions should be prescribed followed by frequent follow-up visits. In some, there may be permanent diminution of vision secondary to corneal scarring.

PATHOLOGY

Sendele and colleagues used specimens obtained from the superior bulbar conjunctiva to demonstrate evidence of acute and chronic inflammatory cell reaction along with pseudoepithelialmatous hyperplasia.[68] In addition, they noted an absence of goblet cells in these specimens along with alterations in the surface macrovilli in the form of flattening, as well as the presence of granular inclusions suggestive of lipoproteins. These pathologic features are nonspecific and did not provide any further insight into specific etiology.

ETIOLOGY

The etiology of superior limbic keratoconjunctivis in contact lens wearers is not clear. It does not appear to be similar to giant papillary conjunctivitis in its origin, but the adsorption of materials such as thimerosal may lead to this problem.[48,68,80,81] In one series, 61 patients who developed this problem were found to be using a topical medication that contained thimerosal.[80] Of the 21 patients in this series who have had skin tests performed, only one had a positive response to thimerosal. Of the 10 patients with a negative skin test, all had a rapid response when a challenging dose of 0.005% thimerosal and normal saline was instilled into the inferior conjunctival cul-de-sac. In another series of 40 patients, all of whom had been exposed to thimerosal preservative solutions, 5 out of the 15 patients who were tested had a positive response to thimerosal on the conjunctival challenge patch testing and intradermal testing. None of the 10 remaining patients showed a conjunctival or skin response to thimerosal. In the study by Miller and colleagues, only one of the six patients who were skin tested had a reaction to thimerosal.[48] In another study of 31 patients, a positive response was seen in 27 eyes tested with 0.004% thimerosal preservative. However, it is intriguing that thimerosal in the absence of contact lenses does not seem to develop the picture of superior limbic syndrome. Once this syndrome occurs, exposure to solutions containing thimerosal produces recurrence. It appears that the combination of the presence of a contact lens and thimerosal exposure is needed to develop this clinical problem.

TREATMENT

Once superior limbic syndrome is recognized, contact lens wear should be discontinued. Most patients respond favorably to this measure with complete resolution of the problem. In those cases where the problem has been chronic, resolution requires a longer period of time. Refitting of contact lenses should be deferred until corneal surface irregularity, neovascularization, and infiltration of the superficial part of the cornea are completely resolved. One has to be sure that the patient is instructed in the use of a different care regimen and solutions that do not contain thimerosal, followed by frequent follow-up care.

CORNEAL COMPLICATIONS

Almost every form of corneal problem can occur following the use of contact lenses, ranging from the most subtle superficial punctate keratopathy to corneal ulcers. The manifestation of corneal problems is probably a reflection of a contact lens-induced alteration in corneal status, which may be either physiological or anatomical. Even though the exact pathogenesis of many of these problems is still to be elucidated, it is important for the practitioner to recognize the different forms of corneal involvement and their management. In general, the physiologic alterations include changes in epithelium and endothelium. Hypoxia, allergy, or infection appear to be the underlying causes for most of the problems.

SUPERFICIAL PUNCTATE KERATOPATHY

Superficial punctate keratopathy of diverse morphology can occur with different types of contact lens wear.[65] It may manifest in patients who wear hard contact lenses as the classic staining at the 3-o'clock and 9-o'clock positions, or it may be a diffuse form of punctate keratopathy covering the entire surface of the cornea. In cases where there is a fitting problem, apical staining pattern may be seen (Color Fig. 9-3).

Clinical Picture

The clinical picture of superficial punctate keratopathy does not differ significantly from any other type of punctate keratopathy. Positive fluorescein staining is typical, with multiple punctate lesions scattered throughout the cornea or confined to a particular region of the cornea. Sometimes in contact lens overwear syndromes, a confluent area of punctate staining can be seen in the central part of the cornea. Irregular patterns somewhat resembling pseudodendritic forms have been described recently in soft contact lens wearers.[43,76] In contrast to dendrites of herpes simplex, these lesions are slightly raised, gray, and irregular epithelial plaques that stain variably with fluorescein and rose bengal (Fig. 9-6). Bilaterality of these lesions is another characteristic that differentiates them from herpes simplex. The differential diagnosis of dendritic lesions include herpes zoster keratitis, healing erosions, use of timolol, and tyrosinemia.

The patients may complain of no symptoms or may have extreme symptoms of chronic irritation, foreign body sensation, and a marked decrease in visual acuity because of the changes in the corneal surface secondary to the epithelial irregularity.

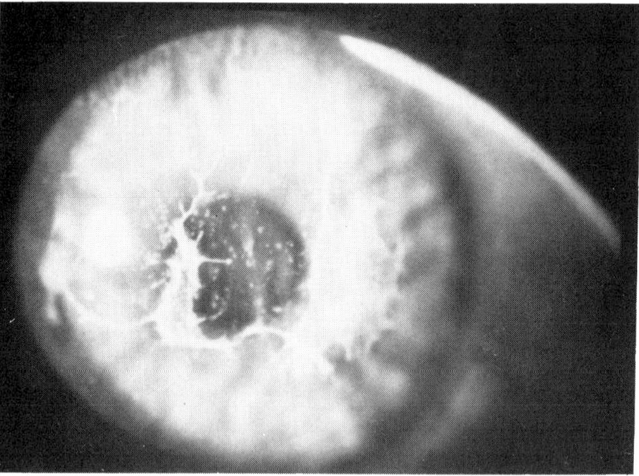

Figure 9-6 Appearance of pseudodendrite in soft contact lens wearer. (Courtesy of Dr. Jeffrey K. Harris)

Pathogenesis

The exact pathogenesis of superficial punctate keratopathy in most instances is not clear. However, it can occur as a mechanical factor following the use of contact lenses, as a toxic reaction to contact lens solution, or as a hypoxic phenomenon.[61] Very often, these are secondary to epithelial hypoxia compounded by mechanical trauma or decreased corneal sensitivity. A number of preservatives in contact lens solutions may produce a similar picture. Tear film abnormalities and fitting problems may be additional factors. Contact lenses were shown to induce diverse epithelial changes as described in Chapter 1, and these changes may be the underlying factors for some forms of epitheliopathy.

Treatment

Resolution occurs with simple discontinuation of the contact lenses. In some instances, however, treatment requires several months before the cornea can regain its normal smooth appearance. The use of topical lubricant solutions may provide symptomatic relief occasionally. Some corneas may be left with residual haze. Refitting of lenses can be done after the resolution of acute phenomena; however, preservative-free cleaning solutions should be used.

EPITHELIAL MICROCYSTS

A recently described phenomenon secondary to contact lens wear is the development of epithelial microcysts (Fig. 9-7).[28,65,82] This is rarely observed in daily-wear contact lens wearers, but is quite common with extended-wear

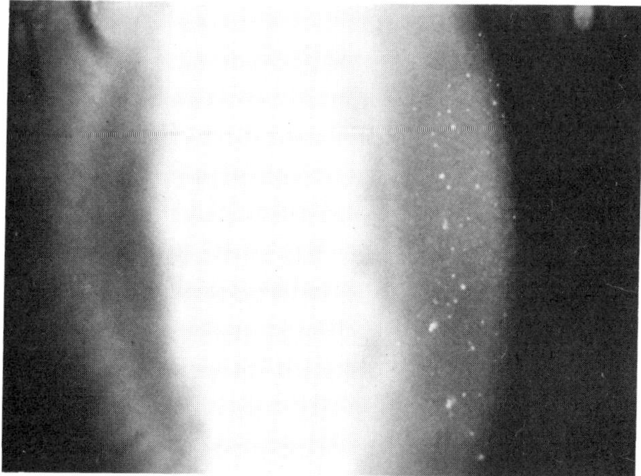

Figure 9-7 Slit lamp photomicrograph demonstrating the appearance of epithelial microcysts (low magnification) in the paracentral area of the cornea. (Courtesy of Dr. Steve Zantos)

lens wearers. In a recent study, Kenyon and Polse observed these cysts in 100% of extended-wear lens patients.[32] However, the clinical significance of these changes is not clear at this time. Whether they are a response to hypoxia in a subtle form is still to be determined. In persons who develop microcysts, other complications may also be seen, such as alterations in the morphologic appearance of corneal endothelium. These patients may not have any subjective symptoms. The most effective treatment in these cases is the cessation of contact lens use, which leads to reversal of these changes within a few weeks.

SUBEPITHELIAL KERATITIS

Several reports in the literature have described the appearance of subepithelial opacities that are akin to lesions seen in cases of viral keratoconjunctivitis.[7–9] The clinical appearance is in the form of multiple concentric, round, grayish-white opacities in the superficial stroma of the cornea as well as the subepithelial region and distributed throughout the cornea. These may sometimes be limited to the periphery, but the involvement of the central part of the cornea can lead to visual impairment. There usually is no associated inflammatory reaction, but in some cases, where it is due to toxic conjunctivitis or toxic reaction, one can see considerable degree of conjunctival reaction. However, the anterior segment will be quiet in most instances.

Pathogenesis

The exact pathogenesis of subepithelial keratitis is not clear. Although the changes may be due to viral infection of the eye, a differential diagnosis has to be made and every attempt should be made to eliminate this possibility. Very often the resolution of the changes by simple discontinuation of contact lens use suggests their etiology. There is evidence to suggest that this may represent an antigen–antibody reaction of some nature, or that this might be a toxic reaction to some of the preservative materials in the contact lens solutions.[7,51,52]

Treatment

The most effective treatment of subepithelial keratitis is the discontinuation of the contact lens, by which the contact lenses as well as preservatives are eliminated. In those cases where the patient is very symptomatic and the vision is threatened, the use of topical steroids may be indicated.

CORNEAL EDEMA

Although corneal edema is a very rare complication associated with the use of the current generation of contact lenses, particularly the gas-permeable and high water content hydrogel lenses, it still remains a cause for concern in contact lens wearers. The manifestation of corneal edema can vary from subtle changes in corneal thickness, which may not manifest clinically, to overt corneal edema.

Clinical Picture

Corneal edema confined to the stroma may not present any symptoms. However, slit lamp evaluation can reveal the existence of stromal edema in the form of an increase in corneal thickness, which can be measured more accurately by using the technique of pachymetry. Once the edema becomes more advanced, the involvement of the epithelium leads to a marked decrease in visual acuity. Epithelial edema alters the normal surface, resulting in distortion of vision with an ultimate decrease in visual acuity. The patient may also complain of pain from surface irregularity, as well as breakdown of bullae. Vertical striae also have been reported in cases with corneal edema.[59] The major complaint is of changes in visual acuity. Early recognition of corneal edema is possible only by serial documentation of the status of the cornea and by employing the technique of pachymetry.

Pathogenesis

Although the exact pathogenesis of corneal edema in contact lens wearers is still a matter of debate, a number of factors have been implicated.

1. The presence of a contact lens that induces corneal hypoxia may lead to the development of corneal edema. The change to anaerobic metabolism stimulates the accumulation of large quantities of lactate in the corneal stroma, which by osmotic action imbibes large quantities of fluid into the corneal stroma, increasing the thickness of the stroma with resulting corneal edema. A number of biochemical alterations can occur. The exact sequence of these changes and the possible mechanisms have already been described in Chapter 1.

2. Tear flow under the contact lens is one of the important sources of oxygen to the cornea. Very minimal tear flow occurs under a contact lens.[30,58] If tear flow is impaired by any mechanism, corneal edema can ensue.

3. Any change in the integrity of the corneal epithelial surface may also lead to corneal edema. Corneal epithelial defects as well as erosions secondary to contact lens wear can lead to corneal edema.

4. There have been numerous reports in the recent past of changes that occur in corneal endothelium following the use of contact lenses. Long-term wear of PMMA lenses has been shown to produce significant change in morphology, showing greater degrees of polymegethism.[5,14,67] A similar phenomenon has also been reported with the use of soft contact lenses as well as extended-wear contact lenses.[29,45] This phenomenon tended to be relatively stable, and did not show any trend towards recovery to normal even after several months of cessation of lens wear. The exact significance of this was not clear. Studies by Sweeney and co-workers and O'Neal and Polse have shown that patients with polymegethous corneal endothelium produced greater changes in the corneal thickness compared with patients with normal corneal endothelium when stressed with contact lenses. A similar observation by Rao and colleagues of patients with endothelial polymegethism found them to be more vulnerable to develop corneal edema following intraocular surgery.[61,62] A cornea with low endothelial cell density may also be more likely to develop corneal edema following the use of a contact lens.[11] Nirankari and co-workers reported development of corneal edema in aphakic eyes both with daily- and extended-wear contact lenses.[54] Based on these findings, alterations in the corneal endothelium may indeed be responsible for corneal edema in at least a segment of the population. Precontact lens assessment of the corneal endothelium may be helpful in eliminating some of the problems in these patients.

The development of corneal edema is much more common with tight-fitting PMMA lenses, hydrogel lenses when the lens fit is steep, or lenses with low oxygen transmissibility. The problem has been minimized to a great degree with the current generation of gas-permeable contact lenses.

Treatment

The mainstay of treating corneal edema is again the cessation of lens use. Once the edema clears, the entire situation has to be reassessed before the patient is refitted with contact lenses. Careful evaluation of possible causes is mandatory. The problem can be averted by careful screening and follow up of patients after initial fit. In patients (such as aphakic patients) where the corneal endothelium has a marked decrease in cell density along with other alterations, one has to pay special attention to the recognition of early signs of endothelial distress. Once the problem has been resolved, contact lens use can be resumed by changing to a lens with a flatter fit and greater oxygen transmissibility. In patients where edema occurs when using extended-wear lenses, switching to a daily-wear regimen may alleviate the problem.

CORNEAL ULCERS

The development of corneal ulcer is one of the most dreaded complications of contact lens wear. Numerous reports in the recent literature have suggested that the incidence of ulcers has escalated with the use of soft contact lenses.[13,17,39,78] The corneal ulcers that occur in contact lens wearers can be either sterile or infective. Although sterile corneal ulcers are associated with less corneal morbidity, such a diagnosis is often difficult to make without microbiological investigations. A corneal ulcer should be considered infective unless proven otherwise.

STERILE CORNEAL ULCERS

Sterile corneal ulcers appear to be the extreme clinical expression of an antigen–antibody reaction in the cornea. They can occur with the use of daily-wear as well as extended-wear soft contact lenses. The ulcers have no predilection to any one part of the cornea, and often resolve without producing any residual corneal scarring. Sometimes they may be associated with acute inflammatory reaction with the presence of hypopyon (Fig. 9-8).

Pathogenesis

Although the exact pathogenesis of aseptic corneal ulceration is not clear, it is believed that this is usually secondary to immune phenomena. Prompt response to steroid therapy may suggest this etiology.

Management

In all cases, corneal scrapings have to be obtained and appropriate microbiological investigations have to be done. The therapeutic considerations should be based on the severity of the clinical picture. Whenever there is clinical suspicion of infective etiology, aggressive treatment with antibiotics, probably employing combination therapy, should be instituted immediately. In cases where no clinical response is seen and where no microorganism could be isolated from the cultures of corneal scrapings, one may initiate judicious administration of topical corticosteroids with close monitoring of the patient. Most patients respond favorably to this therapy.

INFECTIVE CORNEAL ULCERS

Infective corneal ulcers have the greatest potential for sight-threatening sequelae. There has been an alarming increase in the number of cases of bacterial ulcers reported with the use of contact lenses, particularly extended-wear lenses.[1,41] Both myopic patients and aphakic patients can develop this complication. In early stages (Fig. 9-9), it can be corrected

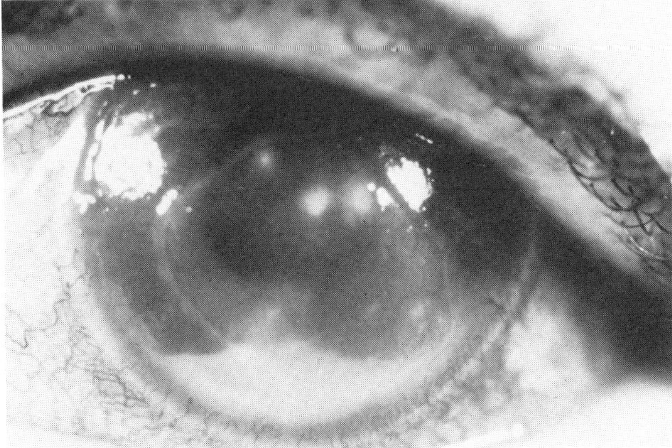

Figure 9-8 Sterile corneal ulcer in the central part of the cornea with considerable anterior chamber inflammatory reaction leading to hypopyon formation.

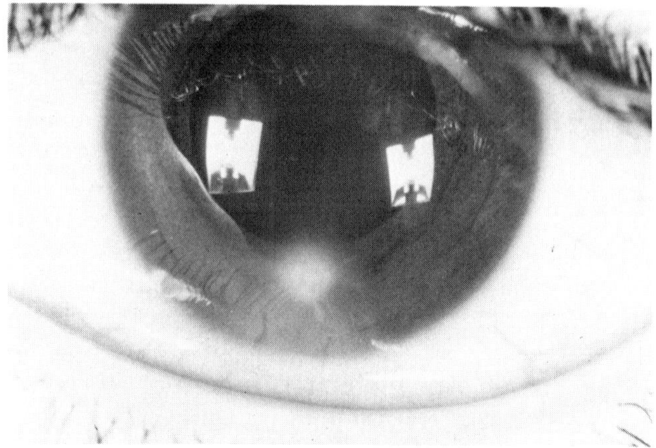

Figure 9-9 Corneal ulcer secondary to daily-wear soft contact lens. The ulcer is in the peripheral part of the cornea; the central cornea is spared.

without any sequelae, although severe involvement in patients with impaired host defenses can lead to corneal scarring (Fig. 9-10). In addition, considerable concern has been expressed about the use of therapeutic lenses in postkeratoplasty patients because the incidence of corneal ulcers appears to be high in this group.[18,40,69] These ulcers tend to progress very rapidly (Fig. 9-11).

Predisposing Factors

Although no clear-cut evidence exists directly incriminating contact lenses in causing corneal ulcers, the incidence of corneal ulcers in these eyes appears to be disproportionately higher. A number of contact lens-related factors may play a role:

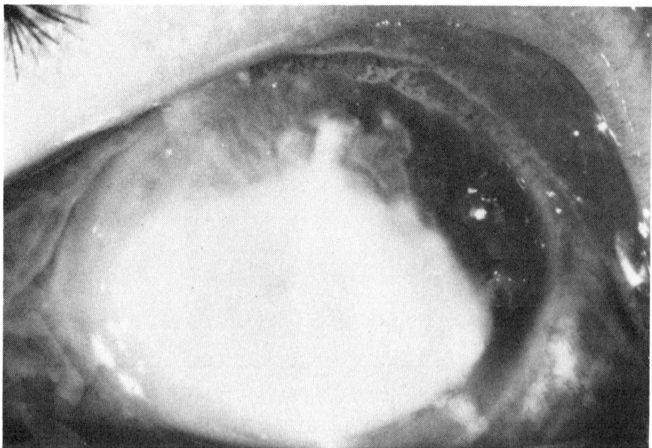

Figure 9-10 Corneal ulcer in a diabetic patient following extended-wear contact lens use. The ulcer involves two thirds to three fourths of the corneal surface.

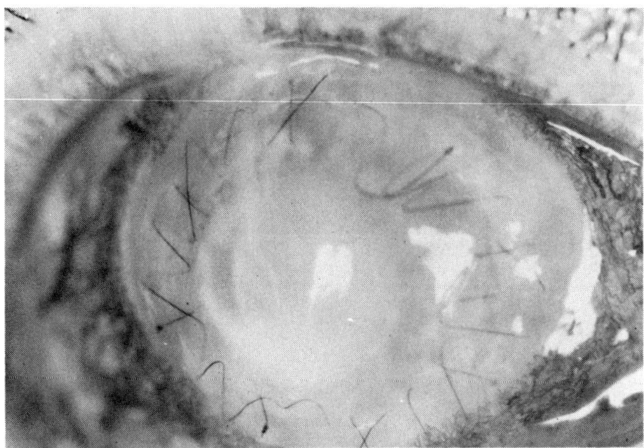

Figure 9-11 *Pseudomonas* corneal ulcer in a corneal graft involved the entire graft within a period of about 24 hours. The initial presentation was of a small infiltrate in the periphery of the graft. This followed the use of a bandage lens for 7 days to treat an epithelial defect.

1. Improper sterilization of the lenses;
2. Use of contaminated solutions or contact lens cases;
3. Poor patient compliance;
4. Infected contact lenses harboring microorganisms;
5. Lens spoilage; and
6. Improper patient selection.

One of the important considerations is appropriate patient selection and screening prior to contact lens fitting, particularly for extended-wear lenses. It is imperative that the clinician be cognizant of potential danger signals and look for them. Proper assessment of the integrity of the external eye is of paramount importance. This includes the following:

1. Evaluating the condition of the eyelids, specifically looking for any evidence of blepharitis and meibomitis, defects in lids, improper closure, and blink response;
2. Evaluating the precorneal tear film, because eyes with tear film dysfunction run a higher risk of infections;
3. Evaluating corneal epithelial integrity by fluorescein or rose bengal staining;
4. Assessing corneal sensitivity; and
5. Measuring corneal thickness.

An appropriate evaluation of the cornea and anterior segment may help to minimize the incidence of these complications. Patient instruction is also a factor of paramount importance for successful contact lens wear. The patient should be made aware of the common symptoms suggestive of a problem (such as increasing irritation, redness, intolerance to the contact lens, or blurring of vision) and should be advised to report to the clinician immediately. In cases where access to a clinician is a problem, the patient should be instructed to remove the lens from the eye as the first step.

In certain eyes, bacterial ulcers have been traced to the patient's hygenic factors and solutions that were used to clean the lens. In a few reports, bacteria isolated from the ulcer was also cultured from the contact lens solution. Here again, patient instruction can minimize such problems. Adams and co-workers have traced the development of ulcers to a recent manipulation of the contact lens.[1]

Clinical Picture

The clinical picture of bacterial ulcers following contact lens wear does not differ significantly from any other type of bacterial corneal ulcer.

Pathogenesis

Although the transportation of different organisms into the eye may be by different routes, their ability to produce corneal infections is dependent on both their virulence and host factors.

Certain host factors probably favor the development of this problem. For a corneal ulcer to develop, a break in the epithelial surface is a prerequisite for all but a few organisms. Several factors in contact lens wearers may compromise the epithelial surface and thereby its barrier effect. Contact lenses alter the surface epithelial morphology and decrease corneal sensitivity. In aphakic patients, the epithelial surface is compromised.[63] A number of epithelial alterations have been described (see Chapter 1) that lead to an impairment of epithelial barrier function. The chronic subclinical insult from contact lenses may aggravate this situation further. These factors, together with lid infections and tear film dysfunction, can make the cornea highly susceptible to infections. In all postoperative eyes, this situation is compounded by further epithelial alteration and greater hypoesthesia. In addition, there may be local immunosuppression with the use of steroids. The cumulative effect of a number of these factors may lead to the greater incidence of corneal ulcers in eyes that have been subjected to intraocular surgical procedures.

Treatment

The most important factor is early recognition along with prompt and aggressive treatment. Such a course can minimize the chances of sight-threatening sequelae. Once the infection occurs, the treatment is based on the same lines as that for any other type of bacterial corneal ulcer, such as the use of intensive topical and subconjunctival antibiotics in appropriate dosages and combinations.

CORNEAL NEOVASCULARIZATION

Clinical Appearance

Corneal neovascularization may be superficial or deep. The patient is very often asymptomatic until the visual axis is threatened. However, in the instance of deep vascularization, the deposition of lipids in the stroma and scar tissue produces visual difficulties (Color Fig. 9-4).[31] This phenomenon causes greater concern in eyes with corneal transplants, where corneal vascularization may be a factor in triggering corneal graft rejection.[40]

Incidence

Neovascularization of the cornea occurs, to a varying degree, in the majority of patients using soft contact lenses. Although most of the patients with extended-wear contact lenses develop this problem, the neovascularization is superficial. Deep stromal vascularization is very rare with high water contact lenses.

Although this complication is more commonly seen with extended wear of soft contact lenses compared to the daily wear of contact lenses, it can occur with both modalities of contact lens wear.[19,23,33,40,55,60,72,77] Deep stromal vascularization leads to greater morbidity than superficial vascularization does. The introduction of high water contact lenses and other lenses with high oxygen permeability has alleviated the problem to a considerable degree.

Pathogenesis

Although the exact pathogenesis of corneal vascularization is not clear, the relative anoxia that is induced by the presence of the contact lenses may be responsible.

Treatment

Although superficial neovascularization (extending to less than 2 mm inside the cornea) is not a major cause of visual loss, the problem should be managed promptly. Usually, discontinuation of lens wear alone produces regression of the process. If neovascularization is associated with evidence of inflammatory reaction, treatment with topical corticosteroids is often effective.

After complete regression of these changes, patients on an extended-wear schedule may have to be switched to a daily-wear regimen, or be refitted with a flatter lens or with one that has greater oxygen permeability.

CONCLUSION

Contact lenses are increasingly popular for the correction of different refractive errors, as well as for the management of corneal diseases. Although the advantages are obvious, the risk of complications[31] is real. A proper appraisal of the risk–benefit ratio is crucial to obtain optimal results and to minimize the potential for sight-threatening sequelae.

REFERENCES

1. Adams CP, Cohen EJ, Laibson PR et al: Corneal ulcers in patients with cosmetic extended-wear contact lenses. Am J Ophthalmol 96:705, 1983
2. Allansmith MR, Baird RS, Greiner JV: Vernal conjunctivitis and contact lens associated giant papillary conjunctivitis compared and contrasted. Am J Ophthalmol 87:544, 1979(b)
3. Allansmith MR, Korb DR, Greiner JV et al: Giant papillary conjunctivitis in contact lens wearers. Am J Ophthalmol 83:697, 1977
4. Allansmith MR, Korb DR, Greiner JV: Giant papillary conjunctivitis induced by hard or soft contact lens wear: Quantitative histology. Ophthalmology 85:766, 1978
5. Barr JT, Schoessler JP: Corneal endothelial response to rigid contact lenses. Am J Optom Physiol Opt 57:267, 1980
6. Berger RO, Streeten BW: Fungal growth in aphakic soft contact lenses. Am J Ophthalmol 91:630, 1981
7. Binder PS: Complications associated with extended wear of soft contact lenses. Ophthalmology 86:1093, 1979
8. Binder PS: Extended wear of three soft contact lenses. Contact Intraocular Lens Med J 5:456, 1979
9. Binder PS: The extended wear of soft contact lenses. JCE Ophthalmol 15:32, 1979
10. Binder PS, Rasmussen DM, Gordon M: Keratoconjunctivitis and soft contact lens solutions. Arch Ophthalmol 99:87, 1981
11. Binder PS, Woodward C: Extended wear hydrocurve and sauflon contact lenses. Am J Ophthalmol 90:309, 1980
12. Binder PS, Worthen DM: Clinical evaluation of continous-wear hydrophilic lenses. Am J Ophthalmol 83:549, 1977
13. Brown SI, Bloomfield S, Pearce DB et al: Infections with the therapeutic contact lens. Arch Ophthalmol 91:275, 1974
14. Caldwell DR, Kastl PR, Dabezies OH et al: The effect of long-term hard lens wear on corneal endothelium. Contact Intraoc Lens Med J 8:87, 1982
15. Cavanagh HD, Bodner BI, Wilson LA: Extended wear hydrogel lenses: Long term effectiveness and costs. Ophthalmology 87:871, 1980
16. Cioletti KR: Determination of thimerosal content in contact lens polymers. Int Contact Lens Clin 13:3, 1980
17. Cooper RL, Costable IJ: Infective keratitis in soft contact lens wearers. Br J Ophthalmol 61:250, 1977
18. Cowden JW: Continuous wear aphakic soft contact lenses following keratoplasty. Ann Ophthalmol 12:579, 1980
19. Dohlman DH, Boruchoff SA, Mobilia EA: Complications in the use of soft contact lenses in corneal disease. Arch Ophthalmol 90:367, 1973
20. Doughman DJ, Mobilia EA, Drago D et al: The nature of "spots" on soft lenses. Ann Ophthalmol 7:345, 1975
21. Fichman S, Baker VV, Horton HR: Iatrogenic red eyes in soft contact lens wearers. Int Contact Lens Clin 15:202, 1978
22. Fowler SA, Greiner JV, Allansmith MR: Attachment of bacteria to soft contact lenses. Arch Ophthalmol 97:569, 1979
23. Gasset AR, Lobo L, Houde W: Permanent wear of soft contact lenses in aphakic eyes. Am J Ophthalmol 83:115, 1977

24. Gasset AR, Mattingly TP, Hood I: Source of fungus contamination of hydrophilic soft contact lenses. Am J Ophthalmol 11:1295, 1979
25. Greiner JV, Covington HI, Allansmith MR: Surface morphology of giant papillary conjunctivitis in contact lens wearers. Am J Ophthalmol 85:242, 1978
26. Greiner JV, Fowler SA, Allansmith MR: Giant papillary conjunctivitis. In Dabezies OH (ed): Contact Lenses: The CLAO Guide to Basic Science and Clinical Practice, pp 43.1–43.11. New York, Grune & Stratton, 1984
27. Greiner JV, Korb DR, Allansmith MR: Pathogenesis of contact lens papillary conjunctivitis: A hypothesis. In Silverstein A, O'Conner S (eds): Immunology and Immunopathology of the Eye. New York, Masson & Cie, in press
28. Humphreys JA, Larke JR, Parrish ST: Microepithelial cysts observed in extended wear contact lens wearing subjects. Br J Ophthalmol 64:888, 1980
29. Holden BA, Sweeney DF, Vannas A et al: Contact lens induced endothelial polymegethism. Invest Ophthalmol (supp) 26:275, 1985
30. Josephson JE, Caffery BE: Infiltrative keratitis in hydrogel lens wearers. Int Contact Lens Clin 16:223, 1979
31. Kaufman HE: Problems associated in the prolonged wear of soft contact lenses. Ophthalmology 86:411, 1979
32. Kenyon KR, Polse KA: Influence of wearing schedule on extended wear complications. Invest Ophthalmol 23:143, 1985
33. Kersley HJ, Kerr C, Pierse D: Hydrophilic lens for "continuous" wear in aphakia: Definitive fitting and problems that occur. Br J Ophthalmol 61:38, 1977
34. Klintworth GK, Reed JW, Hawkins HK et al: Calcification of soft contact lenses in patient with dry eye and elevated calcium concentration in tears. Invest Ophthalmol 16:158, 1977
35. Korb DR, Allansmith MR, Greiner JV et al: Biomicroscopy of papillae associated with hard contact lens wearing. Ophthalmology 88:1132, 1981
36. Korb DR, Allansmith MR, Greiner JV et al: Prevalence of conjunctival changes in wearers of hard contact lenses. Am J Ophthalmol 90:336, 1980
37. Korb DR, Greiner JV, Allansmith MR et al: Biomicroscopy of papillae associated with wearing of soft contact lenses. Br J Ophthalmol 67:733, 1983
38. Korb DR, Greiner JV, Finnemore VM et al: Treatment of contact lenses with papain: Increase in wearing time in keratoconic patients with giant papillary conjunctivitis. Arch Ophthalmol 101:48, 1983
39. Krachmer JH, Purcell JJ, Jr: Bacterial corneal ulcers in cosmetic soft contact lens wearers. Arch Ophthalmol 96:57, 1978
40. Lemp MA: The effect of extended-wear aphakic hydrophilic contact lenses after penetrating keratoplasty. Am J Ophthalmol 90:331, 1980
41. Lemp MA, Blackman J, Wilson LA: Gram-negative corneal ulcers in elderly aphakic eyes with extended wear lenses. Ophthalmology 91:60, 1984
42. Lohman LE, Tripathi RC, Tripathi BJ et al: Correlation of specular microscopic and laboratory evaluation of soft contact lens spoilage. Invest Ophthalmol ARVO Supp 25:320, 1984
43. Margolies LJ, Mannis MJ: Dendritic corneal lesions associated with soft contact lens wear. Arch Ophthalmol 101:1551, 1983
44. McCarey BE, Wilson LA: pH osmolarity and temperature effects on the water content of hydrogel contact lenses. Contact Intraoc Lens Med J 83:3, 1982
45. McRae S, Matsuda M, Yee R et al: The effect of contact lenses on corneal endothelium. Invest Ophthalmol (suppl) 23:275, 1985
46. Meisler DM, Berzins UJ, Krachmer JH et al: Cromolyn treatment of giant papillary conjunctivitis. Arch Ophthalmol 100:1608, 1982

47. Meisler DM, Laret CR, Stock EL: Tranta's dots and limbal inflammation associated with soft contact lens wear. Am J Ophthalmol 89:66, 1982

48. Miller RA, Brightbill FS, Slama S: Superior limbic keratoconjunctivitis in soft contact lens wearers. Cornea 1:293, 1982

49. Miranda M, Garcia-Castineiras S: Effects of *pH* and some common topical ophthalmic medications on the contact lens Permalens. CLAO J 9:43, 1983

50. Mondino BJ, Groden LR: Conjunctival hyperemia and corneal infiltrates with chemically disinfected soft contact lenses. Arch Ophthalmol 98:1767, 1980

51. Mondino BJ, Salamon SM, Zaidman GW: Allergic and toxic reactions in soft contact lens wearers. Surv Ophthalmol 26:337, 1982

52. Morgan JF: Complications associated with contact lens solutions. Ophthalmology 86:1107, 1979

53. Mullen W, Shephard W, Labovitz J: Ophthalmic preservatives and vehicles. Surv Ophthalmol 17:469, 1973

54. Nirankari VS, Baer JC: Persistent corneal edema in aphakic eyes from daily-wear and extended wear contact lenses. Am J Ophthalmol 98:329, 1984

55. Nirankari VS, Karesh J, Lakhanpal V et al: Deep stromal vascularization associated with cosmetic, daily-wear contact lenses. Arch Ophthalmol 101:46, 1983

56. O'Neal MR, Polse KA: Decreased rate of corneal hydration recovery with aging reduced endothelial function. Invest Ophthalmol (suppl) 23:53, 1985

57. Pitts RE, Krachmer JH: Evaluation of soft contact lens disinfection in the home environment. Arch Ophthalmol 97:470, 1979

58. Polse KA: Tear flow under hydrogel contact lenses. Invest Ophthalmol Vis Sci 18:409, 1979

59. Polse KA, Sarver MD, Harris MG: Corneal edema and vertical striae accompanying the wearing of hydrogel lenses. Am J Optom Physiol Opt 52:185, 1975

60. Rao GN, Norton SW: Extended wear lenses for aphakic correction (experience with Cooper Permalens). Contact Lens 6:258, 1980

61. Rao GN, Shaw EL, Arthur EJ et al: Endothelial cell morphology and corneal deturgescence. Ann Ophthalmol 11(6):885, 1979

62. Rao GN, Aquavella JV, Goldberg SH et al: Pseudophakic bullous keratopathy: Relationship to preoperative corneal endothelial status. Ophthalmology 91:1135, 1984

63. Rao GN: Corneal surface in aphakic eye. CLAO Journal (in press)

64. Refojo MF, Holly FJ: Tear protein absorption hydrogels: A possible cause of contact lens allergy. Contact Intraoc Lens Med J 3:23, 1977

65. Ruben M: Acute eye disease secondary to contact lens wear. Lancet 1:138, 1976

66. Ruben M, Tripathi RC, Winder AR: Calcium deposition as a cause of spoilation of hydrophilic soft contact lenses. Br J Ophthalmol 59:141, 1975

67. Schoessler JP, Woloschak MJ: Corneal endothelium in veteran PMMA contact lens wearers. Int Contact Lens Clin 8:19, 1981

68. Sendele DD, Kenyon KR, Mobilia EF et al: Superior limbic keratoconjunctivitis in contact lens wearers. Ophthalmology 90:616, 1983

69. Smith SG, Lindstrom RL, Nelson JD et al: Corneal ulcer–infiltrate associated with soft contact lens use following penetrating keratoplasty. Cornea 3(2):131, 1984

70. Smolin G, Kumato M, Nozik RA: The microbial flora in extended wear soft contact lens wearers. Am J Ophthalmol 88:543, 1979

71. Spring TF: Reaction to hydrophilic lenses. Med J Aust 1:499, 1974

72. Stein HA, Slatt BJ: Extended wear of soft contact lenses in perspective. Int Contact Lens Clin 14:35, 1977

73. Sweeney DF, Holden BA, Vannas A et al: The clinical significance of corneal endothelial polymegethism. Invest Ophthalmol (suppl) 23:53, 1985
74. Tripathi RC, Ruben M: Degenerative changes in a soft hydrophilic contact lens. Ophthalmol Res 4:185, 1973
75. Tripathi RC, Tripathi BJ, Ruben M: The pathology of soft contact lens spoilage. Ophthalmology 87:365, 1980
76. Udell IJ, Mannis MJ, Meisler DM et al: Pseudodendrites in soft contact lens wearers. CLAO J 11(1):51, 1985
77. Weinberg RJ: Deep corneal vascularization caused by aphakic soft contact lens wear. Am J Ophthalmol 83:121, 1977
78. Weissman BA, Mondino BJ, Pettit TH et al: Corneal ulcers associated with extended wear soft contact lenses. Am J Ophthalmol 97:476, 1984
79. Wilson LA, Schlitzer RL, Ahearn DG: Pseudomonas corneal ulcers associated with soft contact lens wear. Am J Ophthalmol 92:546, 1981
80. Wright P, McKie I: Preservative-related problems in soft contact lens wearers. Trans Ophthalmol Soc UK 102:3, 1982
81. Wright P: Superior limbic keratoconjunctivitis. Trans Ophthalmol Soc UK 92:555, 1972
82. Zantos SG, Holden BA: Transient endothelial changes soon after wearing soft contact lenses. Am J Physiol Opt 54:856, 1977

SOLUTIONS FOR CLEANING, DISINFECTION, AND STORAGE

JEFFREY K. HARRIS

Successful contact lens wear depends on many factors. It is important to conceive of the contact lens as only one part of a lens system. The other parts are lens care solutions and patient environment. After consideration of factors that relate to indications and contraindications for lens wear, the practitioner must carefully select a lens polymer and care solutions appropriate to the patient's needs, fit the lens, and supply necessary instruction and follow up. Control over the lens system is maintained until the patient leaves the office, at which point the patient takes over. At this time, problems related to contact lens wear will be minimized if a good job has been done.

This chapter will concentrate on the solutions used for cleaning, disinfecting, and storing contact lenses. If correctly chosen, solutions can enhance vision, comfort, and safety in a convenient and economical fashion. Solution/solution, solution/polymer, and solution/patient interactions will be considered.

SOLUTION TERMINOLOGY

An understanding of solution terminology is basic to an understanding of this chapter. A *solution* is a homogeneous mixture of one or more substances (*solutes*) dispersed in a dissolving medium (the *solvent*). *Solubility* refers to the degree to which the solute dissolves. A *suspension* is one type of solution and consists of small particles of a solid dispersed in a liquid. An *emulsion* consists of small globules of one liquid dispersed in another liquid.

Solvents are classified into three groups: polar, consisting of strong dipolar molecules and forming hydrogen bonds (*e.g.,* water); semipolar, consisting of strong dipolar molecules but not forming hydrogen bonds (*e.g.,* acetone); and nonpolar, consisting of molecules with little or no dipolar character (*e.g.,* mineral oil).

Important interactions occur at the contact lens/tear boundary, cornea/ tear boundary, solute/solvent boundary, and so on. The nature of some of these boundary or interface interactions falls under the general category of *interfacial* phenomena. Examples include wetting, adsorption, surface tension reduction, and micelle formation. These will each be discussed under the appropriate section in this chapter.

Numerous factors must be considered when a solution is formulated for use with contact lenses or in the eye. These factors include tonicity, viscosity, hydrogen ion concentration (*p*H), stability, corneal contact time, preservative, sterility, and effect on tissue regeneration.[105]

The eye tolerates a wide range of tonicity. The sodium chloride (equivalent) concentration of an ophthalmic solution may safely range from 0.7% to 1.5%. A wide *p*H range is tolerated as well because of the following factors: (1) tears have a neutralizing action; (2) most ophthalmic solutions have a low buffer capacity when compounded in distilled water or isotonic saline; (3) there is rapid tear production on instillation of an irritating substance into the eye; and (4) there is a relatively small amount of medication normally instilled into the eye.[145]

WETTING AND SURFACTANTS

SORPTION

Adsorption is a process by which a gas, liquid, or solid concentrates on the surface of a contiguous liquid or solid surface.[142] It is a surface phenomenon. It may occur within a porous material, but it occurs on the surface of the pores. Molecules dissolved in solution may adsorb onto solid surfaces if they have chemical groups that can interact with those of the solid surface or if they are surface-active and the surface area of the solid is large. Adsorption will be discussed further in the section on cleaning. *Absorption* differs in that it involves a penetration of one substance into another. Adsorption may be followed by absorption, and the two are often difficult to distinguish. The term *sorption* may refer to either process.

WETTING

Wetting describes the spread of a liquid over the surface of a solid.[33] It is of interest to us because it pertains to the spread of tears or solutions over a contact lens or over the cornea. Spreading of a liquid over a surface depends on the relationship between the forces of adhesion and cohesion. *Adhesion* refers to the force of attraction between molecules of one substance and those of another. *Cohesion* refers to the force of attraction between molecules of the same substance. If the force of adhesion is greater than that of cohesion, then a liquid will wet a solid surface.

In the center of a drop of water, the force of cohesion acts equally on all molecules in all directions so that there are no resultant forces acting on any one molecule. At the surface, however, this force produces a net inward pull because there is no balancing outward pull. Thus, a drop of water tends to bead up and achieve the smallest surface area for its volume. The energy present at the surface is called *surface tension.*[142] It is defined as the force in dynes perpendicular to a line 1 cm long on the surface. *Surface free energy* is a similar unit based on surface area rather than on linear measurement. The *critical surface tension* of a surface is the surface tension of a liquid that will just wet the surface and spread, instead of just forming droplets on the surface.[8]

Substances that contain exposed polar groups, such as metals, have high surface tension and are *hydrophilic* (water-loving). Nonpolar substances, such as Teflon, have low surface tension and are *hydrophobic* (water-hating). *Interfacial tension* occurs at the interface between a solid and a liquid, and is the sum of the surface tension of the solid plus the surface tension of the liquid minus the intermolecular forces of attraction between the solid and the liquid.

SURFACTANTS

Water has a high surface tension. Solids with a low surface tension are incompletely wet by water. *Surface-active* materials (surfactants) can be used to achieve complete wetting.[86] They lower the surface tension of water, thus enabling it to wet low surface tension solids or to mix with water-insoluble substances.[84] The molecules or ions of a surface-active substance contain a hydrophobic tail (*e.g.,* alkyl chain) and a hydrophilic head (*e.g.,* carboxyl group). When dissolved in water, this substance locates at the surface with its hydrophilic head buried in the water and its hydrophobic tail pointing outward. This forms a low energy surface and enhances wetting of a solid that has low surface tension. In general, the more water-soluble a molecule is, the less surface activity it shows.

Surfactants can be classified as *ionic* or *nonionic* depending on whether the polar group is charged. The ionic surfactants can be further classified as *anionic* (surface-active ion bears a negative charge), *cationic* (surface-active ion bears a positive charge), or *amphoteric* (surface-active ion bears either a positive or negative charge or both, depending on the *p*H of the solution).

Many anionic detergents cause the dissociation of sheets of corneal epithelium into single cells. Cationic and nonionic detergents have no significant effect. Thus, anionic surfactant use is infrequent in the eye.[25]

Nonionic surfactants are used frequently because of good compatibility, stability, and generally low toxicity. This group includes compounds such as tyloxapol, propylene glycol, polyvinyl alcohol, and others.

Cationic agents are often used as surface-active agents when dissolved in water. However, their use in pharmaceutical preparations is as antimicrobial preservatives rather than surfactants because cations adsorb readily at cell membrane structures and lead to lysis. Benzalkonium chloride is a good example of this group.

Surfactants can influence the rate and extent of absorption of certain drugs.[67] Enhancement as well as inhibition of absorption and pharmacologic activity may occur and depends on interaction with biologic membranes and modification of membrane permeability, interaction with drug, interaction with dosage form, and interaction with the organism itself.

Three major pharmaceutical uses of surfactants are as wetting, solubilizing, and emulsifying agents. They will be discussed further under Cleaning and under Disinfection and Storage.

MICELLES

Molecules may aggregate into small soluble units known as *micelles*.[142] Micelles in water consist of many molecules oriented in a near-spherical structure such that the polar groups are oriented outwards toward the water and the nonpolar groups are oriented inward toward each other. The reverse situation may occur in a nonaqueous solvent. Micellar solutions can solubilize substances not ordinarily soluble in a given solvent, and may increase the amount of drug in solution as well as its biologic availability and chemical stability. Micelle formation occurs with molecules that exhibit interfacial activity, and thus may occur whenever surfactants are used. Micelles do not lower surface tension. The *critical micelle concentration* (CMC) is the minimum concentration of the surfactant in a solution at which micelle formation occurs. An example of the use of micelles occurs in Allergan's Cleaning and Disinfecting Solution.

WETTING ANGLE

The angle between a liquid and a solid surface gives an indication of the relative values of the forces of adhesion and cohesion that result in interfacial tension. It is known as *angle theta* or the *contact angle*. In contact lens work, it is referred to as the *wetting angle*. This angle is measured in degrees, and gives some idea of the ability of a certain solid to be wet by a certain liquid under defined conditions. Wettability is inversely proportional to the wetting angle. If the solid is completely wet by the liquid, then theta is zero and a uniform film of liquid will result. If no wetting is present, then theta is 180°. A liquid will not spread over a surface if theta is greater than 90°; a "bead" will result. Hydrophobic surfaces have a low wetting angle and wet poorly with water. Hydrophilic surfaces have a high wetting angle and wet well with water. Pure silicon is hydrophobic; polymethylmethacrylate (PMMA) is relatively hydrophobic; hydroxyethylmethacrylate (HEMA) is hydrophilic.

Many factors affect the wetting angle.[116] These include cleanliness of the sample tested, soaking of the sample, and the technique of measurement. Therefore, if a practitioner wishes to compare wetting angles of different materials, it is important to know the measurement technique and conditions used. Three basic testing methods have been used: the Sessile Drop, Captive Bubble, and Wilhelmy Plate techniques. The interested reader is referred to literature on the subject for further details.[11,107,116]

Specifics of wetting angle measurements cannot be directly correlated to function of the contact lens in the eye, but have some value in predicting patient comfort and acceptance of a material and the need for specific care solutions to enhance comfort.

Wettability is required for superior lens function.[131] Lack of wetting at the tear/lens interface results in light scattering and in rupture of the tear film over the lens, both of which result in poor vision. Oxygen transport and metabolic waste disposal may be impeded.[86] Additionally, comfort and tolerance by the cornea are decreased.

Wettability of a contact lens surface depends on the nature of the molecules present in the surrounding tears or contact lens solution, and on the interaction between them. Wettability may be enhanced by (1) appropriate alteration of the lens surface to increase the surface tension; (2) using a lens solution that has a low surface tension; or (3) using a lens solution that lowers the interfacial tension with the lens surface. Wetting agents may be placed in solutions used on the lens in the eye, but are of limited value because they are rapidly washed away.

The primary function of a wetting solution is to increase wettability of the lens. This is done by coating the lens with a hydrophilic substance. Other functions include providing a protective coating over the lens surface so that it does not directly contact the finger during insertion, preventing the transfer of oily deposits to the lens surface, stabilizing the lens on the fingertip, and promoting easier insertion.[33,115]

Wetting will decrease if the lens surface is contaminated. Deposits and exposure to petroleum-based compounds and cream soaps will decrease wettability of the lens.[116] Ivory soap is composed of animal fat, is not water soluble, and can leave a film on contact lenses. Deodorant and beauty soaps contain oils that are not water soluble. Heavy-duty abrasive soaps may leave particles on the fingertips that could damage contact lenses. A handsoap for lens care should be water soluble, should produce a good lather, should have no fragrance or oily additives, should remove oil, grease, and dirt, and should contain an antimicrobial agent.[65]

All lenses should be dispensed in their fully hydrated state. In addition to comfort, hydration can affect lens parameters. A lens that is not fully hydrated may not fit as expected. Silcon and Silsoft lenses may never wet properly again if they are ever allowed to dehydrate.[11]

CLEANING

Cleaning can decrease deposit buildup as well as decrease complications caused by deposits. It also aids the disinfection process by removing bacteria and fungal remnants and deposits that can harbor microorganisms and perhaps inactivate the preservatives in cold disinfection solutions.[32] Protein can bind to preservatives and disinfectants and block their action. The protein coat on a lens can prevent the action of these agents by blocking their access to an organism.[46] Thus, appropriate lens care can help prevent and remove deposits as well as enhance preservation and disinfection.

DEPOSITS

Deposits are a significant and perhaps the main cause of lens problems. Morgan showed that, after 6 months of daily soft contact lens wear, 50% of troubles could be traced to deposits.[120] This figure increased to 80% after 8 months of lens wear. Problems that are attributed to preservatives may often be due instead to inadequate cleaning.[27] Deposits decrease comfort and wearing time, decrease visual acuity, increase the risk of infection, and may cause giant papillary conjunctivitis. They enhance the binding of preservatives, which may lead to increased irritation, and offer binding sites to bacteria. They can reduce tear breakup time, alter physical parameters of the lens (and thus alter fit), serve as a nutritional source for organisms, decrease oxygen permeability of the lens, and cause other problems.[37,54,170]

During the first hours of soft contact lens wear, cells and bits of mucus adhere to the lens surface. As wear continues, more mucus is deposited and is ground into an amorphous coating. Extended-wear lenses have thicker but smoother coatings than do daily-wear lenses. Deposits and bacteria build up on the coating. Rubbing with surfactant may remove deposits without changing the character of the coating. Enzyme cleaner produces an "eaten granular" appearance in the coating. Combined used of surfactant and enzyme gives the most effective cleaning, but leaves 25% of the lens surface area still coated.[52]

Various types of deposits occur. The elements that contribute to soft contact lens deposits have been grouped by Tripathi under four headings: (1) organic elements (protein, lipid, mucin, organic pigments); (2) inorganic elements (calcium salts, mercury, iron); (3) mixed elements of the above; and (4) manufacturing and physical defects, polymer impurity, aging, and decay.[169]

Deposit formation may be affected by systemic factors. For example, contraceptive pills may lead to lipid deposits and mucin deposits on hydrogel lenses.[169,170]

The frequency of different deposit types is polymer-specific and relates to interactions between deposits and the lens surface. For example, lipid is a more significant problem with silicone, silicone/acrylate, and cellulose acetate butyrate lenses, whereas protein is a more significant problem with hydrogel lenses.[151] Hydrogel lenses absorb and adsorb proteins.[99] Most tear proteins carry a negative electrical charge at physiologic pH. Lysozyme carries a positive charge and probably interacts strongly with the negative charge on the surface of the hydrogel lens. Thus, it forms one of the most common and difficult to remove deposits. Increased lysozyme uptake is noted with increasing acid content in the HEMA polymer of the hydrogel lens.[163] There are fewer deposits on polymethylmethacrylate lenses, and they are generally easier to remove. Ease of removal is partially related to the fact that one can clean these lenses much more vigorously than other types of lenses.

Contact lens care systems also affect the types of deposits seen. For example, protein is more of a problem in hydrogel lenses disinfected with heat than when chemical disinfection is used. This is particularly so when the protein has been inadequately cleaned from the lens prior to heating. Lenses from a chemical disinfection system that are saturated with chlorhexidine adsorb lipid to their surfaces.[5] In either system, lipid and protein deposits are best solubilized in an alkaline environment.[103]

CLEANING AGENTS

Three basic types of cleaning agents are used: surfactant, oxidative, and enzymatic.[44]

Surfactant Agents

Surfactant agents are meant to be used on a daily basis with daily-wear lenses and whenever the lens is removed with extended-wear lenses. These agents are particularly important when heat disinfection is used. Their use is enhanced by mechanical cleaning with the fingers or by insertion with the contact lens into a mechanical agitation device. Their action may be potentiated by altering pH or osmolarity of the solution to cause surface stress and distortion, cracking deposits away from the lens.[81,93] The cleaning properties of a surfactant depend on its ability to lower surface tension. These agents are particularly useful against lipid and deposits other than denatured protein. Regular use is helpful in decreasing deposition.

Surfactant cleaners should be rinsed from the lens before heat disinfection is used; otherwise, they may produce a coating on the lens.

Recently, the effectiveness of surfactant agents has been enhanced by adding abrasive particles (Boston Lens Cleaner) or polymeric (nylon) beads (OptiClean) to surfactant solutions. Particulate matter increases the mechanical cleansing effect and may allow removal of deposits bound to the surface in addition to the usual surface debris removed by surfactants. Solutions using them must be shaken prior to use. They are effective on PMMA and gas-permeable hard lenses. Use of surfactant solutions that contain particulate matter may decrease the need to use enzyme.[53,161]

The Boston Lens cleaner should not be used with the Silcon (100% silicone) lens because it decreases wettability.[10] The nylon beads in OptiClean have a more rounded surface and are probably safe on this material. However, OptiClean should not be used on SilSoft lenses because it may break down the hydrophilic surface.

Potential problems from abrasive particle use include the possibility of a negative effect on the surface of silicone lenses or on surface-treated lenses, scratches on the lens surface that could enhance deposition, eye irritation if the particles are not rinsed from the lens, and lack of effectiveness if the bottle is not shaken before it is used.[73] The abrasive material must be chosen carefully by the manufacturer with regard to hardness, particle size, and particle sharpness.

Oxidative Agents

Oxidative cleaning systems are able to remove previously formed deposits from hydrogel lenses. These agents include persulfates, perborates, hypochlorites, hydrogen peroxide, and others. Their action is enhanced by heating. Their disadvantages include the necessity to detoxify the lens after their use and the deleterious effect they may have on hydrogel lens structure. They can oxidize the polymer that makes up the hydrogel; this damage becomes worse with use. Protein deposition may be enhanced by routine use of a severe oxidative system, probably due to surface damage.

Hydrogen peroxide penetrates hydrogel lenses and is said to provide deep cleaning through oxidation of foreign matter.[14] It can remove organic and inorganic deposits. Proteins are oxidized to smaller molecular weight compounds that are more easily soluble.[81] Hydrogen peroxide is hypotonic and causes swelling of the lens secondary to osmosis. This results in surface expansion and breaking of some protein and lipid bonds and may aid in the removal of trapped debris.[88] Later, lens shrinkage continues to rupture bonds (the "accordion effect"). This may decrease the necessity or at least the frequency of enzyme use with hydrogel lenses.

Hydrogen peroxide that is available at the supermarket but that is not specifically intended for use with contact lenses should not be used. These products may have varying concentrations of hydrogen peroxide as well as colorants and other adulterants.[90] They may contain components that can adversely affect hydrogel structure. Hydrogen peroxide will be discussed further under Disinfection and Storage.

Enzymatic Agents

Enzymatic action is specific for a certain type of linkage and should not affect lens structure. Enzymes work by cleaving bonds and producing smaller molecular weight substances that are more soluble. Enzymes are the most useful agents against denatured protein. They have been recommended for use with hydrogel and with gas-permeable lenses when protein deposits are a problem.[112]

The two enzymes available at present in the United States are derived from papaya (papain) and from pork pancreas (pancreatin). Papain (Soflens Enzymatic Contact Lens Cleaner) is a sulfhydrylprotease that has specific activity against protein. It is now available in an effervescent tablet. Pork pancreatin (OptiZyme) is an effervescent enzyme tablet with protease, amylase, and lipase activity. It has been used successfully by some of the patients who had not succeeded with Soflens enzymatic cleaner.[27] At the present time, it is not certain which of these two products is superior. There is some suggestion that the protease activity in papain is better than that in pancreatin.[98] The significance of the added amylase and lipase activity in pancreatin is uncertain.

Enzyme may be sensitizing. Though rare, papain has been reported to produce urticaria, angioedema, anaphylaxis, and asthma in susceptible patients.[15] Pancreatin is useful in these patients. There may be patients who are sensitive to pancreatin but not to papain.

It is important to use a surfactant cleaner both before and after the use of an enzymatic cleaner. The surfactant will remove debris on the surface of the deposits, thus enhancing the ability of the enzyme to interact with the deposit. The surfactant should be rinsed off the lens before placement in enzyme solution, or enzyme efficiency may be diminished.[151] After the enzyme has been used, debris is still present on the lens surface. This must be removed, and use of a surfactant at this time is more effective than rinsing alone. This is particularly important prior to heat disinfection, because heat may cause protein lying on the surface to strongly bond to the lens.

OTHER CLEANING AIDS

A *chelating* agent such as EDTA is sometimes incorporated into a cleaning solution. Chelating molecules can bind a metallic ion, such as calcium, within themselves. EDTA has some antibacterial activity and will be discussed further under Disinfection and Storage. Theoretically, this agent will complex calcium and aid in the prevention of crystalline deposits and in their removal. However, this effect is temperature-dependent and primarily useful only at elevated temperatures.[2] Therefore, this effect is more likely to be of value in a heat disinfection system.

Ultrasound provides a method of sonic agitation and may be used to shorten and enhance the cleaning process.[160]

PURGING

Sometimes it is desirable to *purge* a hydrogel lens, that is, to clear it of chemicals to which it has been exposed. This procedure may be useful if fluorescein has accidentally been instilled in an eye wearing a lens, or if a patient is sensitive to one of the chemicals in the care system. A simple purge may be accomplished by surface cleaning with surfactant, and enzyme if necessary, followed by multiple soaks with unpreserved saline.[81] The success of the procedure is related to surface cleanliness, length of time the lens has been used, water content, and polymer type.[141]

A more complicated purging procedure may be used if the lenses are not easily replaced, for example, if they are not readily available or if it is not economically feasible to replace the lens. This is performed as follows: (1) clean the surface of the lens with a slurry of baking soda and surfactant; (2) rub each surface vigorously for 30 seconds and rinse thoroughly with a strong stream of distilled water; (3) check lens clarity and condition when dry under a magnifier; (4) wash and rinse the lens by placing it in a 30 ml or 40 ml Pyrex beaker with 25 ml of distilled water to cause swelling; place the beaker on a hot plate with a magnetic stirrer for 1 hour; (5) remove the lens, rinse thoroughly with distilled water while rubbing between the fingers, and repeat for an additional hour with fresh distilled water; (6) allow the lens to cool, then transfer to a beaker with 25 ml of unpreserved normal saline for a minimum of 1 hour; (7) place the lens in a new case or vial with unpreserved saline and heat disinfect.[141] If this procedure is used, the lens should not be replaced in the eye until the symptoms have resolved. This may be useful for a toric lens, or any custom, expensive lens, or for an office which self-insures.

Purging may also be useful if a patient has a reaction to Flexsol and the practitioner wishes to switch to heat disinfection without replacing the lens. If the high molecular weight polymers in Flexsol are not cleaned completely from the lens, they will elongate on heating and change the lens polymer.[104,160]

CONCLUSION

Historically, PMMA lenses have tolerated cleaning by a variety of methods. These include the use of Polident, detergents, shampoos, toothpaste, lighter fluid, carbon tetrachloride, beer, scouring powder, steel wool, silver polish, baby oil, benzine, calamine lotion, and douche powder.[21,103,110,115] No other lens material has provided this kind of latitude in resistance to insult. The lens materials in use today offer many advantages over PMMA, but require more careful handling to maintain those advantages. It is vital that solutions to be used to clean (or disinfect and store) a contact lens be approved for the specific lens material.

DISINFECTION AND STORAGE

TERMINOLOGY

There is some confusion among patients and practitioners about the terms *disinfection* and *sterilization*. It is important that these terms and their implications be understood, because infectious processes present serious challenges to the practitioner and serious consequences to the patient.

Sterilization is a process that destroys any form of viable organism. The process may be either physical or chemical. *Disinfection* is a process that destroys pathogenic organisms or renders them inert. This process may not destroy spores, tubercle bacilli, and certain viruses.[20] The term disinfection is usually used in reference to a process applied to an inanimate object,[69] for example, a contact lens. The Food and Drug Administration requires disinfection but not sterilization.[155] The term *preservation* is applied to a solution, and refers to the ingredients of the solution that destroy or inhibit the multiplication of microorganisms. Solutions used to disinfect contact lenses contain preservatives to prevent organism growth. The preservative ingredient(s) may be the same as the disinfecting ingredient(s). The United States Pharmacopeia requires that ophthalmic solutions "contain a suitable substance or mixture of substances to prevent the growth of or to destroy microorganisms accidentally introduced when the container is opened during use."[171] *Asepticization* is a term associated with the Bausch & Lomb moist heat unit and refers to its disinfection process.

DESIRABLE PROPERTIES

The following properties are desirable in a disinfectant: high efficacy, wide antimicrobial spectrum, rapid lethal action, ability to penetrate into crevices and beneath films of organic matter, ability to achieve lethal concentrations in the presence of organic matter, compatibility with chemical substances present in solution, chemical stability, good tolerance, low cost, and satisfactory esthetics (odor, color).[69]

Desirable properties in a preservative include effectiveness in low concentration against a wide variety of organisms; solubility in formulation at required concentration; nontoxic and nonsensitizing in required concentration; compatible with a wide variety of drugs and agents; satisfactory esthetics; active with long-term stability over a wide range of pH and temperature; inexpensive; nonreactive with the container; and low surface tension when used topically.[9,16,69,108] Unfortunately, the chemical properties that give many preservatives their broad spectrum of activity may make them not only toxic to human tissue but also allergenic.

Ideally, we need agents that are physiological bacteriostatic agents (*e.g.*, lysozyme) and are known to be well tolerated in the body.[40] We would also like an agent that does not affect the tear film. Benzalkonium chloride (0.01%), propylparaben (0.03%), and chlorhexidine (0.01%) have been shown to increase tear film drying, whereas thimerosal and phenylmercuric nitrate showed no change.[41] The tear film effect seems related to the surface activity of the preservative.

As applied to soft contact lens disinfecting solutions, we are looking for a solution that disinfects within 4 to 6 hours, is not easily inactivated by small amounts of tear components such as protein or lipid, does not bind to protein or other surface lens deposits, does not react with or adsorb to the lens, and is not irritating or toxic to the eye.[32] The antimicrobial efficiency of such a solution depends on various factors including preservative concentration, initial level of microorganism, pH, temperature, ionic strength, and presence of formulatory adjuvants.[36]

SIGNIFICANCE OF PRESERVATION

Why should ophthalmic solutions be preserved? A contamination rate of 58% has been noted in preparations lacking preservatives.[1] Twenty-four percent of patient lens problems may be related to the presence of pathogenic organisms.[170] About 30% of patients fitted with hydrogel lenses carry such organisms.

One study found a 13% incidence of bacterial contamination of multidose eyedrop bottles. In 2% of the cases, the bacteria were considered to be clinically and microbiologically significant. Bottle contents were sterile, but 21% of the tips yielded bacteria on culture.[87]

Contamination is more likely to be seen in a squeeze bottle than in a bottle that uses a pipette-type dispenser.[28] After contamination, the cap of a squeeze bottle receives little exposure to preservatives from the bottle. A recent case of *Serratia* ulcer was caused by an eyedropper bottle that had sterile contents but a contaminated cap. The moisture collected in the dead space between the cap and bottle apparently acted as a culture medium.[165] This highlights the potential for and serious consequences of contamination of multidose dispensers.

Contamination of the lens storage case has resulted in *Pseudomonas* ulcers.[68] In one study of 29 asymptomatic contact lens wearers, 10 (35%) had contaminated cases. These were all patients who used heat disinfection, and many of the lens cases were defective.[138] Clearly, mechanical cleansing of the lens case should be part of a care system. This decreases the microbial load presented to the preservative or disinfecting solution.

Fungi do not penetrate a soft lens under normal conditions.[45] In fact, one group of patients wore lenses with a mycelium present (*Candida*) on the lens for weeks to months without any change in corneal health.[97] However, *Aspergillus* organisms may penetrate and degrade lens material under more severe conditions. In one report, 1% of returned hydrogel lenses had fungi growing in them.[97] Mechanical cleansing reduces the likelihood of protein coagulation on the lens surface in the course of heat disinfection and thus reduces the potential to serve as an organism-harboring site.[49]

Patients who use cosmetics are at higher risk for infection. Cosmetics may be contaminated during use with saprophytic molds, animal-associated yeasts, and various bacteria. In a study of 428 samples from 235 patients, 12% had fungal growth and 43% had bacterial growth.[175] The potential for problems is staggering.

Perhaps the main source of ophthalmic solution contamination is inadequate instillation techniques.[128] Patient compliance with directions from the lens fitter and from the solution manufacturers is another source of significant problems.[160] We need to demonstrate drop instillation to our patients and spend the time with them to reinforce the importance of proper lens care. Other suggestions to decrease the possibility of infection include restricting bottle use to one person, limiting the length of time of use (this can be done partially by restricting bottle size), and perhaps recommending only single-dose containers.[9]

EVALUATION OF PRESERVATIVES

Contradictions are present in the literature regarding evaluation of various preservative agents. These may occur because of differences in test variables: preservative agent (concentration and supplier), test organisms (strain, growth conditions, level of inoculum), test solutions (water, buffered solution, final ophthalmic formulation, interaction with container), test temperature, contact time, inactivators employed for the agent, solution pH, and criteria by which the agent is judged.[128]

Solutions tested in animal eyes may show species differences. The rabbit eye is more sensitive to chemical irritation than the eye of higher primates or man, perhaps because of a lower blinking rate and lesser lacrimal response to irritation.[22]

Solution/container interactions may represent a significant problem. The FDA has recommended that chemical disinfection systems be tested in the containers that hold the lenses. Studies have shown that both the hydrophilic lenses and polyethylene lens cases have increased the time needed for killing a standard inoculum over that needed in a glass tube.[134] The interactions between preservatives and plastic containers that reduce antimicrobial activity are a function of formulation, preservative concentration, surface area to volume ratio of the container, storage time, and temperature. Chlorhexidine and benzalkonium chloride interact by surface adsorption, whereas thimerosal and chlorobutanol penetrate the plastic matrix. Thus, solutions containing thimerosal and chlorobutanol are more likely to show preservative loss with long-term storage.[143] Lens/preservative interactions represent a complicated area for study, but there is no doubt that both lens surface and matrix interactions are important.[144,154,157,160]

CHEMICAL VERSUS HEAT DISINFECTION

Chemical disinfection was the first system used with contact lenses. It was applied to PMMA lenses, and was successful and generally well tolerated. PMMA soaks up little if any preservative and is easily rinsed. Chemical disinfection also works well for CAB and silicone/acrylate lenses. However, because of lens surface considerations, the solutions must be specially formulated. Recommendations of the lens manufacturer must be followed closely, and the patient should be instructed not to use standard hard contact lens solutions with silicone/acrylate materials.

Unfortunately, hydrogel lenses absorb the preservatives and disinfectants originally used for hard lenses. The hydrophilic surface and porosity of the gel lens present difficulties in the development of cold sterilizing storage solutions.[19] These materials concentrate chemicals and protract the contact time between cornea and chemical. Thus, it is not possible to use the same kind of disinfection solution for both hard and soft lenses. The first system approved for hydrogel disinfection in the United States was a heat disinfection system.[48] This was followed by a system from Burton, Parsons & Com-

pany that combined thimerosal, chlorhexidine, and EDTA in the storage/
disinfecting solution.

Microbiologically, heat and chemical disinfection are roughly equivalent.[75] Heat disinfection requires about 80° C for 10 minutes for disinfection
of hydrophilic lenses.[26] The advantages of heat disinfection include uniform
distribution of heat throughout the case, lower frequency of allergic reactions, and lack of development of bacterial resistance. Its disadvantages
include shorter lens life and increased likelihood of deposits and deposit-
related problems, such as giant papillary conjunctivitis.[5,19] Modern heat
units are simple and, when combined with a nonpreserved saline or sorbate-
preserved saline, offer a simple, low cost, effective system for low water
content hydrogel lenses. However, heat decontamination is not totally se-
cure when unpreserved normal saline is used.[127]

In late 1978 the FDA required that only antimicrobial-preserved saline
solutions be used because of reports of *Pseudomonas* conjunctivitis.[58,95]
Pseudomonas organisms can grow in distilled water without visible turbid-
ity. Other bacteria, such as *Achromobacter, Flavobacterium,* and *Serratia,*
have also been shown to grow in distilled water.[47,136] When sodium chloride
tablets were withdrawn from the market, an increase in contact lens-related
ocular inflammation was noted by practitioners. Sodium chloride tablets
were approved and reintroduced again in 1980–1981 in a kit that allowed
the preparation of only a one-day supply of saline at one time. However,
other problems with patient preparation of saline exist.[79] The distilled water
used may have unwanted mineral and microbial impurities. Salt and pH
concentrations may alter hydrogel lens fit (see discussion of Changes in Lens
Parameters and Fit under Solution-Related Complications). Lack of filtra-
tion may cause particulate contamination of patient-prepared saline. Hard
particulate matter larger than 10 μm may cause corneal injury.[104]

Preserved solutions for chemical disinfection may be more foolproof
than heat disinfection, but neither system can prevent misuse or lack of use.
The commonest failure in compliance with chemical disinfection is the
attempt to economize on the use of chemical disinfectant by not replacing
the storage solution in the case.[127]

CATEGORIES OF PRESERVATIVE AGENTS

There are five major categories of antimicrobial preservative agents[128]: (1)
quaternary ammonium compounds; (2) mercurials; (3) alcohols;
(4) esters of parahydroxybenzoic acid; and (5) miscellaneous. Each group
will be discussed separately.

Quaternary Ammonium Compounds

The quaternary ammonium compounds ("quats") include *benzalkonium
chloride* (BAC) and *alkyl triethyl ammonium chloride* (ATEAC). These are
surface-active, cationic disinfectants. They may be neutralized and possibly

precipitated by anionic agents.[109] They are equally effective against many gram-negative and gram-positive bacteria, and they work in a similar fashion. The mode of antimicrobial action is thought to be due to surface activity on living cell surfaces or to interference with respiration and glycolysis of the organisms.[33] On PMMA, BAC can form a hydrophobic surface; thus, its concentration is kept at a minimum in wetting and soaking solutions. BAC may decrease wettability of silicone–acrylate surfaces by interacting with hydrophilic groups.[12] Though controversial, this effect probably exists. BAC binds to hydrogel lenses, possibly through an interaction with negatively charged polar regions at the lens surface.[60] This strong binding (adsorption) limits its use with hydrogels.

BAC is bacteriostatic at low concentration and bactericidal at higher concentrations.[16] There is some evidence that suggests greater activity against gram-positive bacteria. Its activity against gram-negative organisms is increased by EDTA. It is thought that the di-cations of calcium and magnesium have a blocking effect on BAC due to competition for active sites in the cell membrane. EDTA sequesters these divalent cations so that the positively charged BAC can fit into the vacant sites.[128]

BAC is rapid in action and is extremely effective when used properly. Its antibacterial action can be reduced by soaps, serum, organic matter, metallic ions, rubber, and cotton.[72,145]

When applied to the eye, BAC produces disruption of the tear film, a decrease in the breakup time, changes in the epithelial surface with separation of adjacent surface cells and premature desquamation, and an increase in corneal permeability.[29] The increase in corneal permeability enhances the absorption of various drugs applied to the corneal surface. Strong concentrations can retard the healing of corneal epithelium.[33]

ATEAC is a relatively new preservative. It is formulated with Polysorbate 80. The positively charged ATEAC is surrounded by the Polysorbate 80 and forms a micelle that is too large to penetrate a hydrogel lens. Thus, ATEAC is unable to adsorb to the lens and is less likely to cause chemical injury to the cornea, but it is still able to interact with microorganisms as a preservative. Polysorbate 80 acts as a surfactant daily cleaner, so this combination works as both a preservative/disinfectant and daily cleaner.[78,149] Polysorbate 80 cannot be used with BAC; it inactivates BAC due to binding or association.[101]

Mercurials

The mercurial agents include *thimerosal, phenylmercuric acetate* (PMA), and *phenylmercuric nitrate* (PMN). These compounds are primarily bacteriostatic.[16] Thus, there is the potential for subsequent *in vivo* infection because of neutralizing agents associated with blood and body tissue. Their mechanism of action appears to be through inhibition of sulfhydryl enzymes by the mercuric ion. The mercuric ion may also interact with other chemical moieties. Interaction with sulfhydryl groups near cell surfaces causes permeability changes and cell lysis. Resistance can occur.

The mercurials are degraded by hydrogen peroxide, light, and heat.[16] Glutathione and compounds containing sulfhydryl groups tend to decrease the activity of thimerosal.[72] Phenylmercuric salts are lost from solution when they are in contact with polyethylene, and they are readily absorbed by rubber.

Thimerosal is sodium ethylmercuric thiosalicylate, better known as merthiolate. It has been used in tincture form as a topical antiseptic in the United States. Because it acts slowly when used alone, it is often combined with other preservatives. It is a medium to strong allergen in humans. Thimerosal is a basic salt of a weak organic acid, and thus can be used only in alkaline and neutral solutions.[16] Early binding experiments showed that thimerosal did not bind to HEMA, whereas PMA and PMN did.[155] Thus, the phenylmercuric compounds may be used only with non-HEMA lenses. Thimerosal does not bind to HEMA. It equilibrates with the water phase and passes freely in and out. Thus, HEMA lenses absorb an amount of thimerosal equivalent to their water content.[15] Thimerosal may bind to protein left on the lens surface, resulting in concentration and possibly a toxic or allergic response (see discussion of Adverse Ocular Response under Solution-Related Complications).[181]

PMN has been associated with the deposition of mercury in the cornea and in the lens (see discussion of Mercurialentis under Solution-Related Complications).

Alcohols

The alcohols include *chlorobutanol* and *phenylethyl alcohol.* Comments about one alcohol generally apply to the other. Chlorobutanol is bacteriostatic and is less commonly used because it is unstable with long-term storage.[126] It can be absorbed by rubber stoppers or lost through plastic containers, and is volatile and unstable except under acid conditions.[16] Its concentration in solution is dependent on the method of formulation. Its mode of action is that of an epitoxoid, and it is lethal only after it permeates into the bacterial cell.[72] Both chlorobutanol and phenylethyl alcohol may have a slight anesthetic effect.[17,128] They are best used in combination with other agents because of their slow onset of action. Both of these agents can bind to hydrogel and silicon materials, and may cause discomfort when released.[46,81] Phenylethyl alcohol is more effective against gram-negative bacteria than it is against gram-positive bacteria.[111]

Parabens

The *parabens* are all esters of parahydroxybenzoic acid. They should not be used as sole agents because they are slow in effect and are susceptible to development of resistant organisms. They are incompatible with certain chemicals, including polyvinylpyrrolidine, polyethyleneglycol, and methylcellulose.[128] However, for concentrations in which polymers are usually employed, binding of parabens is not sufficient to prohibit their application as a preservative.[123] Their decomposition is accelerated by heat and alkaline *p*H, and they are inactivated by surfactants and certain fungi.[175]

Parabens are more effective against molds and fungi than against bacteria, and are more effective against gram-positive bacteria than against gram-negative bacteria. They are effective only at concentrations near their limit of solubility, and these concentrations may irritate the eye.[9] Solutions containing these agents would be expected to lose antiseptic efficacy with time due to hydrolytic breakdown of the agents.[103] Their chemical structure is related to the ester type of local anesthetics (*e.g.,* procaine and tetracaine), and they may cross-react antigenically with these agents.[94] They are common preservatives in eye makeup.

Different paraben esters are additive or perhaps synergistic with each other.[70] Their usefulness is limited by water solubility. This problem may be overcome by using different members, such as methylparabens and propylparabens. The water solubility decreases, the lipid solubility increases, and activity and toxicity increase with an increase in the alkyl chain length up to a maximum at the butyl ester.[16] These agents are potent sensitizers in topical application, but this does not appear to be a problem in ophthalmic use.

Miscellaneous

The group that may be classified as miscellaneous includes many different agents. The following drugs will be discussed: chlorhexidine, hydrogen peroxide, sorbic acid, EDTA, trimethoprim, and iodine.

CHLORHEXIDINE

Chlorhexidine was approved by the FDA in 1976 for use in preoperative scrubbing and soft contact lens disinfection. It binds to HEMA, but with an affinity of about 10% of that of BAC. Its active moiety is cationic, and it is synergistic with thimerosal in the concentration used for hydrogel lens disinfection.[155] It acts by binding to the cell surface, disrupting membrane integrity, and causing leakage of cellular proteins and nucleic acids.[134]

Chlorhexidine has high bacteriostatic and bactericidal activity against a variety of bacteria and fungi,[148] exceeding that of BAC.[16] This activity is reduced by organic substances such as blood, pus, and serum.

Chlorhexidine can interact with anionic detergents, resulting in deposition of a water-insoluble film on contact lenses.[22,154] It will precipitate most bicarbonates, borates, phosphates, and sulfates.[128] It may also bind to protein on lenses, causing significant irritation when placed on the eye. The combination of chlorhexidine with denatured protein may result in a new antigen that can provoke giant papillary conjunctivitis.[96,114,169]

The dermal patch test shows that chlorhexidine is highly sensitizing.[1,15] However, delayed hypersensitivity reactions are less likely to develop than with thimerosal, because chlorhexidine is less widely used and has a lower concentration in the tear film (unless there has been protein binding).[126]

Chlorhexidine has been shown to have no effect on epithelium or endothelium when used as a soft lens disinfectant, and is considered by some to be the most effective ophthalmic preservative available.[76,128]

Chlorhexidine should not be used in solutions that are used on the Opus III lens. This lens contains butyl styrene copolymerized with other monomers, one of which contains silicone. It will complex to the hydrophilic surface.[74]

HYDROGEN PEROXIDE

Hydrogen peroxide is an oxidizing agent that has some cleaning properties, previously discussed. Its mechanism of action as a disinfectant is thought to involve free oxygen radicals released by metallic ions originating from the bacteria. These oxygen radicals act on the cell wall of the organism and result in cell rupture and death.[14,89] The kill rate is enhanced by elevated temperature.[16]

Defense mechanisms against free radicals have evolved in all respiring organisms and consist of the enzymes catalase and peroxidase, which inactivate hydrogen peroxide, and of superoxide dismutase, which scavenges the superoxide radical.[16] Hydrogen peroxide can also be neutralized by sodium pyruvate (which reacts to form sodium acetate, carbon dioxide, and water), sodium bicarbonate (which reacts to form sodium carbonate, carbon dioxide, and water), sodium thiosulfate, and platinum.[14,63] High temperature catalyzes hydrogen peroxide into oxygen and water. Organic material reduces the microbiological activity.[75]

Uptake of hydrogen peroxide from solution differs with contact lens materials. In one study, the Softcon lens imbibed hydrogen peroxide more quickly than did the Soflens.[63]

Many common pathogens are rendered harmless with 10 minutes of exposure to hydrogen peroxide, but other organisms, such as *Candida albicans,* may require much longer exposure times, perhaps as long as 1 hour.[14,135] This data may force a lengthening of currently recommended exposure times.

The first approved hydrogen peroxide system in the United States was the Septicon system, which requires two steps. The first step consists of a 20-minute rinse in Lensept (3% hydrogen peroxide). The second step is an overnight rinse in a cup containing a platinum catalytic disk and saline. The minimum life of this catalytic disk should be 6 months. After 180 cycles with the disk, an assay showed an average of 7.6 ppm peroxide in the contact lens.[89]

The two-step system lacks some convenience. The Aosept Catalytic Disinfection System, just released in the United States, disinfects and neutralizes in one step.[66]

Residual peroxide must be removed from the lens, otherwise it can cause corneal discomfort. Removal of the lens from hydrogen peroxide and transfer to a saline soak carries about 3000 ppm of residual peroxide. Over 100 ppm has a high risk of discomfort and below 50 ppm has rare discomfort.[90] The threshold for awareness is 20 ppm, and 60 ppm has no detrimental short-term effect on corneal integrity.[89]

Drops of 3% hydrogen peroxide on the human eye cause pain but no damage. Damage is seen in the rabbit, probably due to a species difference.[63] Wearing a Hydrocurve II lens that was inadvertently stored in 3% hydrogen peroxide produced pain, tearing, and mild keratopathy, but no serious problems.[100]

Hydrogen peroxide offers many advantages over other chemical care systems. It is safe, effective, and does not contain sensitizing ingredients. It has some apparent inherent cleansing activity. It is particularly valuable when a patient has developed sensitization to other preservative/disinfecting agents, and may represent the "agent of the future."[14,75]

SORBIC ACID

Sorbic acid (2,4-hexadienoic acid) is a mold and yeast inhibitor and is also used as a fungistatic agent for foods, especially cheese. *Potassium sorbate* is a water-soluble salt of sorbic acid.[142] Sorbic acid is a naturally occurring compound and may be obtained from the berries of the mountain ash. Its active form is the nonionized acid, which is more effective at *p*H 4 or below.[16] It has a broad range of activity against fungi, attributed to inhibition of dehydrogenase systems. Its antibacterial properties are more selective, showing greater activity against catalase-positive organisms than against catalase-negative organisms.[16] Sorbic acid is stable for 2 years and is compatible with all hydrogel lenses. It is not taken up and is not concentrated. Its ability to inhibit enzymatic processes is enhanced by EDTA.[42] The metabolic endproducts are carbon dioxide and water.[139] The FDA has allowed the use of sorbic acid or potassium sorbate as preservatives in soft contact lens solutions since 1983.[156]

Sorbic acid and potassium sorbate may discolor certain lenses. This is more likely to occur at higher sorbate concentrations, when the lenses are older and have deposits on them, when the solution is old, and when directions are not properly followed.[75,113,156] This reaction may be patient-specific.

The sorbate products were developed for hydrogel lenses recommended for heat disinfection (*i.e.,* those lenses with a water content of 35% to 45%). When higher water content extended-wear lenses are heated in a sorbate-preserved solution without proper cleaning, discoloration may occur. This is caused by a reaction between oxidation products (aldehydes) of sorbic acid and dirt or amino acids (possibly lysine from tear protein) on the lens.[75,156] Discoloration is said to be less when the lenses are disinfected in hydrogen peroxide before soaking in a sorbate-preserved saline, probably due to oxidative cleavage of protein on the lens.[75] The rate of sorbic acid oxidation is dependent on temperature, *p*H, light, and the presence of oxygen and trace metal ions. Degradation decreases with increasing *p*H and is negligible above *p*H 7. EDTA complexes metal ions, thus decreasing oxidation rate.[156]

Discoloration may be avoided by thorough lens cleansing before soaking, limitation of heat exposure, and by not mixing solutions from different manufacturers. A discolored lens usually can be decolorized with cleaning and bleaching solutions, such as 0.25% sodium hypochlorite or 3% hydrogen peroxide, followed by purging the lens.[156]

EDTA

EDTA is *Ethylenediaminotetraacetate,* also known as edetate. EDTA refers to any salt of edetic acid, such as sodium edetate or calcium edetate. It is a chelating agent that increases the activity of cationic antimicrobials such as BAC and chlorhexidine, presumably by removing calcium or magnesium from microbial cell membranes and increasing cell permeability.[16,33,72,134,140] It may also enhance the effect of chlorobutanol.[72] Some believe that the antimicrobial activity is due to a detergent-like action rather than to EDTA's chelating properties.[128] EDTA has been shown to be effective in preventing *Pseudomonas* organisms from becoming resistant to various bactericidal agents.[71] It may decrease the antimicrobial effect of phenylmercuric nitrate and thimerosal.[103,154] EDTA is antagonized by magnesium and calcium ions.[18]

TRIMETHOPRIM

Trimethoprim has recently been marketed as the preservative in Sof/Pro Clean II. This is the first time this preservative has been used in an ophthalmic preparation. It does not cause irritation or sensitization, and reputedly will not discolor or adsorb onto the lens. It is said to be compatible with HEMA, CAB, silicone, and related polymer groups.[106,159] It is a folic acid antagonist that inhibits the reduction of dihydrofolic acid to tetrahydrofolic acid. It is synergistic with the sulfas. *In vitro,* it is active against most gram-positive cocci and most gram-negative rods except for *Pseudomonas* and *Bacteroides* organisms. Further use and testing will define the value of this agent as a preservative.

IODINE

Use of various solutions of *iodine* for disinfection has been reported.[30,32,91] Elemental iodine is a potent and rapidly acting preservative. Its efficacy is reduced in the presence of organic matter because of binding and complex formation. Toxicity is relatively low. This agent, perhaps in a new formulation, offers potential for further research. Potential problems might include hypersensitivity and teratogenicity. Povidone-iodine is known to be capable of altering DNA in living cells and may result in mutagenesis.[180]

WET VERSUS DRY STORAGE

The problem of wet versus dry storage for hard lens materials has been discussed for many years, with proponents of both sides. This is not an issue for hydrogel lenses, where wet storage is a must. The proponents of dry storage for PMMA lenses claimed that lens cases were frequently contaminated when wet storage was used and that dry storage was safer.[38,130] If dry storage is used, some recommend a ventilated case, because moisture present on the lens might be sufficient to encourage bacterial growth.[179] Proponents of wet storage (in a preserved solution) believe that there is higher sterility, increased comfort, and better visual performance.[7,13,34,35,118]

The wetting properties of PMMA lenses may be enhanced by soaking.[6,12] A lens that wets poorly is less comfortable and is more likely to develop deposits. Silicone lenses must never be allowed to dehydrate, because they may never wet properly again.[11] Because of certain solution/lens incompatibilities, the manufacturer's recommendations must be followed closely when specifying a set of solutions for a given lens.[10]

CONCLUSION

At the present time, there is no ideal preservative or disinfectant. Each agent has some limitation in the area of toxicity or lack of broad-spectrum coverage or both. Manufacturers handle these difficulties by using lower concentrations and combining agents for maximum effectiveness and minimum toxicity. Research into physiological agents and into other modes of disinfection such as the use of microwaves may provide answers to these problems.

SOLUTION-RELATED COMPLICATIONS

A variety of problems have been attributed to solutions and their components. Because solutions are only one part of the system consisting of the lens, solutions, and patient environment, it is often difficult to distinguish a problem caused by one part from a problem caused by another. Additionally, interactions may be present between solutions used, between solutions and a specific lens polymer, and so on. This complicates the picture and may make definitive diagnosis impossible.

Much work has been done in the basic sciences to evaluate effects of various components of solutions on cells. Preservative effects have been reported and are significant, particularly when the preservative is used in a solution that will be applied topically to the eye. BAC is probably the worst offender of the ophthalmic preservatives. It is capable of producing effects on cell membranes at 0.001% levels.[1,23,24,62,77,137,167,168,177] Other preservatives cause problems as well.[76,164]

This section will concentrate on certain clinical complications. The reader interested in basic science aspects should seek further information in the references noted above. Solution-related complications to be covered will be classified as follows: adverse ocular response, nonallergic keratopathy, carcinogenic/mutagenic, mercurialentis, and changes in lens parameters and fit.

ADVERSE OCULAR RESPONSE

Drug-related complications are frequent. In hospitalized patients, estimates range from 6% to 15%.[132] The causes of these complications include direct toxicity, alterations in host response (immunologic impairment or modification of normal flora), drug interactions, and idiosyncratic responses. True allergic or immunologic reactions probably account for 25% or fewer of these reactions.

Adverse ocular response is a nonspecific term that includes both immune and nonimmune reactions.[93] The response may be either toxic or allergic. A toxic (or irritative or nonimmune) response is dependent on dose level (concentration, length of exposure) and host response. In this case, both the chemical and solution characteristics (*e.g.,* tonicity, *p*H, osmolarity) can initiate inflammation. Toxic microbial or degradation products may also cause irritation.[174] An allergic or immune response (the terms are used here interchangeably) is initiated by binding of gamma globulin and subsequent binding of complement or by direct binding of complement. This is followed by activation of the immune cascade.

Patients may be exposed to allergens by ocular or nonocular routes (*e.g.,* preserved vaccines, skin tests).[126] Thus, an allergic response may occur to a contact lens solution even though the patient has no apparent history of exposure to that solution. In fact, the exposure of mucous membranes such as conjunctiva to simple organic molecules is more likely to produce tolerance than sensitization.[57]

Toxic reactions may be very difficult to distinguish from allergic reactions. Generally, the toxic reaction occurs on first exposure to the agent, is limited to the site of contact, and causes burning or stinging. An allergic reaction requires previous exposure, may spread beyond the site of contact, is usually associated with itching, and can cause a true positive patch test. Typically, it takes longer to develop than the toxic reaction.[133,174]

Symptoms of the adverse ocular response include burning, itching, irritation, redness, tearing, swelling, and loss of lens tolerance. Signs include conjunctival injection, chemosis, papillary and follicular hypertrophy, corneal edema, punctate keratitis, corneal ulcers and infiltrates, discharge, and excess lens movement.[93,117] A toxic reaction is more likely to cause punctate epithelial erosions and bright red conjunctival injection, whereas an allergic response is more likely to be associated with epithelial and stromal edema, infiltrates, and pale red conjunctival injection.[133]

In the contact lens wearer, tear protein that is bound to the lens surface may cause an allergic response.[117] Adsorbed protein molecules may become more antigenic, possibly because the most polar amino acids are involved in adsorption and the more hydrophobic groups, which are exposed, are involved in immune reactions.[173] Alternating dry/wet and hot/cold conditions, as well as mechanical rubbing from lids and fingers, may enhance the antigenic potential.[174] Additionally, antigenic deposits are often difficult to remove; thus, the eye is exposed to them over a long period of time. Patients with a history of seasonal hay fever, eczema, vernal conjunctivitis, ocular reactions to cosmetics, food allergy, or drug reactions are at increased risk.[117]

The most common reactions to preservatives include contact dermato-conjunctivitis, punctate keratopathy, and papillary conjunctivitis.[174] Most drugs are small molecules with molecular weight less than 1000 daltons. They are haptens and are not antigenic unless they are bound to a carrier protein.[117,132] This antigen combines with lymphocytes from the thymus, resulting in drugs (lymphokines) that mediate the inflammatory response. Sensitization occurs when a sufficient dose of antigen reaches regional lymph nodes. This requires anywhere from 5 days for a strong allergen to years for a weak allergen. After the patient has been sensitized, re-exposure to the antigen causes appearance of the clinical disease within 12 to 72 hours. In the eye, binding of hapten and carrier protein probably occurs in the superficial conjunctival stroma. Thus, drugs with low molecular weights (less than 1000 daltons) and high lipid permeability are more likely to cause an allergic response. Lipid-soluble vehicles, such as ointments, and detergents facilitate the entrance of drugs into the conjunctiva.[174]

The two response modes for allergic reactions caused by these chemicals are immediate (type I hypersensitivity) and delayed (type IV hypersensitivity). Delayed hypersensitivity occurs more frequently and is of more significance in contact lens-associated allergy.[126]

The patch test is the standard test used to make a diagnosis of delayed hypersensitivity. In a study of 1200 Americans, reaction rates were relatively high for some common ophthalmic preservatives. These include thimerosal (8%), EDTA (7%), and parabens (3%).[147] About 40% of patients allergic to thimerosal are also allergic to mercury. Reactions may also occur to sorbic acid, chlorhexidine, chlorobutanol, phenylmercuric acetate, and vehicles such as propylene glycol.[50,126]

The route of challenge is very important. Challenge of a contact-hypersensitive patient through oral ingestion or injection is ineffective, and patch testing must be performed.[158] There is low reliability in skin testing patients to determine immediate sensitivity to local anesthetics (which are chemically related to parabens); intracutaneous testing is suggested in this setting.[94]

Reaction frequency differs among patients from different parts of the world. These differences are due to mode of use and availability of the allergen in a specific area.[124] For example, a very high incidence of thimerosal sensitivity is noted in Sweden. This is felt to be due to TB testing of children and young adults with a solution that was preserved with thimerosal.[146]

The patch test is performed by soaking a gauze pad with the antigen, applying it to the forearm, covering it with impermeable tape for 48 hours, and reading it at 48, 72, and 96 hours for induration, erythema, and vesicles. An intradermal test can be performed with a TB syringe and a 30-gauge needle. This is examined at 24 and 48 hours for erythema and induration.[126]

Problems with skin testing include false-positive and false-negative reactions. False-positive reactions may occur when the substance produces direct irritation rather than an immune response. False-negative reactions may occur with the patch test when the skin is relatively resistant to development of contact dermatitis.[174]

Treatment of the adverse ocular response requires discontinuing exposure to the inciting agent. Thorough review of all lens care solutions and other solutions being used in the eye is necessary. Examination of the lens for deposits should be carried out at the slit lamp. This is facilitated if the patient is instructed to keep the eye open so that the lens surface may be observed to dry. The surface is then much easier to evaluate. The fit of the lens also should be assessed. Irritation from the care system must be differentiated from that due directly to the lens. Contact lenses may cause peripheral epithelial staining if they decenter, epithelial erosions, corneal edema, and foreign body tracks.[127]

If lens deposits are noted, the lens should be cleaned and replaced if satisfactory cleaning is not possible. These deposits may be causing the irritation or may be binding solution preservatives that are causing the irritation. The care system should be reviewed at the same time for possible anomalies. Deposits suggest that the cleansing routine is inadequate or that the lens is too old to cleanse properly. A change from chemical to heat disinfection with nonpreserved saline or a change to a hydrogen peroxide disinfection system sometimes may be helpful. If these procedures fail, the practitioner should change the lens to another polymer in the hope that it will be less likely to interact with the patient's ocular milieu to cause deposits.

If the lens is irritating immediately on placement in the eye, thorough rinsing of solutions from the lens or even placement of the lens in a soaking solution of unpreserved saline before insertion may be required.

Topical steroids may be used to enhance resolution of inflammation, but are not usually required. If used, the patient must be monitored more carefully for steroid side-effects. The practitioner must be certain that an infection is not the source of the irritation.

Sometimes, a patient is unable to tolerate contact lens wear with any care regimen. In these cases, if the patient is highly motivated towards lens wear, refitting should be attempted 4 to 6 months later. Some of these patients will be successful at this time.[150]

Any of the preservatives in use may potentially cause an irritative response in the eye. Thimerosal is the most common cause of irritation and may cause problems in 2% to 50% of users.[95,125,176] This is probably due to delayed hypersensitivity, though some workers disagree.[57,181] Mercury is sensitizing, but many patients who react to thimerosal do not react to mercury. The thiosalicylate portion of the thimerosal molecule seems to be the cause of most of these reactions; specifically, the thiophenol fraction.[1,43,146] Patch testing may be negative early, and should be read at 96 hours.[146] An intradermal test may help to make the diagnosis. This test may be negative if the antigenic source is a combination of thimerosal and either contact lens or adsorbed surface protein.[1] Thus, conjunctival "inoculation" may sometimes be necessary. Some studies have found a low rate of positive skin tests, but a high rate of response to thimerosal on conjunctival challenge.[176,181] Placement of a HEMA lens soaked in thimerosal on the eye can be used as an ocular patch test.[95]

Thimerosal can cause many false-positive skin tests.[57] This seems to be more common in young adult males without skin disease, and may be specific to this substance and to the young skin.[82] Contact dermatitis on the hands of a patient who used soft lens solutions has been reported in the absence of eye or lid involvement.[153]

Nine patients using disinfecting solutions containing thimerosal were examined because of redness and corneal epithelial problems that began after taking tetracycline. The problems cleared on a nonthimerosal regimen, and most patients were able to resume using thimerosal-containing solutions after tetracycline was discontinued.[31] This suggests the possibility of an otherwise unknown reaction, and should be considered in any patient presenting with a red eye who has previously shown good tolerance to thimerosal products.

Other preservatives may cause problems, but usually with lower frequency. Chlorhexidine, chlorobutanol, EDTA, parabens, and BAC may all cause contact dermatitis, but true ocular delayed hypersensitivity is infrequent or nonexistent.[126] Using the patch test, chlorhexidine has been demonstrated to be the most highly sensitizing of the preservatives.[15] It binds (adsorbs) to the lens more than other preservatives, but releases slowly and seems to cause little problem if the lenses are clean. Chlorhexidine may be released rapidly from lens debris, thus causing more irritation in patients with a lens deposit problem.[104] It can cause a positive patch test reaction.[172]

EDTA has been reported to cause an acute allergic conjunctivitis and periorbital dermatitis. In a report of three cases, two patients cross-reacted with ethylenediamine, known to be a potent sensitizing agent. This is a chemical that has many uses, and can be found in such common substances as salad oil and wine. It has been used to prevent discoloration due to traces of metals in various preparations, to prevent oxidation catalyzed by trace metals in cosmetics, to stabilize solutions, and as a systemic treatment for urinary calculi, hypercalcemia, and lead poisoning.[140]

The parabens can sensitize skin and cause a cutaneous allergic response. Allergy from oral and parenteral administration has not been reported.[142]

BAC also has been reported to produce an allergic conjunctivitis. Patients may be sensitized to BAC by systemic administration of agents that are chemically related to quaternary ammonium compounds, such as cholinergic agents, hypotensive drugs (*e.g.,* tetraethylammonium chloride), and neuromuscular blocking agents (*e.g.,* decamethonium bromide).[51] BAC is the most potentially irritating preservative of those in ophthalmic use.[174]

There is little information in the ophthalmic literature on sorbate-preserved products because their use in this area is so recent. The incidence of adverse responses appears to be the same as that of thimerosal, but the response appears to be much less severe.[92]

Giant papillary conjunctivitis (GPC) is an allergic conjunctivitis that has been seen in several clinical settings, including patients who wear contact lenses of any type, postoperative patients (due to suture irritation), and patients who wear an ocular prosthesis. The contact lens patients typically complain of blurred vision, mucus, decreased lens tolerance, and erythema, and are found to have papillary changes of the upper tarsal conjunctiva. Rarely, punctate keratitis or a superior white arcuate infiltrate may be seen. Early in the course of the disease the papillae are barely visible, but as the disease progresses the papillae enlarge to greater than 1 mm in diameter.[4]

GPC seems to be due to deposits on the lens. Deposits on lenses from GPC patients appear similar to deposits on lenses from patients who do not have GPC, suggesting that the disease is dependent more on the individual patient response than on the deposit.[55] It is probably not related to a particular type of deposit, but may be related to amount, because reducing deposits reduces symptoms. There is a lower incidence of GPC in PMMA lens wear, probably because these lenses are easier to clean and tend to have fewer deposits (because of the smaller surface area and less adherent material).[56] GPC in hydrogel lens patients is more common among those using heat disinfection because of the increased problem of deposits, though some authors disagree.[79]

GPC is similar in many ways to vernal conjunctivitis. A recent case report of vernal-like limbal inflammation and Trantas dots associated with soft contact lens wear adds to the belief that these diseases share a common pathogenesis.[19]

Treatment includes discontinuing lens wear until the symptoms and perhaps signs have resolved, thorough lens cleaning or lens replacement, and use of a new lens design or polymer if the disease recurs.[39] In a study of keratoconus patients wearing PMMA lenses who developed GPC, treatment with papain was shown to increase lens wearing time.[102] Topical steroids are rarely indicated, and probably should be considered only if symptoms are crippling. Cromolyn may be of some value. Its disadvantage, however, is that it may suppress symptoms but not suppress pathology, thus allowing more significant changes to occur. If cromolyn is used, these patients should be followed more closely and observed for continuing conjunctival changes.

NONALLERGIC KERATOPATHY

Various types of corneal problems can be induced by solutions. These problems may be due to a direct toxic effect of the solution components, to an indirect effect such as enhancing evaporation of the tear film, or due to confusion and use of the wrong solution.

Any surface-active compound may result in punctate gray areas in the corneal epithelium. Overuse of drops containing these agents interferes with the tear film and may also accelerate contact lens drying and deposits.[104] The harmful effect of topical solutions can be correlated with the BAC content.[85] BAC can produce a superficial punctate keratopathy and strong concentrations can retard the regeneration of corneal epithelium.[33] Damage produced is dose- and time-dependent.[24] Some of these effects are due to direct toxicity and some are due to secondary effects from an altered tear film. BAC has been shown to decrease the tear breakup time.[129] Deposits on the posterior lens surface may cause a punctate keratopathy.[83]

Calcific band keratopathy can result from long-term use of drops containing phenylmercuric nitrate. The mercury appears to denature protein, resulting in devitalization of tissue and deposition of calcium.[174]

Twelve patients using a combination of CSI soft lenses and Allergan solutions developed a superficial punctate keratitis. Eight of them were switched successfully to solutions that did not contain thimerosal.[64] It is not clear whether thimerosal was the culprit in this setting. It is certainly possible that thimerosal or other ingredients of a solution may interact with a specific lens polymer in such a way as to cause patient-specific problems. These are very difficult cases to track down, but must always be considered when a patient's solution-related problem does not appear to fit easily into a known category of complications.

As has been mentioned, corneal problems may be due to inadvertent use of the wrong solution. One patient switched the caps on the Boston Conditioning Solution and Boston Lens Cleaner. Use of the cleaner as a conditioning solution resulted in keratitis.[80] We need to emphasize strict care to our patients. This can be helped by solution manufacturers, who can make bottles of different sizes and colors and mark them with easily read labels.

Numerous reports have been published about a syndrome associated with contact lens wear that is similar in many respects to superior limbic keratoconjunctivitis of Theodore.[59,121,152,162] This syndrome may be associated with thimerosal and other preservatives, or it may be seen in patients who have used unpreserved products; thus, its etiology is uncertain. Symptoms include redness, foreign body sensation, blurred vision, photophobia, and tearing. Signs include superior bulbar conjunctival injection, superior limbal epithelial irregularity and pannus, superior corneal subepithelial opacity, tarsal conjunctival papillae, and filaments.[152]

Theodore has distinguished between this syndrome and that which he originally reported.[166] The etiology, clinical course, and treatment differ, but clinical manifestations overlap.

Treatment involves discontinuing lens wear till the symptoms have resolved. At that point, the contact lens should be replaced and the care system changed to either heat disinfection with nonpreserved saline or possibly a hydrogen peroxide care system. The patient should avoid using products that are preserved by agents that were associated with the prior episode.

CARCINOGENIC/MUTAGENIC

There appears to be no practical problem with carcinogenesis related to contact lens solutions. As has been mentioned, povidone-iodine has been shown to be capable of altering DNA.[180] This agent is not currently used in contact lens solutions in the United States.

Systemic EDTA has teratogenic effects. Topical 0.1% and 3% solution used six times per day had no teratogenic effect, but the 3% solution was shown to have embryopathic effects in one study.[61] The usual concentration of EDTA in contact lens solutions is less than 0.1%. Thus, it seems unlikely that a clinical problem will develop. However, practitioners should be aware of this potential and should be certain that patient exposure to EDTA is limited during pregnancy, particularly during the first trimester. A woman who is using multiple and frequent contact lens solutions in her eyes, as well as other preserved drops, may be at some risk.

MERCURIALENTIS

Phenylmercuric nitrate can cause mercury deposition in the cornea and in the lens.[174] A concentration of 0.004% has been shown to produce the appearance of mercurialentis in a significant proportion of patients.[3] Thimerosal, which is more soluble, does not appear to cause a similar problem. The mercury is organic in thimerosal and the bonds may be more stable than in PMN, where the mercury is partly inorganically bound. However, Plano T lenses that were soaked with 0.001% to 0.002% thimerosal and placed on corneas prior to penetrating keratoplasty resulted in a significant amount of mercury in the cornea and aqueous after 4 hours.[178]

Thimerosal is able to produce deposits of mercury on a contact lens that has been thermally disinfected. These deposits appear as gray to black pigment on the lens. They may be associated with a similar appearance in the lens case. The main cause seems to be multiple reuse of preserved saline or chemical disinfection solutions.[5] Rubber gaskets can also cause this problem, because rubber causes decomposition of thimerosal.

CHANGES IN LENS PARAMETERS AND FIT

Lens parameters may be incorrect when they are received from the manufacturer, or they may change slowly with age. However, when the fit of a lens changes in a surprising fashion, the practitioner should consider the possibility that this change was caused by solutions.

Lenses made of materials with pendant ionic groups (carboxyl or basic amino groups) are very responsive to *p*H changes. Lenses containing small amounts of methacrylic acid monomers will shrink at less than *p*H 6 and swell above *p*H 6.[104] At low *p*H, the diameter of the Permalens is reduced. This is associated with shrinkage of the polymer, decrease in water content, and steepening of the lens and thus a tighter fit.[122] A low *p*H may be found in distilled water.

Solution tonicity is also an important factor. Hypotonic solutions cause swelling of the lens and loosening of the fit.[79,104] Hypertonic solutions cause shrinkage of the lens and tightening of the fit. Salt solutions made up by patients must be made exactly according to the directions of the company marketing the salt tablets.

Significant deposits or coating on a lens may also alter the fit.

SUMMARY

Contact lens solutions are used to clean, disinfect, store, and enhance the comfort and fit of all types of contact lenses. They contain many different types of components to perform these functions. Each solution is formulated to provide a specific function or functions with a certain type of lens. Manufacturer's recommendations must be followed closely in this regard. The specific components or the way in which the solution is formulated may cause a wide range of problems for the contact lens patient. These problems may result from interactions between the solution and either the patient, contact lens, lens deposits, or other solutions. Their nature has been discussed here.

Often, problems are caused by incorrect use on the part of the patient. This can often be prevented by thorough instruction by the practitioner or assistant prior to dispensing the contact lens. Specific recommendations regarding type and brand of solution use should be made for each patient, after taking into account manufacturer's recommendations, patient history, and so forth. Patients must be cautioned to read instructions and to follow them. Solutions from different manufacturers should not be randomly mixed. Patients should not share their solutions with other patients, including family members.

The importance of proper lens care and follow up should be emphasized to new contact lens patients before fitting. If a patient is unable to bear the cost of continued solution replacement, this factor should be taken into account and discussed. Patients who call to complain of problems should be evaluated by the practitioner as soon as necessary, on the same day if need be.

All solutions and their components have advantages and disadvantages and thus a specific risk/benefit ratio that varies for each patient. Only by thorough evaluation of the patient and current knowledge of available lenses and solutions can the practitioner make the necessary judgment in a specific case. Utilization of information from this chapter plus constant perusal of the current literature will aid in both making the proper solution choice and evaluating solution-related complications.

REFERENCES

1. Abelson M, Butrus S, Weston J: Thimerosal update. Excerpta Medica, 1983
2. Abrahams, R. Soft and rigid lenses and recent innovations. Presented at CLAO Mid-Winter Meeting, 1985
3. Abrams J, Davies T, Klein M: Mercurial preservatives in eyedrops. Observations on patients using miotics containing thimerosal. Br J Ophthalmol 49:146, 1965
4. Allansmith M, Korb D, Greiner J et al: Giant papillary conjunctivitis in contact lens wearers. Am J Ophthalmol 83:697, 1977
5. Allergan Pharmaceuticals: Office Seminars in Ophthalmology: Identification, Prevention and Removal of Contact Lens Deposits, 1984
6. Allergan Pharmaceuticals Report Series 190A: A comparison of the wetting capability of Wet-N-Soak and Soaclens with Polycon gas permeable contact lenses
7. Bailey N: Contact lens storage: A bacteriological study. Am J Optom 43:244, 1966
8. Baker D, Tighe B: Polymers in contact lens applications. VIII. The problem of biocompatibility. Contact Lens J 10(3):3, 1981
9. Barkman R, Germanis M, Karpe G et al: Preservatives in eye drops. Acta Ophthalmol 47:461, 1969
10. Barr J, Hettler D: Effects of emulsion cleaners on Silcon lenses. Contact Lens Forum 9(11):45, 1984
11. Benjamin W, Ghormley N: Wettability of silicone and silicone–acrylate contact lens materials. Int Contact Lens Clin 10(2):94, 1983
12. Benjamin W, Simons M: Contact angle update: Care regimens and their effect on a rigid silicone–acrylate surface. Int Contact Lens Clin 11(8):500, 1984
13. Bettman Jr J: Contact lens storage, wet or dry? A bactcrial analysis. Am J Ophthalmol 56:77, 1963
14. Billig H, Bailey N, Fleischman W et al: A new, rapid hydrogen peroxide system for contact lens disinfection. CLAO J 10:341, 1984
15. Binder P, Rasmussen D, Gordon M: Keratoconjunctivitis and soft contact lens solutions. Arch Ophthalmol 99:87, 1981
16. Block S (ed): Disinfection, Sterilization, and Preservation, 2nd ed. Philadelphia, Lea & Febiger, 1977
17. Brewer J, Goldstein S, McLaughlin C: Phenylethyl alcohol as a bacteriostatic agent in ophthalmic solutions. J Am Pharm Assoc Sci Ed 42:584, 1953
18. Brown M, Richards R: Effect of ethylenediamine tetraacetate on the resistance of pseudomonas aeruginosa to antibacterial agents. Nature 207:1391, 1965
19. Browne R, Anderson II A, Charvez B et al: Ophthalmic response to chlorhexidine digluconate in rabbits. Toxicol Appl Pharmacol 32:621, 1975
20. Bruck S: Sterilization problems of synthetic biocompatible materials. J Biomed Mater Res 5:139, 1971
21. Burns C, Rarey R: Polident as a contact lens cleaning solution. Am J Ophthalmol 65:251, 1968

22. Burstein N: Corneal cytotoxicity of topically applied drugs, vehicles and preservatives. Surv Ophthalmol 25:15, 1980
23. Burstein N: Preservative cytotoxic threshold for benzalkonium chloride and chlorhexidine digluconate in cat and rabbit corneas. Invest Ophthalmol Vis Sci 19:308, 1980
24. Burstein N, Klyce S: Electrophysiologic and morphologic effects of ophthalmic preparations on rabbit cornea epithelium. Invest Ophthalmol Vis Sci 16:899, 1977
25. Buschke W: Studies on intercellular cohesion in corneal epithelium. J Cell Comp Physiology 33:145, 1949
26. Busschaert S, Good R, Szabocsik J: Evaluation of thermal disinfection procedures for hydrophilic contact lenses. Appl Environ Microbiol 35:618, 1978
27. Carmichael C: Safety and efficacy of a new enzyme cleaner. Int Contact Lens Clin 10(5):286, 1983
28. Coad C, Osato M, Wilhelmus K: Bacterial contamination of eyedrop dispensers. Am J Ophthalmol 98:458, 1984
29. Collin H, Grabsch B, Carroll N et al: The effects of benzalkonium chloride on in vitro corneal endothelium and keratocytes. Int Contact Lens Clin 9(4):237, 1982
30. Conn H, Langer R: Iodine disinfection of hydrophilic contact lenses. Ann Ophthalmol 13:361, 1981
31. Crook T, Freeman J: Tetracyclines and hypersensitivity to thimerosal in contact lens solutions. Am J Optom Physiol Optics 59(10):17, 1982
32. Cureton G, Sibley M: Soft contact lens solutions: past, present, and future. J Am Optom Assoc 45(3):285, 1974
33. Dabezies O: Contact lenses and their solutions: a review of basic principles. Part 1. EENT Monthly 45:39; Part 2, 45:68; Part 3, 45:82, 1966
34. Dabezies O: Wet vs. dry storage of corneal contact lenses: A statistical evaluation. Am J Ophthalmol 59:684, 1965
35. Dallos J, Hughes H: Sterilization of hydrophilic contact lenses. Br J Ophthalmol 56:114, 1972
36. Davies D, Richardson N, Norton D et al: The antimicrobial efficiencies of contact lens solutions. J Pharm Pharmacol 27(supp):24, 1975
37. Davis R: Animal versus plant enzyme. Int Contact Lens Clin 10(5):277, 1983
38. Dixon J, Lawaczeck E, Winkler C: Pseudomonas contamination of contact lens containers. Am J Ophthalmol 54:461, 1962
39. Donshik P, Ballow M, Luistro A et al: Treatment of contact lens-induced giant papillary conjunctivitis. CLAO J 10:346, 1984
40. Dreifus M, Wobmann P: Influence of soft contact lens solutions on rabbit corneae. A clinical and electron microscopical study. Ophthalmic Res 7:140, 1975
41. Duncan A, Wilson W: Some preservatives in eyedrop preparations hasten the formation of dryspots in the rabbit cornea. Br J Pharmacol 56:359P, 1976
42. Dvorak D, Mandt L, Reidhammer T: Investigating B&L's Sensitive Eyes Solution. Contact Lens Forum 9(12):49, 1984
43. Ellis F: The sensitizing factor in merthiolate. J Allergy 18:212, 1947
44. Eriksen S: Cleaning hydrophilic contact lenses: An overview. Ann Ophthalmol 7:1223, 1975
45. Eriksen S: Hydrophilic soft lens sterility and disinfection. In Ruben M (ed):

Soft Contact Lenses: Clinical and Applied Technology, Chap 23. New York, John Wiley & Sons, 1978

46. Eriksen S, Dabezies Jr O: Preservatives. In Dabezies Jr O (ed): Contact Lenses: The CLAO Guide to Basic Science and Clinical Practice, Chap 28. Orlando, FL, Grune & Stratton, 1984

47. Favero M, Carson L, Bond W et al: Pseudomonas aeruginosa: Growth in distilled water from hospitals. Science 173:836, 1971

48. Fichman S: A simplified cold disinfection procedure for hydrophilic contact lenses. Contact IOL Med J 5(2):39, 1979

49. Filppi J, Pfister R, Hill R: Penetration of hydrophilic contact lenses by aspergillus fumagatus. Am J Optom 50:553, 1973

50. Fisher A, Pascher F, Kanof N: Allergic contact dermatitis due to ingredients of vehicles: A "vehicle tray" for patch testing. Arch Dermatol 104:286, 1971

51. Fisher A, Stillman M: Allergic contact sensitivity to benzalkonium chloride. Arch Dermatol 106:169, 1972

52. Fowler S, Allansmith M: The effect of cleaning soft contact lenses: A scanning electron microscopic study. Arch Ophthalmol 99:1382, 1981

53. Fowler S, Allansmith M: Removal of soft contact lens deposits with surfactant–polymeric bead cleaner. CLAO J 10:229, 1984

54. Fowler S, Allansmith M: The surface of the continuously worn contact lens. Arch Ophthalmol 98:1233, 1980

55. Fowler S, Greiner J, Allansmith M: Soft contact lenses from patients with giant papillary conjunctivitis. Am J Ophthalmol 88:1056, 1979

56. Fowler S, Korb D, Finnemore V et al: Surface deposits on worn hard contact lenses. Arch Ophthalmol 102:757, 1984

57. Franklin R: Discussion of "Delayed hypersensitivity to thimerosal in soft contact lens wearers." Ophthalmology 88:808, 1981

58. Fraunfelder F: Which type of saline solution for soft contact lenses is best? Am J Ophthalmol 91:540, 1981

59. Fuerst D, Sugar J, Worobec S: Superior limbic keratoconjunctivitis associated with cosmetic soft contact lens wear. Arch Ophthalmol 101:1214, 1983

60. Gasset A: Benzalkonium chloride toxicity to the human cornea. Am J Ophthalmol 84:169, 1977

61. Gasset A, Akaboshi T: Embryopathic effect of ophthalmic EDTA. Invest Ophthalmol Vis Sci 16:652, 1977

62. Gasset A, Ishii Y, Kaufman H et al: Cytotoxicity of ophthalmic preservatives. Am J Ophthalmol 78:98, 1974

63. Gasset A, Ramer R, Katzin D: Hydrogen peroxide sterilization of hydrophilic contact lenses. Arch Ophthalmol 93:412, 1975

64. Gero G: Superficial punctate keratitis with CSI contact lenses dispensed with the Allergan Hydrocare Cold Kit. Int Contact Lens Clin 11(11):674, 1984

65. Ghormley R: Contact lens care—hand soap? Int Contact Lens Clin 11(6):318, 1984

66. Ghormley R: Hydrogen peroxide—the hydrogel disinfection system of the future? (Part 1). Int Contact Lens Clin 11(11):714, 1984

67. Gibaldi M, Feldman S: Mechanisms of surfactant effects on drug absorption. J Pharmaceut Sci 59:579, 1970

68. Golden B, Fingerman L, Allen H: Pseudomonas corneal ulcers in contact lens wearers. Epidemiology and treatment. Arch Ophthalmol 85:543, 1971

69. Goodman L, Gilman A (eds): The Pharmacological Basis of Therapeutics, 5th ed. New York, Macmillan, 1975
70. Gottfried N: Alkyl p-hydroxybenzoate esters as pharmaceutical preservatives: A review of the parabens. Am J Hosp Pharm 19:310, 1962
71. Gould H: Rationale in the use of contact lens solutions. EENT Monthly 41:359, 1962
72. Gould H, Inglima R: Corneal contact lens solutions. EENT Monthly 43:39, 1964
73. Greco A: Breaking the protein bonds: The use of particles in daily cleaners. Int Contact Lens Clin 11(11):655, 1984
74. Greco A: Freedom of choice: A gas-permeable materials overview. Int Contact Lens Clin 11(11):720, 1984
75. Greco A: A review and update of contact lens care systems. Int Contact Lens Clin 11(5):266, 1984
76. Green K, Livingston V, Bowman K et al: Chlorhexidine effects on corneal epithelium and endothelium. Arch Ophthalmol 98:1273, 1980
77. Green K, Tonjum A: The effect of benzalkonium chloride on the electropotential of the rabbit cornea. Acta Ophthalmol 53:348, 1975
78. Greenberger M: A chlorhexidine-free chemical regimen for hydrophilic contact lenses. Int Contact Lens Clin 8(1):13, 1981
79. Gruber E: Hot or cold care systems for hydrophilic lenses? Contact IOL Med J 7:339, 1981
80. Gruber E: An unusual case of keratitis. Contact Lens Forum 9(10):68, 1984
81. Hales R: Contact Lenses: A Clinical Approach to Fitting, 2nd ed. Baltimore, Williams & Wilkins, 1982
82. Hansson H, Moller H: Patch test reactions to merthiolate in healthy young subjects. Br J Dermatol 83:349, 1970
83. Hesse R, Kneisser G, Fukushima A et al: Soft contact lens cleaning: A scanning electron microscopic study. Contact IOL Med J 8(1):23, 1982
84. Holly F: Surface chemical evaluation of artificial tears and their ingredients. I. Interfacial activity at equilibrium. Contact IOL Med J 4(2):14, 1978
85. Holly F: Surface chemical evaluation of artificial tears and their ingredients. II. Interaction with a superficial lipid layer. Contact IOL Med J 4(3):52, 1978
86. Holly F: Surface chemistry of contact lens wear. Int Ophthalmol Clin 13(1):279, 1973
87. Hovding G, Sjursen H: Bacterial contamination of drops and dropper tips of in-use multidose eye drop bottles. Acta Ophthalmol 60:213, 1982
88. Janoff L: AO Technical Report. Clinical results using the Septicon system without supplemental enzymes.
89. Janoff L: The effective disinfection of soft contact lenses using hydrogen peroxide. Optician 178:24, 1979
90. Janoff L: The Septicon system: A review of pertinent scientific data. Int Contact Lens Clin 11(5):275, 1984
91. Johnson D, Littlewood T: A clinical study to determine patient acceptance and efficiency of a new regimen of soft lens care. Contact IOL Med J 3(3):17, 1977
92. Josephson J: Letter to the Editor. Int Contact Lens Clin 11(10):586, 1984
93. Josephson J, Caffery B: Hydrogel lens solutions. Int Ophthalmol Clin 21(2):163, 1981
94. Kahn G, Aldrete A, Ryan S: A comparison of dermal sensitivity to preservative and local anesthetic drugs. Ann Allergy 29:480, 1971

95. Kame R: Adverse ocular response to soft lens solutions. Contact Lens Forum 9(1):97, 1984

96. Kaufman H: Problems associated with prolonged wear soft contact lenses. Ophthalmology 86:411, 1979

97. Keates R (mod): Panel discussion on cleaning and sterilizing rigid and flexible lenses. In Bitonte J, Keates R (eds): Symposium on the Flexible Lens: The Future of Flexible Lenses Versus Rigid Lenses, Chap 24. St Louis, CV Mosby, 1972

98. Kjellsen T, Kiral R, Eriksen S: Single-enzyme versus multi-enzyme contact lens cleaning system: Speed and efficiency in removing deposits from hydrogel contact lenses. Int Contact Lens Clin 11(11):660, 1984

99. Klein P: A review of deposits on extended wear hydrophilic lenses. Int Contact Lens Clin 10(3):161, 1983

100. Knopf H: Reaction to hydrogen peroxide in a contact-lens wearer. Am J Ophthalmol 97(6):796, 1984

101. Kohn R, Gershenfeld L, Barr M: Effectiveness of antibacterial agents presently employed in ophthalmic preparations as preservatives against pseudomonas aeruginosa. J Pharmaceut Sci 52(10):967, 1963

102. Korb D, Greiner J, Finnemore V et al: Treatment of contact lenses with papain. Increase in wearing time in keratoconic patients with papillary conjunctivitis. Arch Ophthalmol 101:48, 1983

103. Krezanoski J: Contact lens products. J Am Pharmaceut Assoc NS10(1):13, 1970

104. Krezanoski J: A new look at soft lenses and their solutions. Am Pharm NS21(5):12, 1981

105. Krishna N, Brow F: Polyvinyl alcohol as an ophthalmic vehicle. Effect on regeneration of corneal epithelium. Am J Ophthalmol 57:99, 1964

106. Lamberts D, Buka T, Knowlton G: Clinical evaluation of trimethoprim-containing ophthalmic solutions in humans. Am J Ophthalmol 98:11, 1984

107. Lamberts D, Sibley M, Dabezies Jr O: Wetting. In Dabezies Jr O (ed): Contact Lenses: The CLAO Guide to Basic Science and Clinical Practice, Chap 8. Orlando, FL, Grune & Stratton, 1984

108. Lawrence C: An evaluation of chemical preservatives for ophthalmic solutions. J Am Pharmaceut Assoc Sci Ed 44(8):457, 1955

109. Lawrence C: Inactivation of the germicidal action of quaternary ammonium compounds. J Am Pharmaceut Assoc Sci Ed 37:57, 1948

110. Lewis E: A new method of cleaning contact lenses. EENT Monthly 45:43, 1966

111. Lilley B, Brewer J: The selective antibacterial action of phenylethyl alcohol. J Am Pharmaceut Assoc Sci Ed 42(1):6, 1953

112. Lowther G: Caring for hard GP lenses. Int Contact Lens Clin 11(2):75, 1984

113. Lowther G: Disinfection of extended wear lenses. Int Contact Lens Clin 11(1):14, 1984

114. MacKeen D, Green K: Chlorhexidine kinetics of hydrophilic contact lenses. J Pharm Pharmac 30:678, 1978

115. Mandell R: Contact Lens Practice, 3rd ed. Springfield, IL, Charles C Thomas, 1981

116. Mandell R: Is there an angle to wetting? Contact Lens Forum 9(8):45, 1984

117. McMonnies C: Allergic complications in contact lens wear. Int Contact Lens Clin 5(4):57, 1978

118. Medicornea. Contact lenses—wet vs. dry storage.

119. Meisler D, Zaret C, Stock E: Trantas dots and limbal inflammation associated with soft contact lens wear. Am J Ophthalmol 89:66, 1980

120. Miller B: Observations of deposits on soft contact lenses by different methods of light microscopy, scanning microscopy, and electron microprobe analysis. Int Contact Lens Clin 7(2):22, 1980

121. Miller R, Brightbill F, Slama S: Superior limbic keratoconjunctivitis in soft contact lens wearers. Cornea 1(4):298, 1982

122. Miranda M, Garcia-Castineiras S: Effects of pH and some common topical ophthalmic medications on the contact lens Permalens. CLAO J 9:43, 1983

123. Miyawaki G, Patel N, Kostenbauder H: Interaction of preservatives with macromolecules. III. Parahydroxybenzoic acid esters in the presence of some hydrophilic polymers. J Am Pharmaceut Assoc Sci Ed 48(6):315, 1959

124. Moller H: Why thimerosal allergy? Int J Dermatol 19:29, 1980

125. Mondino B, Groden L: Conjunctival hyperemia and corneal infiltrates with chemically disinfected soft contact lenses. Arch Ophthalmol 98:1767, 1980

126. Mondino B, Salamon S, Zaidman G: Allergic and toxic reactions in soft contact lens wearers. Surv Ophthalmol 26:337, 1982

127. Morgan, J. Complications associated with contact lens solutions. Ophthalmol 86:1107, 1979

128. Mullen W, Shepherd W, Labovitz J: Ophthalmic preservatives and vehicles. Surv Ophthalmol 17:469, 1973

129. Norn M, Opauszki A: Effects of ophthalmic vehicles on the stability of the precorneal film. Acta Ophthalmol 55:23, 1977

130. Obear M, Winter F: Bacteriologic culture of wet and dry contact lens storage cases. Am J Ophthalmol 57:441, 1964

131. Olson A: Surface properties: Wettability and adsorption. Contact Lens J 10(10):11, 1982

132. Patterson R, Anderson J: Allergic reactions to drugs and biologic agents. JAMA 248(20):2637, 1982

133. Paugh J, Caywood T, Peterson S: Toxic reactions associated with chemical disinfection of soft contact lenses. Int Contact Lens Clin 11(11):680, 1984

134. Penley C, Ahearn D, Schlitzer R et al: Laboratory evaluation of chemical disinfection of soft contact lenses. II. Fungi as challenge organisms. Contact IOL Med J 7(3):196, 1981

135. Penley C, Llabres C, Wilson L et al: Efficacy of hydrogen peroxide disinfection systems for soft contact lenses contaminated with fungi. CLAO J 11:65, 1985

136. Penley C, Schlitzer R, Ahearn D et al: Laboratory evaluation of chemical disinfection of soft contact lenses. Contact IOL Med J 7(2):101, 1981

137. Pfister R, Burstein N: The effects of ophthalmic drugs, vehicles, and preservatives on corneal epithelium: A scanning electron microscope study. Invest Ophthalmol Vis Sci 15(4):246, 1976

138. Pitts R, Krachmer J: Evaluation of soft contact lens disinfection in the home environment. Arch Ophthalmol 97:470, 1979

139. Puls D, Lindgren L, Cosgrove F: Sorbic acid as a fungistatic agent for certain pharmaceutical preparations. J Am Pharmaceut Assoc Sci Ed 44(2):85, 1955

140. Raymond J, Gross P: EDTA: Preservative dermatitis. Arch Dermatol 100:436, 1969

141. Remba M: Purging soft contacts. Contact Lens Forum 4(11):56, 1979

142. Remington's Pharmaceutical Sciences, 14th ed. Easton, Mack Publishing, 1970

143. Richardson N, Davies D, Meakin B et al: The preservative content of contact lens solutions on storage. J Pharm Pharmacol 27 (supp):27P, 1975
144. Richardson N, Meakin B, Davies D: The interaction of preservatives with PolyHEMA. J Pharm Pharmacol 27(supp):26P, 1975
145. Riegelman S, Vaughan Jr, D: A rational basis for the preparation of ophthalmic solutions. Surv Ophthalmol 3:471, 1958
146. Rietschel R, Wilson L: Ocular inflammation in patients using soft contact lenses. Arch Dermatol 118:147, 1982
147. Rudner E, Clendenning W, Epstein E et al: Epidemiology of contact dermatitis in North America: 1972. Arch Dermatol 108:537, 1973
148. Rye R, Wiseman D: Release of phosphorus-32-containing compounds from Micrococcus lysodeikticus treated with chlorhexidine. J Pharm Pharmacol 16:516, 1964
149. Scheffel C: Clinical testing of Allergan Cleaning and Disinfecting Solution. Allergan Pharmaceuticals Report Series No 172, 1980
150. Schwaderer K: Letter to the Editor. Int Contact Lens Clin 10(1):6, 1983
151. Seidner L, Sharp S: Surface deposits with gas permcable lenses. Contact Lens Forum 9(10):55, 1984
152. Sendele D, Kenyon K, Mobilia E et al: Superior limbic keratoconjunctivitis in contact lens wearers. Ophthalmology 90:616, 1983
153. Sertoli A, DiFonzo E, Spallanzani P et al: Allergic contact dermatitis from thimerosol in a soft contact lens wearer. Contact Dermatitis 6:292, 1980
154. Shively C: Accessory solutions utilized in contact lens care and practice. In Ruben M (ed): Soft Contact Lenses: Clinical and Applied Technology, Chap 25. New York, John Wiley & Sons, 1978
155. Sibley M: Disinfection solutions. Int Ophthalmol Clin 21(2):237, 1981
156. Sibley M, Chu V: Understanding sorbic acid-preserved contact lens solutions. Int Contact Lens Clin 11(9):531, 1984
157. Sibley M, Yung G: A technique for the determination of chemical binding to soft contact lenses. Am J Optom 50:710, 1973
158. Silverstein A, Welter S, Zimmerman L: Studies on experimental ocular hypersensitivity to simple chemicals. Am J Ophthalmol 50:937, 1960
159. Sposato P: Lens care products: Marching to industry's beat. Contact Lens Forum 9(8):25, 1984
160. Stein H (mod): Symposium: How to solve flexible lens care problems. Contact IOL Med J 7(2):89, 1981
161. Stein H, Harrison K: The safety and effectiveness of Polyclens, an all purpose cleaner for hydrophilic soft contact lenses. CLAO J 9:39, 1983
162. Stenson S: Superior limbic keratoconjunctivitis associated with soft contact lens wear. Arch Ophthalmol 101:402, 1983
163. Stone R, Mowrey-McKee M, Kreutzer P: Protein: A source of lens discoloration. Contact Lens Forum 9(9):33, 1984
164. Takahashi N: Cytotoxicity of mercurial preservatives in cell culture. Ophthalmic Res 14(1):63, 1982
165. Templeton III W, Eiferman R, Snyder J et al: Serratia keratitis transmitted by contaminated eyedroppers. Am J Ophthalmol 93:723, 1982
166. Theodore F: Letter to the Editor. Arch Ophthalmol 101:1627, 1983
167. Tonjum A: Effects of benzalkonium chloride upon the corneal epithelium studied with scanning electron microscopy. Acta Ophthalmol 53:358, 1975
168. Tonjum A: Permeability of rabbit corneal epithelium to horseradish peroxi-

dase after the influence of benzalkonium chloride. Acta Ophthalmol 53:335, 1975

169. Tripathi R, Tripathi B: Soft lens spoilage: Nature, etiology, and pathogenesis. Ophthalmic Forum 2(2):80, 1984
170. Tripathi R, Tripathi B, Ruben M: The pathology of soft contact lens spoilage. Ophthalmology 87:365, 1980
171. United States Pharmacopeia, 20th rev. Rockville, United States Pharmacopeial Convention, 1980
172. Van Ketel W, Melzer-Van Riemsdijk F: Conjunctivitis due to soft lens solutions. Contact Dermatitis 6:321, 1980
173. Vroman L, Adams A, Klings M: Interactions among human blood proteins at interfaces. Fed Proc 30(5):1494, 1971
174. Wilson II F: Adverse external ocular effects of topical ophthalmic medications. Surv Ophthalmol 24:57, 1979
175. Wilson L, Kuehne J, Hall S et al: Microbial contamination in ocular cosmetics. Am J Ophthalmol 71:1298, 1971
176. Wilson L, McNatt J, Reitschel R: Delayed hypersensitivity to thimerosal in soft contact lens wearers. Ophthalmology 88:804, 1981
177. Wilson W, Duncan A, Jay J: Effect of benzalkonium chloride on the stability of the precorneal tear film in rabbit and man. Br J Ophthalmol 59:667, 1975
178. Winder A, Sheraidah G, Astbury N et al: Penetration of mercury from ophthalmic preservatives into the human eye. Lancet 2(8188):237, 1980
179. Winkler Jr C, Dixon J: Bacteriology of the eye. III. (A) Effect of contact lenses on the normal flora. (B) Flora of the contact lens case. Arch Ophthalmol 72:817, 1964
180. Wlodkowski T, Speck W, Rosenkranz H: Genetic effects of povidone-iodine. J Pharmaceut Sci 64(7):1235, 1975
181. Wright P, Mackie I: Preservative-related problems in soft contact lens wearers. Trans Ophthalmol Soc UK 102:3, 1982

APPENDIX: BIBLIOGRAPHY

Allansmith M, et al: Giant papillary conjunctivitis in contact lens wearers. Am J Ophthalmol 83:697, 1977

Dabezies OH, Jr (ed): Contact Lenses: The CLAO Guide to Basic Science and Clinical Practice. New York, Grune & Stratton, 1984

Hales R: Contact Lenses: A Clinical Approach to Fitting, 2nd ed. Baltimore, Williams & Wilkins, 1982

Harold CE (ed): Contact Lens Care Guide—1985; Review of Ophthalmology. Radnor, PA, Chilton, 1985

Hartstein J (ed): Extended Wear Contact Lenses for Aphakia and Myopia. St Louis, CV Mosby, 1982

Mandell R: Contact Lens Practice, 3rd ed. Springfield, IL, Charles C Thomas, 1981

Miller D, White P (eds): Complications of contact lenses. Int Ophthalmol Clin 21(2), 1981

Mondino B et al: Allergic and toxic reactions in soft contact lens wearers. Surv Ophthalmol 26(6):337, 1982

Montague R (ed): Soft Contact Lenses: Clinical and Applied Technology. New York, John Wiley & Sons, 1978

Morgan J: Complications associated with contact lens solutions. Ophthalmology 86:1107, 1979

Physicians' Desk Reference for Ophthalmology. Oradell, NJ, Edward R Barnhart, 1985

Richmond P, Allansmith M: Giant papillary conjunctivitis. Int Ophthalmol Clin 21(2):54, 1981

Tripathi R, et al: The pathology of soft contact lens spoilage. Ophthalmology 87(5):365, 1980

Tyler's Quarterly Soft Contact Lens Parameter Guide 2, No. 4, Sept 1985

INDEX

Page numbers in italics indicate figures; numbers followed by t indicate tabular material.

Abrasions, corneal, therapeutic lenses
        with, 147–148
Absorption, 227
Acugel lens
    manufacturing information for, 56t
    parameters for, 58t
Adhesion, 227
Adhesive, cyanoacrylate, with
        therapeutic lenses, 148, *150*
Adsorption, 227
Age, extended-wear lenses and, 191
Airlens, parameters for, 42
Alcohols, as preservatives, 241
Alkyl triethyl ammonium chloride
        (ATEAC), 239–240
Allergan solutions, adverse reactions to,
        252
Allergic reactions. *See also*
        Conjunctivitis, allergic
    to solutions, 247–251
Alternating vision bifocal lenses. *See*
        Bifocal lenses, alternating vision
Amphoteric surfactants, 228
Angle
    contact, 229
    wetting, 229–230
Angle theta, 229
Anionic surfactants, 228
Anterior peripheral curve radius,
        minus-lenticular aphakic lens
        fitting and, 180, *181*
Aphakia. *See also* Hydrogel lenses, in
        aphakia
    corneal physiology in, 48–51
    microbiology of eye in, 51

rigid lenses in, fitting, 177–182
    therapeutic lenses in, 154
Appearance, in trial fitting of
        gas-permeable lenses, 45
Aquaflex lens, 84t, 89t
    manufacturing information for, 56t
Aquaflex Standard lens, parameters for,
        58t
Aquaflex Standard Minus lens, 86
Aquaflex Super Thin Minus lens, 86
Asepticization, defined, 236
Aspheric bifocal lenses, rigid, *121,*
        121–122
Astigmatism
    high corneal, 168–172
        correcting, 169–172, *171*
    irregular, 175–177
    postoperative
        as contraindication to extended-wear
            lenses, 53
        as indication for hydrogel lenses, 52
    residual, 164–168
        correction of, 165–168
        estimating, 165
    toric hydrogel lenses for, 91–96, 92–93t
        fitting, 94
ATEAC, 239–240
Autofocal lens, 121

BAC. *See* Benzalkonium chloride
Base curve, 73
    minus-lenticular aphakic lens fitting
        and, 179

Bausch & Lomb HO-4 lens, 85
Bausch & Lomb PA 1 lens, 122–124
Bausch & Lomb 70 lens, 96t
Bausch & Lomb Toric lens, 92–93t,
     95–96
Bedewing, endothelial, 25
Benzalkonium chloride (BAC), 239–240
   adverse ocular reactions and, 250–251,
     252
   interaction with plastic containers, 238
   tear film drying and, 236
Bicon lens, 126, *127*
Bifocal lenses, 118–137
   alternating vision, 124–137, *125*
     hydrogel, 130–135, *131, 132, 133*
       fitting, 134–135, *135*
       patient selection and, 135–137
     rigid, 126–130
       concentric, 126–127, *127*
       fitting, 130
       segment, 127–130, *128, 129*
   fitting, 184–186
   indications and contraindications for,
     185
   simultaneous vision, *118,* 118–124, *119*
     120, 121, 123, 182–183, *183*
     hydrogel, 122–124, *123*
     rigid, *120,* 120–122, *121*
       aspheric simultaneous, *121,*
        121–122
       concentric simultaneous, *120,*
        120–121
       fitting, 122
   translating, 183–184, *184*
Bi-Site lens, 130
Blebs, endothelial, 22, *23*
Blend, 75
Blepharitis, with therapeutic lenses, 146,
     152–153, *153*
Blinking, 27–28
   extended-wear lenses and, 192
Boston Lens Cleaner, 232
Boston lens II, parameters for, 41, 42t
Boston lens IV, parameters for, 41, 42t
Bullous keratopathy, therapeutic lenses
     in, 147, 153

Cabcurve lens, parameters for, 40, 41t
CAB lenses. *See* Cellulose acetate
     butyrate lenses
Camp fused bifocal lens, 130
Carbon dioxide
   diffusion through hydrogel lenses, 49
   restriction of outflow of, 8–9, *9*
   transport in normal cornea, 4
Cataract. *See* Aphakia; Hydrogel lenses,
     in aphakia
Cationic surfactants, 228
Cell density, endothelial, 23
Cellular debris
   disposal of, in normal cornea, 5
   restriction of outflow of, 9
Cellulose acetate butyrate (CAB) lenses,
     parameters for, 40, 41t
Cellusoft lens
   manufacturing information for, 56t
   parameters for, 58t
Central posterior curve (CPC), in
     gas-permeable lens fitting, 43
Centration, in trial fitting of
     gas-permeable lenses, 44
Chelating agents, in cleaning, 234
Chemosis, with limbal hyperemia, 202,
     203
Chlorhexidine, 242–243
   adverse ocular reactions and, 250
   interaction with plastic containers, 238
   tear film drying and, 236
Chlorobutanol, 241
   interaction with plastic containers, 238
Ciba Bi-Soft lens, 118, 123–124, 133
Cibasoft Minus lens, 84t, 85
Cinefro Bicentric bifocal lens, 128
Cleaning. *See* Disinfection; Solutions,
     cleaning
CMC, 229
Cohesion, 227
Combination extended-wear lenses,
     190–191
Combination lens fitting. *See* Piggyback
     lenses
Comfort, in trial fitting of gas-permeable
     lenses, 45

Compliance, poor, as contraindication to
  extended-wear lenses, 53
Concentric bifocal lenses, rigid, *120,*
  120–121
Conjunctiva, 26–27
  clumping of microvilli and, 27
  defects of, therapeutic lenses and, 146
  giant papillary conjunctivitis and,
    26–27
  hyperemia and, 26
  superior limbic keratoconjunctivitis
    and, 27
Conjunctivitis. *See also*
    Keratoconjunctivitis, superior
    limbic
  allergic, 202–203
    management of, 203
    pathogenesis of, 202
    symptoms and signs of, 202
  giant papillary, 26–27, 203–208, *205*
    as adverse reaction to solutions, 251
    pathogenesis of, 206–207
    pathology of, 206
    treatment of, 207–208
  infective, 208
    management of, 208
    symptoms and signs of, 208
  toxic, 209
    clinical picture in, 209
Contact angle, 229
Contour Comfort lens, 130
Cornea
  aphakic, physiology of, 48–51
  evaluation of surface of, extended-wear
    lenses and, 193
  protection of, by therapeutic lenses,
    155
Corneal abrasions, therapeutic lenses
  with, 147–148
Corneal complications, 211–221
Corneal diameter, in gas-permeable lens
  fitting, 43
Corneal edema, 214–216
  clinical picture in, 215
  pathogenesis of, 215–216
  stromal, 15–19, *17, 18, 19*

treatment of, 216
Corneal endothelium, 22–25
  bedewing and, 25
  bleb response in, 22, *23*
  cell density in, 23
  disease of, as contraindication for
    extended-wear lenses, 52
  polymegathism and, 23–24, *24, 25*
Corneal environment
  alteration induced by contact lenses,
    6–10
  normal, 1–6
Corneal epithelium, 10–15
  corneal sensitivity and, 13–15
  fragility of, 15
    therapeutic lenses and, 146
  metabolic changes in, 10–11
  microcysts and, 13, *214, 15,* 213–214
  mitosis and, 11
  oxygen consumption by, 12–13, *13*
  physical changes in, 11
  thinning of, 12–13, *12*
  transcorneal potential and, 11
Corneal erosions, therapeutic lenses with,
    147–148
Corneal infection, as complication of
    therapeutic lens use, 158–159,
    159
Corneal neovascularization, 220–221
  clinical appearance of, 220–221
  as complication of therapeutic lens use,
    160
  incidence of, 221
  pathogenesis of, 221
  stromal, 21–22
  treatment of, 221
Corneal pathology, as indication for
    hydrogel lenses, 51
Corneal perforations, therapeutic lenses
    with, 148, *149*
Corneal sensation, 13–15
  alterations in, as contraindication to
    extended-wear lenses, 53
  extended-wear lenses and, 192
  use of therapeutic lenses and, 160
Corneal stroma. *See* Stroma

Corneal ulcers, 216–220
  infective, 217–220, *218, 219*
    clinical picture in, 220
    pathogenesis of, 220
    predisposing factors for, 218–220
    treatment of, 220
  sterile, 216–217, *217*
    management of, 217
    pathogenesis of, 217
Cosmesis, bifocal lenses and, 136
Cosmetics, risk of infection and, 237
CPC, in gas-permeable lens fitting, 43
Crescent lens, 130
Critical micelle concentration (CMC), 229
Critical surface tension, 228
CSI High Plus lens
  manufacturing information for, 56t
  parameters for, 58t
CSI lens, 64–65, 84t, 86, 89t, 144
  adverse reactions to solutions and, 252
CSI T lens, 96t, 100–101
CW-79 lens
  manufacturing information for, 56t
  parameters for, 58t
Cyanoacrylate adhesive, with therapeutic
    lenses, 148, *150*
Cycloplegics, with therapeutic lenses, 146

Damage, to lens, 196
Debris. *See* Lens debris
DeCarle bifocal lens, 120–121
Diagnostic lens method of fitting, 78–79
Diameter, 73
  corneal, in gas-permeable lens fitting,
    43
  minus-lenticular aphakic lens fitting
    and, 179
Disinfection, 235–245
  chemical versus heat, 238–239
  preservatives in solutions for
    categories of, 239–245
    evaluation of, 238
    significance of, 237
  properties desirable in solutions for,
    236

sterilization differentiated from,
    235–236
  terminology for, 235–236
  of therapeutic lenses, 157–158
DK, 49–50
Drug(s). *See* Topical medications; *specific
    drugs*
Drug delivery, by therapeutic lenses,
    156–157
Dry eye syndromes
  as contraindication to extended-wear
    lenses, 52
  therapeutic lenses in, 148, 152–153
DuraSoft lens, 84t, 89t
  manufacturing information for, 56t
  parameters for, 58t
Durasoft TT lens
  manufacturing information for, 56t
  parameters for, 58t
DuraSoft 2 Custom lens, 92–93t
DuraSoft 2 lens, 89, 133
  manufacturing information for, 56t
  parameters for, 58t
DuraSoft 2 Toric Standard lens, 92–93t,
    94
DuraSoft 3 lens, 64, 83–84, 96t, 97t,
    98–99t, 103
  manufacturing information for, 56t
  parameters for, 58t

Edema, corneal. *See* Corneal edema
EDTA. *See* Ethylenediaminetetraacetate
Embden-Meyerhof anaerobic glycolysis, 4
Emulsion, 226
Endothelium, corneal. *See* Corneal
    endothelium
Entropion, spastic, therapeutic lenses in,
    155, *155*
Enzymatic agents, in cleaning, 200,
    233–234
EOP, 49
Epinephrine, therapeutic lens
    discoloration by, 151, *151*
Epithelium, corneal. *See* Corneal
    epithelium

Equivalent oxygen percent (EOP), 49
Erosions, corneal, therapeutic lenses
        with, 147–148
Ethylenediaminetetraacetate (EDTA),
        245
    adverse ocular reactions and, 250,
        253
    teratogenic effects of, 253
Expectations, bifocal contact lenses and,
        137
Extended-wear lenses, 96t, 96–103, 97t,
        98–99t, 188–194. *See also*
        specific lenses
    in aphakia
        contraindications to, 52–53
        indications for, 51–52
    combination, 190–191
    complications of, 194
        corneal edema as, 17, 19
    follow-up schedule for, 193–194
    and health, 53, 191–192
    hydrophilic, 190
    for hyperopia, 102–103
    indications for, 51
    insertion and removal of, 192
    lens-related factors and, 189–191
    for myopia, 96t, 98–102
    oxygen transmission and, 190
    patient selection for, 191 194
        evaluation of corneal surface and,
        193
        factors influencing, 191–192
    physiology of extended wear and,
        188–189
    surface characteristics and, 189
    thin membrane, 190
Eyelids, 27–28
    bifocal contact lenses and, 137
    blinking and, 28
    defects of, therapeutic lenses and, 146
    microbial flora on, 192
    postsurgical dysfunction of, as
        contraindication to
        extended-wear lenses, 52
    sensitivity of, 27–28
        fitting of hydrogel lenses with, 85,
        90

"First fit" method
    for hyperopia, 90, *91*
    for myopia, 87, *88*
Filamentary keratitis, therapeutic lenses
        in, 148
Fit
    changes in, 253–254
    evaluation of, 55, 79–82, 80t, *81, 82, 83*
    flat, 55, 80, 81, *81*
    steep, 55, 80, 81, *81*
Fitting
    adjustments in, 55, 57
    of bifocal lenses, 184–186
    of gas-permeable lenses, 42–45
        refraction and keratometry in, 42
        selection of parameters in, 43–44
        trial fitting in, 44–45
    of hydrogel lenses, 77–103
        in aphakia, 53–61
            guidelines for, 54–55, 57, 61
            lens selection for, 54
            prefit evaluation for, 53–54
            timing of, 57, 61
        astigmatic, 94
        avoidance of contact lenses and, 78
        choice of lens in, 77–78
        for daily wear, 82–96
        diagnostic lens method of, 78–79
        evaluation of fit and, 79–82, 80t, *81,*
            82, 83
        for extended wear, 96–103
        inventory lens method of, 79
        objectives in, 77
        prefitting evaluation and, 78
        technique of, 79
    in keratoconus, 172–175
    of monovision lenses, in presbyopia,
        116–117
    of piggyback lenses, 175–177
    of rigid lenses in aphakia, 178–182
        lenticular minus-carrier, 179–182
        single-cut, 179
    of therapeutic lenses, 161–162
Flat fit, 55, 80, 81, *81*
Flexlens
    manufacturing information for, 56t
    parameters for, 58t

Flexsol, 234
Fluid permeability, of therapeutic lenses,
        150–151
Follow-up
    in fitting hydrogel lenses, in aphakia,
        61
    schedule for extended-wear lenses,
        193–194
Fragility. *See* Corneal epithelium, fragility
        of
Ful-Range lens, 121
Fulsite lens, 121
Fungal contamination, 237

Gas-permeable lenses, 39–45
    advantages over soft lenses, 39
    cellulose acetate butyrate, parameters
        for, 40, 41t
    cleaning agents for, 233–234
    design of, 39–40
    fitting techniques for, 42–45
        refraction and keratometry in, 42
        selection of parameters in, 43–44
        trial fitting and, 44–45
    siloxanyl/methacrylate combinations,
        parameters for, 41–42, 42t
    styrene, 42
    types of, 39
Genesis-4 lens, 96t
Geo Seg lens, 130
Giant papillary conjunctivitis. *See*
        Conjunctivitis, giant papillary
Glaucoma, as contraindication to
        extended-wear lenses, 52
Glucose supply, to cornea, normal, 2–4
Glycogen supply, to cornea, normal, 2–4

Hard lenses. *See* Rigid lenses
Health, extended-wear lenses and, 53,
        191–192
Heat, chemical disinfection compared
        with, 238–239

HEMA. *See* Hydroxyethyl methacrylate
Herpes simplex keratitis, therapeutic
        lenses in, 148
Hexose monophosphate shunt, 4
Hydracon lens
    manufacturing information for, 56t
    parameters for, 58t
Hydrated polyhydroxyethyl methacrylate
        (PHEMA), 47, 48
Hydrocurve aspheric bifocal lens, 124
Hydrocurve II Daily Wear Spherical lens,
        86
Hydrocurve II lens, 64, 70, 84t, 84–86,
        89t, 92–93t, 95, 96t, 97t, 98–99t,
        99, 102–103, 190
Hydrocurve II$_{45}$ lens
    manufacturing information for, 56t
    parameters for, 59t
Hydrocurve II$_{55}$ lens
    manufacturing information for, 56t
    parameters for, 59t
Hydrogel lenses. *See also specific lenses*
    advantages and disadvantages of, 76–77
    in aphakia, 47–65, 177
        commonly used for extended wear,
            62–65
        compared with lenses for myopia,
            101
        contraindications to, 52–53
        extended-wear lenses for, 62–65
        fitting of, 53–61
        with high water content, 62–63
        indications for, 51–52
        lens care and, 61–62
        lens selection for, 54, 65
        manufacturing information and
            parameters for, 54, 56–57t,
            58–60t
        with medium water content, 63–64
        microbiology of aphakic eye and, 51
        patient selection for, 51–53
        physiology of aphakic cornea and,
            48–51
        prefit evaluation for, 53–54
        ultrathin, 64–65
    application of

by patient, 104–107, *105, 106*
by practitioner, 103, *104*
bifocal, 117–135
  alternating vision, 130–134, *131, 132, 133*
    fitting, 134–135, *135*
  simultaneous vision, 122–124, *123*
    fitting, 124
chemical disinfection of, 238–239
cleaning agents for, 232–234, 244–245
to correct residual astigmatism, 165–166
for cosmetic use, 70–111
design of, 73, *76, 77*
extended-wear. *See* Extended-wear lenses
fitting, 77–103
  in aphakia, 53–61
  avoidance of lenses in, 78
  choice of lens in, 77–78
  for daily-wear lenses, 82–96
  diagnostic lens method of, 78–79
  evaluation of fit and, 79–82, 80t, *81, 82, 83*
  for extended-wear lenses, 96t, 96–103, 97t, 98–99t
  inventory lens method of, 79
  objectives in, 77
  prefitting evaluation for, 78
  technique of, 79
history of, 70
in hyperopia, 87–90, 89t, 102–103
  "first fit" method for, 90, *91*
in irregular astigmatism, 175
manufacture of, 71–73
  lathe-cutting method in, 71–73, *74–75*
  spin-casting method in, 71, *72*
materials and properties of, 47, 48
in myopia, 83–87, 84t, 96t, 98–102
  compared with keratorefractive procedures, 101–102
  compared with lenses for aphakia, 101
  "first fit" method for, 87, *88*
parameters for, 73–75, *76, 77*

purging, 234–235
removal of
  by patient, 107, *107, 108,* 109
  by practitioner, 103, *105*
tinted, 75, 109, *109, 110,* 111, *111*
toric
  for astigmatism, 91–96, 92–93t
  fitting, 94
  manufacture of, 73
  types of, 70
Hydrogen peroxide
  as cleaning agent, 233, 243–244
  disinfection of therapeutic lenses using, 157–158
Hydromarc lens, 96t
Hydromarc Standard lens, 87–88
Hydromarc Toric lens, 92–93t, 95
Hydromarc Ultra-thin lens, 89
Hydron lens, 84t, 89t
  manufacturing information for, 56t
  parameters for, 59t
Hydron Mini lens, 86, 90
Hydron Zero 6 lens, 85
Hydron Zero T lens, 92–93t, 95
Hydrophilic substances, 228
Hydrophobic substances, 228
Hydroxyethyl methacrylate (HEMA), 47, 48
  preservatives and, 241
Hygiene, extended-wear lenses and, 53, 192
Hyperemia
  conjunctival, 26
  limbal, with chemosis, 202, *203*
Hyperopia, hydrogel lenses for. *See* Hydrogel lenses, in hyperopia

Infection. *See also specific infections*
  corneal, as complication of therapeutic lens use, 158–159, *159*
  cosmetics and, 237
Infective conjunctivitis, 208
Infiltrates, into stroma, 20
Interfacial phenomena, 227

Interfacial tension, 228
Interpalpebral area, extended-wear lenses and, 192
Intraocular pressure, use of therapeutic lenses and, 160
Inventory lens method of fitting, 79
Iodine, as disinfectant, 245
Ionic surfactants, 228
Iritis, use of therapeutic lenses and, 160

Jessen Lumicon lens, 130

Keratitis
    punctate, as adverse reaction to solutions, 252
    subepithelial, 214
        pathogenesis of, 214
        treatment of, 214
    therapeutic lenses in, 148
Keratoconjunctivitis, superior limbic, 27, 209–211
    clinical picture in, 209–210
    etiology of, 210–211
    management of, 210
    objective signs of, 210
    pathology of, 210
    treatment of, 211
Keratoconus, 172–175
    fitting lenses in, 172–175
    therapeutic lenses in, 154
Keratometry
    evaluation of hydrogel lens fit and, 80–81, 82
    for gas-permeable lens fitting, 42
Keratopathy
    bullous, therapeutic lenses in, 147, 153
    nonallergic, as adverse reaction to solutions, 251–253
    superficial punctate, 212–213, 212
        clinical picture in, 212
        pathogenesis of, 213
        treatment of, 213

Keratoplasty, therapeutic lenses in, 148–150
Keratorefractive procedures, extended-wear lenses for myopia compared with, 101–102
Kontur Three Angle Bifocal lens, 129
Krebs cycle, 4

Lactate transport, in normal cornea, 4–5
Lagophthalmos, as contraindication to extended-wear lenses, 52
Lathe cutting, 71–73, 74–75, 142, 143
    advantages of, 73
    spin casting contrasted with, 73, 76t
Lens care. See also Solutions
    with hydrogel lenses, 61–62
Lens damage, 196
Lens debris, 196–200
    deposition on therapeutic lenses, 151, 151–152
    removal of, tear pumping and, 48–49
Lens deposits. See also Lens spoilage
    adverse ocular reactions and, 249
    as complication of therapeutic lens use, 159
    composition of, 198–199
    removing, 231–232
Lens handling, difficulties in
    fitting of daily-wear hydrogel lenses and, 85
    fitting of toric lenses and, 95–96
    as indication for extended-wear lenses, 51
Lens loss, 201–202
Lens parameters. See also specific lenses
    changes in, 253–254
    for gas-permeable lenses, 43–44
    for hydrogel lenses, 73–75, 76, 77
Lens splitting, 196
Lens spoilage, 196–200, 197
    clinical manifestations of, 199
    composition of deposits and, 198–199
    diagnosis of, 199
    management of, 200

ocular manifestations of, 199–200
optical manifestations of, 199
predisposing factors in, 198
Lens storage case
contamination of, 237
interactions between preservatives and, 238
Lens thickness, 73
minus-lenticular aphakic lens fitting and, 180
Lenticular minus-carrier lenses, in aphakia, 177, *178*
fitting, 179–182
Lifestyle, extended-wear lenses and, 191
Limbal hyperemia, with chemosis, 202, *203*

Manual dexterity. *See* Lens handling
Medications. *See* Topical medications; *specific medications*
Mercurial(s), as preservatives, 240–241
Mercurialentis, as adverse reaction to solutions, 253
Meso lens, parameters for, 40, 41t
Metabolites
removal of, in normal cornea, 4–5
supply to cornea, normal, 2–4
Metrosoft lens
manufacturing information for, 56t
parameters for, 59t
Micelles, 229
Microbial flora
in aphakic eye, 51
on lid margins, extended-wear lenses and, 192
Microcysts, epithelial, 13, *214, 15,* 213–214
Microvilli, clumping of, 27
Monovision correction of presbyopia, 116–117
fitting and, 116–117
modified, 117–118, 186
Monovision failures, bifocal contact lenses and, 136

Moss-Arner lens, 121
Motivation
for bifocal lenses, 136
poor, as contraindication to extended-wear lenses, 53
Movement
evaluation of hydrogel lens fit and, 80, *81*
in trial fitting of gas-permeable lenses, 45
Myopia, hydrogel lenses for. *See* Hydrogel lenses, in myopia

Neovascularization, corneal. *See* Corneal neovascularization
Neuroparalytic keratitis, therapeutic lenses in, 148
Nonionic surfactants, 228

Occupation, bifocal contact lenses and, 136
Ocular complications, 202–211
of solutions, 247–251
Ocular disease, infectious, as contraindication to extended-wear lenses, 52
Ocular environment, extended-wear lenses and, 192
Ocular surface abnormalities, as indication for hydrogel lenses, 51
O & E 70 lens, 96t
O_3/O_4 Soflens, 96t, 100
Ophthalmic surgery, use of therapeutic lenses in, 148–150. *See also specific procedures*
Optacryl 60 lens, parameters for, 41, 42t
Optic cap size, minus-lenticular aphakic lens fitting and, 180
OptiClean, 232
Optic zones, 73, *76, 77*
diameter of, minus-lenticular aphakic lens fitting and, 179–180

OptiZyme, 234
Oxidative agents, in cleaning, 233
Oxygen
    in closed eye, 7–8
    diffusion through hydrogel lenses,
        49–50
    epithelial consumption of, 12–13, *13*
    in open eye
        diffusion through lens, 6
        tear pumping and, 6–7, *7, 8*
    supply to cornea
        in aphakia, 48–49
        normal, 2, 3t
Oxygen permeability
    of extended-wear lenses, 190
    of therapeutic lenses, 150–151, 152
Oxygen permeability coefficient (DK),
        49–50

Pain relief, with therapeutic lenses, 156
Pancreatin, 233, 234
PA 1 lens, 117–118
Papain, 233, 234
Parabens
    adverse ocular reactions and, 250
    as preservatives, 241–242
Paraperm O₂ lens, parameters for, 41, 42t
Paris SoftSite bifocal lens, 131
Patch test, of solutions, 248–249
Patient instruction
    in fitting hydrogel lenses, in aphakia,
        61
    prevention of solution contamination
        and, 237
    with therapeutic lenses, 161
Patient selection
    evaluation of corneal surface and, 193
    for extended-wear lenses, 191–194
    factors influencing, 191–192
PDC-70 lens, 96t, 97t
Perforation, corneal, therapeutic lenses
        with, 148, *149*
Peripheral curves, 75, *76, 77*
    minus-lenticular aphakic lens fitting
        and, 180

Permaflex lens, 96t
Permalens, 63, 70, 96t, 97t, 99–100, 102,
        144, 190
    manufacturing information for, 56t
    parameters for, 59t
Permeability. *See* Fluid permeability;
        Oxygen permeability
PHEMA. *See* Hydrated polyhydroxyethyl
        methacrylate
Phenylethyl alcohol, 241
Phenylmercuric acetate (PMA),
        240–241
Phenylmercuric nitrate (PMN), 240–241
    tear film drying and, 236
Physiological factors, bifocal contact
        lenses and, 137
Piggyback lenses, 154, *154*
    in irregular astigmatism, 175–177
Pilocarpine, delivery by therapeutic
        lenses, 157
Pinhole lenses, in presbyopia, 117
Plano B lens, 142
Plano O lens, 142, 144
Plano T lens, 142
Plano U lens, 142, 144
PMA, 240–241
PMMA, for therapeutic contact lenses,
        140–141
PMN. *See* Phenylmercuric nitrate
Polycon II lens, parameters for, 42, 42t
Polymegathism, endothelial, 23–24, *24,
        25*
Polymercuric nitrate, adverse reactions
        to, 253
Polymethylmethacrylate (PMMA), for
        therapeutic contact lenses,
        140–141
Potassium sorbate, 244
Power, 73
    in minus-lenticular aphakic lens fitting,
        180–182
    in gas-permeable lens fitting, 43–44
Presbicon lens, 121
Presbiflex lens, 121
Presbyopia, 115–137
    correction with bifocal lenses. *See*
        Bifocal lenses

correction with single vision lenses,
115–118
modified monovision correction and,
117–118
monovision, 116–117
pinhole, 117
Preservation, 236
Preservatives in disinfecting and storage
solutions
categories of, 239–245
evaluation of, 238
significance of, 237
Prism-ballast lenses, 166–168, *167*
Propylparaben, tear film drying and, 236
Punctate keratopathy
as adverse reaction to solutions, 252
superficial, 212–213, *213*
Pupillary diameter, in gas-permeable lens
fitting, 43
Pupil size, bifocal contact lenses and, 137
Purging, 234–235

Quaternary ammonium compounds, as
preservatives, 239–240

Refraction
evaluation of hydrogel lens fit and, 80t,
82
in gas-permeable lens fitting, 42
Refractive error
for bifocal lenses, 136
in gas-permeable lens fitting, 43
Relative sagittal depth (RSD), in fitting
hydrogel lenses, 55, 57
Retinoscopy, evaluation of hydrogel lens
fit and, 81–82, *83*
Revlens, 144
Rigid lenses. *See also specific lenses*
alternating vision bifocal, 126–130
concentric, 126–127, *127*
fitting, 130
segment, 127–130, *128, 129*
in aphakia

fitting, 177–182
lenticular, 177, *178,* 179–182
single-cut, 177, 179–182
cleaning agents for, 232
in irregular astigmatism, 175–177
in residual astigmatism, 166–168
simultaneous vision bifocal, *120,*
120–122, *121*
aspheric, *121,* 121–122
concentric, *120,* 120–121
fitting, 122
wet versus dry storage of, 245–246
RSD. *See* Relative sagittal depth
Rx 56 lens, parameters for, 40, 41t

Safety, in trial fitting of gas-permeable
lenses, 45
Sagittal depth, 75
Saline solution, patient-prepared, 239
Saturn II lens, 191
Sauflon CW-79 lens, 62–63
Sauflon lens, 97t, 102, 190
Sauflon PW lens, 62–63, 70
manufacturing information for, 56t
parameters for, 59t
Sauflon-70 lens, 96t, 100
Secondary curve, minus-lenticular
aphakic lens fitting and, 180
Sensitivity
corneal. *See* Corneal sensation
of eyelids, 27–28
Silcon lens, 232
Siloxanyl/methacrylate combination
lenses, parameters for, 41–42,
42t
SilSoft lens, 232
Simultaneous vision bifocal lenses. *See*
Bifocal lenses, simultaneous
vision
Single-cut aphakic lenses, 177
fitting, 179
Sof-Form II lens
manufacturing information for, 56t
parameters for, 59t

Soflens, 84t, 89t, 141
  "first fit" method of, 87, *88,* 90, *91*
  manufacturing information for, 56t
  parameters for, 59t
Soflens Enzymatic Contact Lens Cleaner,
    233, 234
Softcon EW lens, 63–64
  manufacturing information for, 56t
  parameters for, 60t
Softcon lens, 70, 84t, 85, 89t, 90, 96t, 97t,
    100, 102, 144, 190
  manufacturing information for, 56t
  parameters for, 59t
Softics lens
  manufacturing information for, 56t
  parameters for, 60t
Softics Super Plus lens
  manufacturing information for, 56t
  parameters for, 60t
Soft lenses. *See* Hydrogel lenses
Softlon/PW lens, 144
Softsite lens
  manufacturing information for, 56t
  parameters for, 60t
Solubility, 226
Solutions, 226–255
  change in fit and lens parameters and,
    254
  cleaning, 230–235
    chelating, 234
    deposits and, 231–232
    enzymatic, 200, 233–234
    oxidative, 233
    purging and, 234–235
    surfactant agents as, 232–233
  complications resulting from use of,
    246–255
  disinfectant and storage, 235–246
    categories of preservatives and,
      239–245
    chemical versus heat disinfection
      and, 238–239
    evaluation of preservatives for, 238
    properties desirable in, 236
    significance of preservation of, 237
    terminology for, 235–236
    wet versus dry storage and, 245–246
  micellar, 229
  saline, patient-prepared, 239
  sorption and, 227
  surfactant, 228–229
  terminology for, 226–227
  wetting, 227–228
  wetting angle and, 229–230
Sorbic acid, as cleaning agent, 244–245
Sorption, 227
Spastic entropion, therapeutic lenses in,
    155, *155*
Spin casting, 71, *72,* 141–142, *143*
  advantages of, 71
  lathe cutting contrasted with, 73, 76t
Splinting, by therapeutic lenses, 155–156
Splitting, of lens, 196
Spoilage. *See* Lens spoilage
Steep fit, 55, 80, 81, *81*
Sterilization, disinfection differentiated
    from, 235–236
Storage, wet versus dry, 245–246. *See also*
    Disinfection; Lens storage case
Striae, in posterior stroma, 19–20
Stroma, 15–22
  edema of, 15–19, *17, 18, 19*
    with daily lens wear, 16–17
    with extended lens wear, 17, 19
  infiltrates into, 20
  striae in, 19–20
  thinning of, 20, *21*
  ultrastructural changes in, 20
  vascularization of, 21–22
Styrene lenses, parameters for, 42
Subepithelial keratitis, 214
Superficial punctate keratopathy,
    212–213, *213*
Superior limbic keratoconjunctivitis. *See*
    Keratoconjunctivitis, superior
    limbic
Surface-active materials, defined, 228
Surface free energy, defined, 228
Surface tension
  critical, 228
  defined, 228
Surfactants

classification of, 228
as cleaning agents, 232–233
Surgery, use of therapeutic lenses in, 148–150. *See also specific procedures*
Suspension, 226
Syntex Synsoft bifocal lens, 131
Systemic conditions, extended-wear lenses and, 53, 191–192

Taco test, 107, *108, 109*
TCA, 4
TC-50 lens
  manufacturing information for, 57t
  parameters for, 60t
TC-75 lens, 63
  manufacturing information for, 57t
  parameters for, 60t
Tear(s), inadequate, therapeutic lenses and, 146. *See also* Dry eye syndromes
Tear chemistry
  alteration by contact lens wear, 10
  of normal cornea, 5–6
Tear film drying, disinfecting solution preservatives and, 236
Tear pumping, 48–49
  oxygen restriction and, 6–7
Temperature
  alteration by contact lens wear, 9
  of normal cornea, 5
Therapeutic contact lenses, 140–162
  ancillary therapy and, 145–146
  complications of use of, 158–160
    avoidance of, 160–162
  composition of, 140–141
  contraindications to, 150
  disinfection of, 157–158
  evaluating and refitting, 161–162
  indications for, 147–150
  inherent lens characteristics and, 150–152
  insertion of, 160–161
  lens characteristics and, 142–145

manufacturing techniques for, 141–142, *143*
patient instruction for, 161
physical properties of, 141, *142*
principles of therapeutic efficacy and, 152–158
  drug delivery and, 156–157
  pain relief and, 156
  permeability and, 152
  protection and, 155
  splinting and, 155–156
  visual acuity and, 153–154
  wetting and, 152–153, *153*
Thimerosal, 240–241
  adverse reactions to, 250, 253
  interaction with plastic containers, 238
  tear film drying and, 236
Thin membrane extended-wear lenses, 190
Tight lens syndrome, 144, *145,* 200–201
  clinical manifestations of, 200–201
  pathogenesis of, 201
  treatment of, 201
Tint, 75
Tinted soft lenses. *See* Hydrogel lenses, tinted
Titmus-Eurocon W38E Hydrophilic bifocal lens, 124
Topical medications
  concentration in therapeutic lenses, 152
  therapeutic lens discoloration by, 151, *151*
Toric hydrogel lenses. *See* Hydrogel lenses, toric
Torisoft lens, 92–93t, 95
Toxic conjunctivitis, 209
Transcorneal potential, 11
Tresoft lens
  manufacturing information for, 57t
  parameters for, 60t
Tresoft Thin lens
  manufacturing information for, 57t
  parameters for, 60t
Trial fitting, of gas-permeable lenses, 44–45

Tricarboxylic acid cycle (TCA or Krebs
    cycle), 4
Trimethoprim, 245
Tripol 43 lens
  manufacturing information for, 57t
  parameters for, 60t
TruFocal lens, 131, 133

Ulcers, corneal. *See* Corneal ulcers
Ultracon Prism bifocal lens, 128
Ultracon Three Angle lens, 133
Ultrasound, in cleaning, 234
Uvea, 28
Uveitis, chronic or recurrent, as
    contraindication to
    extended-wear lenses, 52

Variable Focus Lens (VFL), 121
Vascularization. *See* Corneal
    neovascularization
VFL, 121
Vistakon Standard lens
  manufacturing information for, 57t
  parameters for, 60t
Vistamarc lens, 89, 97t
Visual acuity
  evaluation of, with hydrogel lenses, 57
  with therapeutic lenses, 153–154
  in trial fitting of gas-permeable lenses, 45

Wesley-Jessen TruFocal lens, 130–131
Wetting, 227–228
  defined, 227
  of therapeutic lenses, 152–153, *153*
Wetting angle, 229–230